New Insights on Acne, Rosacea, and Hidradenitis Suppurativa: Etiology and Treatment

New Insights on Acne, Rosacea, and Hidradenitis Suppurativa: Etiology and Treatment

Editor

Hei Sung Kim

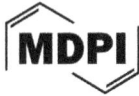

Basel • Beijing • Wuhan • Barcelona • Belgrade • Novi Sad • Cluj • Manchester

Editor
Hei Sung Kim
Incheon St. Mary's Hospital,
The Catholic University of Korea
Seoul
Republic of Korea

Editorial Office
MDPI
St. Alban-Anlage 66
4052 Basel, Switzerland

This is a reprint of articles from the Special Issue published online in the open access journal *Journal of Clinical Medicine* (ISSN 2077-0383) (available at: https://www.mdpi.com/journal/jcm/special_issues/Acne).

For citation purposes, cite each article independently as indicated on the article page online and as indicated below:

Lastname, A.A.; Lastname, B.B. Article Title. *Journal Name* **Year**, *Volume Number*, Page Range.

ISBN 978-3-7258-0127-5 (Hbk)
ISBN 978-3-7258-0128-2 (PDF)
doi.org/10.3390/books978-3-7258-0128-2

© 2024 by the authors. Articles in this book are Open Access and distributed under the Creative Commons Attribution (CC BY) license. The book as a whole is distributed by MDPI under the terms and conditions of the Creative Commons Attribution-NonCommercial-NoDerivs (CC BY-NC-ND) license.

Contents

Ewelina Firlej, Wioleta Kowalska, Karolina Szymaszek, Jacek Roliński and Joanna Bartosińska
The Role of Skin Immune System in Acne
Reprinted from: *J. Clin. Med.* **2022**, *11*, 1579, doi:10.3390/jcm11061579 1

Karolina Chilicka, Monika Rusztowicz, Renata Szyguła and Danuta Nowicka
Methods for the Improvement of Acne Scars Used in Dermatology and Cosmetology: A Review
Reprinted from: *J. Clin. Med.* **2022**, *11*, 2744, doi:10.3390/jcm11102744 11

Yu Ri Woo and Hei Sung Kim
Truncal Acne: An Overview
Reprinted from: *J. Clin. Med.* **2022**, *11*, 3660, doi:10.3390/jcm11133660 24

Karolina Chilicka, Aleksandra M. Rogowska, Renata Szyguła, Monika Rusztowicz and Danuta Nowicka
Efficacy of Oxybrasion in the Treatment of Acne Vulgaris: A Preliminary Report
Reprinted from: *J. Clin. Med.* **2022**, *11*, 3824, doi:10.3390/jcm11133824 38

Monika Rusztowicz, Karolina Chilicka, Renata Szyguła, Wiktoria Odrzywołek, Antoniya Yanakieva, Binnaz Asanova and Sławomir Wilczyński
A Split Face Comparative Study to Evaluate the Efficacy of 40% Pyruvic Acid vs. Microdermabrasion with 40% Pyruvic Acid on Biomechanical Skin Parameters in the Treatment of Acne Vulgaris
Reprinted from: *J. Clin. Med.* **2022**, *11*, 6079, doi:10.3390/jcm11206079 48

Karolina Chilicka, Monika Rusztowicz, Aleksandra M. Rogowska, Renata Szyguła, Binnaz Asanova and Danuta Nowicka
Efficacy of Hydrogen Purification and Cosmetic Acids in the Treatment of Acne Vulgaris: A Preliminary Report
Reprinted from: *J. Clin. Med.* **2022**, *11*, 6269, doi:10.3390/jcm11216269 57

Lennart Ocker, Nessr Abu Rached, Caroline Seifert, Christina Scheel and Falk G. Bechara
Current Medical and Surgical Treatment of Hidradenitis Suppurativa—A Comprehensive Review
Reprinted from: *J. Clin. Med.* **2022**, *11*, 7240, doi:10.3390/jcm11237240 68

Aleksandra Tobiasz, Danuta Nowicka and Jacek C. Szepietowski
Acne Vulgaris—Novel Treatment Options and Factors Affecting Therapy Adherence: A Narrative Review
Reprinted from: *J. Clin. Med.* **2022**, *11*, 7535, doi:10.3390/jcm11247535 95

Nark-Kyoung Rho
Revisiting the Role of Local Cryotherapy for Acne Treatment: A Review and Update
Reprinted from: *J. Clin. Med.* **2023**, *12*, 26, doi:10.3390/jcm12010026 104

Danuta Nowicka, Karolina Chilicka, Iwona Dzieńdziora-Urbińska and Renata Szyguła
Skincare in Rosacea from the Cosmetologist's Perspective: A Narrative Review
Reprinted from: *J. Clin. Med.* **2023**, *12*, 115, doi:10.3390/jcm12010115 122

Yvonne Nong, Nimrit Gahoonia, Julianne Rizzo, Waqas Burney, Raja K. Sivamani and Jessica Maloh
Prospective Evaluation of a Topical Botanical Skin Care Regimen on Mild to Moderate Facial and Truncal Acne and Mood
Reprinted from: *J. Clin. Med.* **2023**, *12*, 1484, doi:10.3390/jcm12041484 132

Julia E. Rymaszewska, Piotr K. Krajewski, Łukasz Matusiak, Joanna Maj
and Jacek C. Szepietowski
Satisfaction with Life and Coping Strategies among Patients with Hidradenitis Suppurativa: A
Cross-Sectional Study
Reprinted from: *J. Clin. Med.* **2023**, *12*, 2755, doi:10.3390/jcm12082755 . . . . **142**

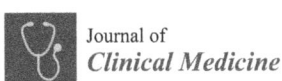

Review

The Role of Skin Immune System in Acne

Ewelina Firlej [1,*], Wioleta Kowalska [2,*], Karolina Szymaszek [1], Jacek Roliński [2] and Joanna Bartosińska [1]

[1] Department of Cosmetology and Aesthetic Medicine, Medical University of Lublin, 20-093 Lublin, Poland; joannabartosinska@umlub.pl (J.B.); 57471@umlub.pl (K.S.)
[2] Department of Clinical Immunology, Medical University of Lublin, 20-093 Lublin, Poland; jacek.rolinski@umlub.pl
* Correspondence: ewelinafirlej@umlub.pl (E.F.); wioleta.kowalska@umlub.pl (W.K.)

Abstract: Acne vulgaris is a skin disease that often occurs in adolescence and in young adulthood. The main pathogenic factors are hyperkeratinization, obstruction of sebaceous glands, stimulation of sebaceous gland secretion by androgens, and bacterial colonization of sebaceous units by *Cutibacterium acnes*, which promotes inflammation. Little is known about the role of skin immune cells in the development of acne lesions. The aim of the study was to try to understand the role of skin immune cells in the course of acne. Recent studies have shown that there are at least four major pathways by which *Cutibacterium acnes* interacts with the innate immune system to induce inflammation: through TLRs, activating inflammasomes, inducing the production of matrix metalloproteinases (MMPs), and stimulating antimicrobial peptide (AMP) activity. Cells of adaptive immune response, mainly Th1 and Th17 lymphocytes, also play an important role in the pathogenesis of acne. It is worth emphasizing that understanding the role of the skin's immune cells in the pathogenesis of acne may, in the future, contribute to the application of modern therapeutic strategies that would avoid addiction to antibiotics, which would alleviate the spectrum of resistance that is now evident and a current threat.

Keywords: acne vulgaris; AMP; MMP; Th1 and Th17 lymphocytes; treatment

1. Introduction

Acne vulgaris is a skin condition commonly affecting adolescents and young adults. The main pathogenic factors of acne include hyperkeratinisation, the secretion from the sebaceous glands stimulated by androgens, dysbiosis of the skin microbiome, and *Cutibacterium acnes* (*C. acnes*); and the overcolonisation of pilosebaceous units, which might provide favourable conditions for perifolliculitis. The clinical presentation of acne ranges from its mild form (mild comedonal acne) to severe inflammatory nodulocystic acne affecting the skin of the face, chest, and back. Based on current findings, it can be stated that the increased activity of sebaceous glands induced by androgens triggers the proliferation of *C. acnes*, anaerobic bacterium present in the sebum accumulating in follicular ducts. The induction of inflammatory reactions by *C. acnes* is the main aetiologic factor contributing to the pathogenesis of acne vulgaris. In particular, the IL-1 family of cytokines plays a key role both in triggering acne lesions and in the inflammatory response in acne. Nonetheless, there is still a lot to be discovered on the importance of the skin immune cells for the development of acne lesions, both in the early stage and in further stages of acne [1,2].

Saurat J.-H. et al. [3] provides models for further understanding the biological events of comedogenesis. The latest knowledge is gained from both lineage tracking experiments in mice and sebaceous responses to xenobiotics in humans. Emphasis is placed on sebaceous stem cells LRIG1+ in the isthmus of the sebaceous duct. LRIG cells can differentiate toward epithelial or sebaceous type and should, therefore, be prime targets for comedogenic factors. This population can, therefore, be a source of blackhead lesions. This may also explain the sentence that "the more comedones, the fewer mature sebocytes" in acne histology [3,4].

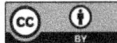

Manfredini M. et al. [5] assessed the evolution of acne lesions from clinically unchanged skin in mild to moderate acne patients using in vivo reflection confocal microscopy (RCM) and dynamic optical coherence tomography (D-OCT). After analyzing seventy complete sets of clinical pictures comrpising RCM and D-OCT, it was shown that the appearance of an acne lesion is preceded by the growth of large follicles in the area corresponding to funnel keratinization. There is an increase in inflammatory parameters, such as the growth of small bright cells in RCM and the vascular network in D-OCT, that return to normal after acute inflammation has subsided [5].

The objective of the paper is to explore the role of the cells of the skin immune system in the course of acne. The paper includes a review and analysis of the literature on the subject published in the period between 2005 and 2021. Without doubt, a better understanding of the pathogenesis of acne might further translate into effective treatments of patients suffering from this skin disease. Acne requires a multidirectional approach and cooperation between physicians specializing in various medical fields, as well as psychologists and cosmetologists. Therapeutic success may be achieved thanks to the understanding and processes accounting for immunology processes taking place in skin and hair follicles.

2. The Aetiology and Pathogenesis of Acne

Acne affects 80 percent of adolescents, yet the condition often persists until early adulthood and may cause scarring and skin discolouration [6–8]. Acne lesions develop in hair follicles on the skin in the areas of cheeks, forehead, chin, mandible, and chest. The combination of increased secretion of the sebum and abnormal excessive proliferation of keratinocytes results in the development of microscopic lesions called microcomedones. The accumulation of the sebum, the enlargement of a sebaceous gland, and the accumulation of the keratin material in the microcomedone area result in the development of comedones. According to the conventional views of acne pathogenesis, C. acnes, which is present on healthy skin, colonize follicular ducts and trigger an innate immune response, resulting in the progression from so-called non-inflammatory comedones to inflammatory papules, pustules, or nodules. However, in the last decade, several pieces of evidence were provided, suggesting that inflammation can occur across the entire life cycle of acne lesions even before comedones develop [7].

Recent studies conducted at molecular and cell level provided a hint of an explanation of how the factors causing acne interact. Inflammation was found in all acne lesions, and for that reason, an inflammation in the area of the pilosebaceous unit can be regarded as a defining characteristic of acne [9]. The acne exposome, which is the total sum of exposure to all environmental factors, also affects the presence, aggravation, and duration of acne. Exposome-related factors include nutrition, psychological and work-related factors, lifestyle, cosmetics, medications, climate-related factors, and pollution. The factors impact on the skin through the interaction with the skin protective barrier, sebaceous glands, innate immunity, and skin microbiota [10]. It was formerly believed that acne skin lesions were developed upon the abnormal sloughing of keratinocytes that line the sebaceous gland, which resulted in excessive keratosis of the pilosebaceous duct and the formation of microcomedones. However, recent years have experienced a shift in the understanding of acne pathogenesis, and it is currently believed that it is a primary inflammatory dermatitis. Studies showed the presence of a subclinical infection in normal skin of patients with acne, before microcomedones developed [11]. Acne lesions are initiated by an obstruction of the opening of the pilosebaceous duct, which might result from the excessive keratosis of the epithelium. The cells accumulate in the sebaceous gland and move to the pilosebaceous duct. Sebaceous glands expand and sometimes burst, causing the escape of contents to the surrounding tissue. The studies showed the presence of inflammation markers in the contents of microcomedones. It was also shown that IL-1 was present in comedonal contents. It is worth noting that the so-called "inflammatory components", i.e., CD4+ T cells and macrophages, are also present in the skin and are unaffected by acne lesions [9]. In the course of inflammation, myeloid cells respond immediately and produce pro-inflammatory mediators that affect the activation of cells located in the closest proximity and facilitate the migration of cells to the area of the ongoing inflammatory process [12]. Myeloid cells of the skin also serve as a connection between innate and adaptive immune responses (Figure 1).

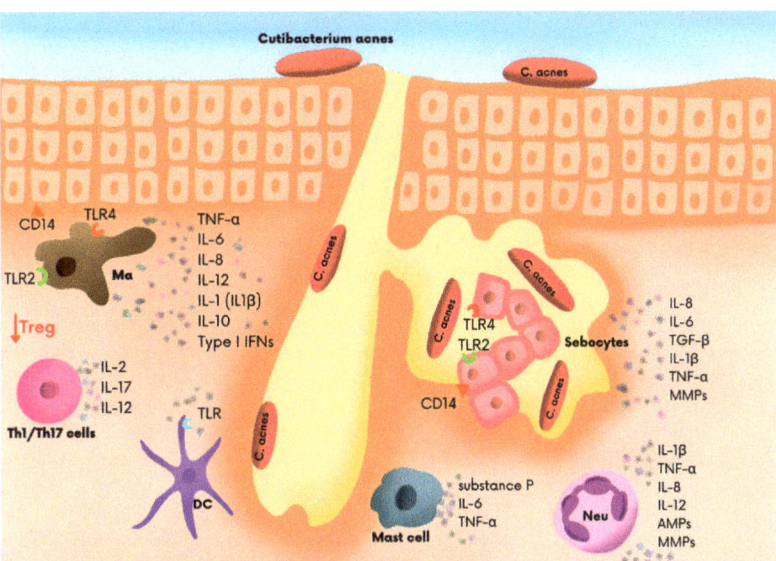

Figure 1. The immune cells in microenvironment of sebaceous gland in acne vulgaris patients. The main skin immune cells, i.e., Langerhans cells, dendritic cells of the dermis, macrophages, mast cells, B and T cells, and keratinocytes [13]. Neutrophils are not cells residing in the skin, but they accumulate in the skin in the course of inflammation. In general, skin cells communicate by secreting large quantities of biologically active cytokines and chemokins, which regulate their function and migration in specific skin layers.

Depending on the morphological characteristics and the intensity of lesions, the following clinical forms of acne were identified: comedonal acne, with the prevalence of closed and/or open comedones; papulopustular acne, characterized by the presence of inflammatory lesions (papules and/or pustules); highly inflammatory acne (including nodular acne and conglobate acne) with the presence of nodules or cysts; acne keloidalis, characterized by scarring; acne fulminans; and acne excoriée [13–15]. The aforementioned disorders were diagnosed on the basis of medical examination and interview both in the clinical and cosmetology practice. As regards clinical practice, acne belongs to most frequent dermatological diseases, and its pathogenesis requires further research [16,17].

Inverse acne (acne inversa, hidradenitis suppurativa; HS) is a severe, chronic inflammatory disease. Normally, the lesions are located in the area of skin folds and are painful nodules with a tendency to fistula formation and scarring. There are discussions to this day as to whether the disease belongs to the acne group. In the course of the disease, hyperkeratosis and destruction of the hair follicles occur, and the involvement of apocrine sweat glands is a secondary phenomenon. The estimated prevalence of HS is 1%, with a predominance of women [18,19].

PAPA syndrome, a hereditary autoinflammatory syndrome caused by mutations in the proline-serine-threonine phosphatase 1 (PSTPIP1) gene, is clinically characterized by purulent arthritis, acne, and pyoderma gangrenosum. PASH and PAPASH syndromes are similar to PAPA syndrome, but the former does not present accompanying arthritis and has a different genetic background, while the latter is characterized by purulent arthritis, acne, pyoderma gangrenosum, and suppurative hidradenitis. PAPA, PASH, and PAPASH are associated with the over-expression of IL-1 and tumour necrosis factor (TNF)-α and may respond to biological drugs that specifically target these cytokines [20–22].

3. Immune Cells Participating in the Pathogenesis of Acne

The pathogenesis of acne vulgaris is complex and involves mutual interactions between hormonal, microbiological, and immunological factors. Nevertheless, the mechanisms behind the causes of acne vulgaris still remain unclear.

The knowledge adapted in the last decade indicates that acne vulgaris is a disease characterized by excessive inflammation in the area of pilosebaceous units and the surrounding skin. It is partially generated by the interaction of *C. acnes* with the cell components of skin, namely keratinocytes, sebocytes, and tissue macrophages. *C. acnes* is a Gram-positive anaerobic bacterium secreting inflammatory substances that can be crucial in acne pathogenesis [23]. The bacteria produce lipase, hyaluronidase, and proteases and activate immune cells, thus causing inflammation [24]. The substances are identified by PRRs. TLRs constitute one of the main categories of PRRs [23]. Various types of TLR-expressing cells are present in the epidermis, including keratinocytes and Langerhans cells. Cells present in the dermis and migrating to this skin layer also demonstrate TLR expression. These include macrophages, dendritic cells, lymphocytes, and mast cells. In a good state of health, immune cells account for 7% of skin cells, of which ca. 3.78% are Langerhans cells, 0.45% are NK cells, 0.24% are macrophages, 0.79% are dendritic cells, 0.41% are T cells, and 1.33% are other immune cells, i.e., innate lymphoid cells (ILC), neutrophils, and macrophages. It is worth noting that 80% of all T cells residing in the skin are memory T cells. CD4+ and CD8+ T_{RM} cells account for 83% and 17% of T cells, respectively, while the share of regulatory T cells (Treg) amounts to approximately 5–10% of all T cells residing in the skin. Yang et al. [25], in their studies, found a high percentage of wandering neutrophils, monocytes, and activated mast cells but a lower infiltration of Treg cells in areas affected by acne lesions. Interestingly, the scholars observed a significantly higher infiltration of Treg cells and resting dendritic cells in non-lesional skin areas of acne patients in relation to the skin of healthy individuals. This suggests immunosuppression in unaffected areas of the skin of acne patients, which might explain, i.e., the absence of papules there. In their studies, Ozlu et al. [26] identified TLR2+ macrophages in acne lesions and around pilosebaceous units and proved that the number of the cells increased as the condition progressed. In turn, Jugeaou et al. [27] described an upregulated expression of TLR2 and TLR4 in keratinocytes in persons with inflammatory acne. It is suspected that, in the course of inflammatory acne, *C. acnes* activates cells by interactions with TLR2 and TLR4. This interaction results in the production of pro-inflammatory cytokines including TNF and IL-1, and IL-8 and Il-12. IL-8 contributes to the recruitment of neutrophils and further damage to the epithelium of sebaceous glands, whereas IL-12 promotes Th1-type response [28]. It was also showed that, as acne was aggravated, the cells demonstrated an increased expression of TLR2. TLR2, also present on the surface of perifollicular macrophages, shows affinity to *C. acnes*, which triggers the secretion of pro-inflammatory cytokines, such as IL-8 and IL-12. These interleukins also create favourable conditions for the chemotaxis of neutrophils and the secretion of lysosome enzymes that take part in the mechanism of intracellular bacteria killing. This probably explains why a higher efficacy to TLR2-targeted drugs, such as topical retinoids, was observed in patients with a more severe form of acne [29]. TLR2 seems to be an effective target for therapeutic intervention based on blocking the inflammatory response in the course of the invasion of *C. acnes*. Therefore, research focused on TLR2 provides valuable information on new therapeutic targets of acne vulgaris. It was also proven that *C. acnes* might also induce the differentiation of monocytes into two separate cell subsets of innate immune response: CD209+ macrophages that more effectively phagocytose and kill *C. acnes* and CD1b+ dendritic cells that activate T cells and release pro-inflammatory cytokines [28]. It is worth stressing that the synthesis of chemokines and cytokines by monocytes is induced by the activation of TLR2 in which *C. acnes* is mediated [26]. Jugeau et al. [27], in their studies aimed at defining the role of *C. acnes* in inflammatory acne, showed an increased expression of TLR2 and TLR4 in the epidermis of acne lesions in vivo. In turn, Selway et al. [30] evaluated the role of TLR2 in the pathogenesis of acne and its significance in comedogenosis. The scholars found the expression of TLR2 in basal and infundibular keratinocytes and sebaceous glands and discovered that its activation provoked the release of IL-1α from primary human keratinocytes in vitro [30]. It was also shown that the increased activation of TLR2 stimulated excessive cornification and comedogenosis in human sebaceous glands ex vivo [26]. Prior studies had shown that some medications applied in the treatment of acne might modify the expression of TLR. In a study performed by Tenaud et al. [31], it was proven that, in acne patients, the expression of TLR2 by keratinocytes was downregulated after 24 h of incubation with adapalene. In turn, Jarrousse et al. [32] found that zinc salts were able to reduce the expression of TLR2, thus demonstrating anti-inflammatory action in the course of acne [26]. Jeoung et al. [33] examined the influence of topical ALA-photodynamic therapy for acne on the level of TLR2 and TLR4 expression. In this study, five out of 10 cases had elevated TLR2 expression before photodynamic therapy. The expression of this receptor was reduced after the application of the therapy. However, no changes in patients with normal immunoreactivity of TLR2 were reported. It was also shown that the expression of TLR4 was increased prior to the therapy in three out of ten patients, and the level of TLR4 expression decreased after therapy was completed [26,33].

In their studies, Bakry et al. [34] showed significant differences in the intensity of TLR2 expressions in pilosebaceous units and inflammatory infiltrations of the skin between acne-affected skin and normal skin. It was found that the expression of TLR2 was more intense in pilosebaceous units and skin infiltrations in areas of inflammatory lesions and severe acne lesions [34]. Moreover, Ozlu et al. [26] showed that the expression of TLR increased in papular and comedonal lesions in relation to nodular lesions in the epidermis area and in papular lesions in comparison with pustular lesions in the inflammation region and in the dermis area. Moreover, TLR4 expression was lower in comedonal lesions than in papular lesions in the dermis [26]. The results suggest that TLRs play a significant role in the development of various clinical presentations of acne. The inflammatory response triggered by *C. acnes*, including the secretion of IL-1 cytokines, constitutes the key pathogenic factor resulting in the manifestation of the disease. *C. acnes* promotes the secretion of IL-1β and IL-18 through the inflammasome pathway with caspase-1 mediation and nucleotide-binding oligomerization domain (NLRP), such as sensor protein. Inflammasomes are a group of intracellular proteins that transform pro-caspase-1 into caspase-1. Caspase-1 activates pro-interleukin-1β to its active form [29]. It is worth noting that both NLRP3 active caspase-1 are expressed by tissue macrophages CD86+ in acne lesions, which also suggests the participation of inflammasome complexes in acne pathogenesis. The exact mechanism related to the activation of NLRP3 inflammasome is still unclear. However, Qin et al. [35] showed in their research that the K+ efflux is necessary to activate NLRP3-dependend caspase-1 in human monocytes and, consequently, to the further release of IL-1β in response to stimulation by *C. acnes*. In light of the potential role of IL-1β in acne pathogenesis, monoclonal anti-IL-1β and/or molecules that could regulate NLRP3, caspase-1, or K+ efflux should be considered in treatments of acne [35].

Additionally, *C. acnes* stimulates the production of matrix metalloproteinases (MMP). These enzymes are related to inflammation and may play a vital role in matrix degradation and in the formation of post-acne scarring [29]. Numerous studies have shown that *C. acnes* triggers the increased activity of several MMPs [29,36]. A few types of MMPs were found in the sebum of acne patients, including MMP-1, MMP-13, and MMP-9. In their studies, Hammam et al. [36] observed that the level of MMP-9 in the blood samples taken from acne patients was significantly higher relative to the control group. Moreover, the scholars observed that the relationship between the level of MMP-9 and the number of face areas affected by inflammatory pustules and nodules, but no interrelation was found between MMP-9 and scarring [36].

Research performed in recent years have demonstrated that antimicrobial peptides (AMP) play a significant role in the pathogenesis of chronic inflammatory skin diseases [26,37]. AMPs are an important component of the innate immune system. AMPs are structures that both ensure basic protection and induce the development of the immune system. They are recognized on the basis of their cutaneous antimicrobial and immunomodulatory properties and demonstrate the ability to inhibit not only bacterial, protozoal, and fungal infections but also viral infections [38]. It is believed that these proteins play their antimicrobial function by binding with the surface of microorganisms and forming pores on their cell membranes. The AMP family includes α- and β-defensins, S100 protein, ribonuclease, and others [26]. Other AMPs, such as β-defensin (hBD)-2 and hBD-3, cathelicidin LL-37 show a low level of expression in healthy skin, but they are induced in the course of a skin inflammation and infection. The release of AMP may be induced by bacteria, bacterial products, TLR, or pro-inflammatory cytokines [39]. In addition to antibacterial action, AMPs are also strongly engaged in the migration of inflammatory cells and the release of cytokines [26]. In recent years, it was proven that the regulation of AMP synthesis was disturbed in acne patients. In in vitro studies, it was observed that C. acnes induce the expression of hBD-2 by keratinocytes and sebocytes. Given that, the increased expression of hBD-2 in acne lesions might be triggered by C. acnes. There is evidence that TLRs, such as TLR2 and TLR4, for which their expressions are upregulated by C. acnes, could mediate in induction. Cathelicidin LL-37 is another AMP demonstrating activity against C. acnes in in vitro conditions. With respect to acne pathogenesis, it has been found that LL-37 limits bacterial growth and shows anti-inflammatory properties; for instance, LL-37 is able to reduce the production of TNF by macrophages stimulated by bacterial components [24]. Medications applied in acne therapy can also modulate AMP expression. Using the ex vivo lipopolysaccharide LPS-induced inflammatory skin explant model, Poiraud et al. [40] demonstrated an increased expression of hBD2 following treatment by zinc gluconate, but no changes were found in hBD4 expression [40]. Boroyava et al. [41] examined the effect of isotretinoin therapy in acne on AMP expression levels with the use of RT-PCR. The scholars measured AMP expression levels before, during, and six months after the commencement of isotretinoin therapy. In relation to the control group, an increased expression of, i.e., cathelicidin, HBD-2, lactoferrin, and lysozyme, and lower expression levels of α-defensin-1 were observed in acne patients prior to the therapy. The expression of cathelicidin, HBD-2, and lactoferrin was reduced in the course of therapy. On the other hand, isotretinoin therapy had no effect on the increased expression of lysozyme and ribonuclease-7, which demonstrate a stronger antimicrobial action than pro-inflammatory action [40,41]. Without doubt, the antibacterial action of AMPs in acne will have a beneficial effect, which has been proven in the application of standard antibiotics and other antibacterial agents in the treatment of acne.

In recent years, emphasis was also placed in the importance of adaptive immune response cells in the course of acne. It was proven that immunogenic proteins of *C. acnes* released to the sebaceous gland duct may be processed by Langerhans cells, which in turn may present antigens to CD4+ T cells in local lymph nodes. Histological studies showed that CD4+ T cells were the most numerous cells of the white blood cell system in early-stage inflammatory infiltrations (6–72 h) in acne lesions, which suggests that they might take part in immune response triggered by the colonization of the sebaceous gland by *C. acnes* [42]. Neutrophils appear in these lesions after 24 and 72 h, when such lesions are clinically identified as pustules. CD8+ cells infiltrate the lesions at a later stage [43]. Recent in vitro studies have shown that *C. acnes* also stimulate adaptive immune response, by inducing Th1 and Th17 lymphocytes to secrete IFN-γ and IL-17A and other pro-inflammatory cytokines [29]. In addition, IL-17$^+$ cells were found in perifollicular infiltrations in biopsy specimens of inflammatory acne lesions [44]. It is worth noting that, cytokines, i.e., IL-1β and IL-6 i TGF-β, were also found in acne lesions, and they play a significant role in the activation of Th17. Hence, acne was called T helper type 17 (Th17)-mediated disease [42]. Th17 cells not only characteristically induce the recruitment of neutrophils, which contribute to antimicrobial action, but also cause tissue injury [44]. In the same studies, it was shown that vitamin A (all-trans-retinoic acid) and vitamin D (1,25-dihydroxyvitamin D3) supressed this inflammatory stimulation. This discovery might be used to develop another acne therapy option in the future. Kistowska et al. [42] also found that *C. acnes* can promote mixed Th17/Th1 responses by inducing the secretion of IL-17A and IFN-γ from specific CD4+ T cells in vitro. Furthermore, it has been shown that both *C. acnes*-specific subpopulations of Th17 and Th17/Th1 cells can be found in the peripheral blood of patients suffering from acne [42]. Kelhala et al. [45] took an attempt to examine an inflammatory response, particularly the IL-23/Th17/IL-17A axis in acne lesions in vivo [45]. IL-17A and IL-17F are the key cytokines for the recruitment and activation of neutrophils, but they can also target different cell types including keratinocytes, endothelial cells, monocytes, and fibroblasts. These cells have the ability to secrete pro-inflammatory mediators, i.e., IL-6, TNF, IL-1β, PGE2, and MMP. All the aforementioned cytokines activate the production of Th17 from naive T cells in the presence of IL-23. TGF-β is a key cytokine in both Th17 and Treg-cell differentiation, while IL-17 and IFN-γ synergize in pro-inflammatory cytokine production in keratinocytes [45]. It is worth noting that Treg cells have not been studied in the context of acne lesions before. Kelhala et al. [45] were the first ones to demonstrate that the number of Foxp3+ cells significantly increased in acne lesions in the papillary dermis based on the results of immunohistochemistry. Regulatory T cells prevent autoimmunity and suppress immune responses. Retinoic acid can regulate reciprocally Tregs and Th17 via TGF-β-dependent generation of Foxp3. It is believed that it is a mechanism that may be of importance in the treatment of acne by isotretinoin. Moreover, elevated serum levels of IL-10 were found in acne patients, and the expression of this cytokine was increased in acne lesions. Although acne is often a chronic disease, a single acne lesion is seldom secondarily infected and is rapidly demarcated. The increased IL-10 expression and Treg cells may demarcate the inflammation of a single acne lesion efficiently [44]. The data provided indicate that acne vulgaris is a primary infectious disease, and histological, immunological, and clinical evidence suggest that inflammation is present at all stages of acne-lesion development [7]. Immune pathways at the core of initiating and propagating inflammation in acne are complex and may be related to *C. acnes*. Furthermore, inflammation may occur in acne lesions independently of these bacteria. The process is mediated by androgens or by neurogenic activation, followed by the secretion in the skin of pro-inflammatory neuropeptides [45,46].

4. Genetic Factors in Pathogenesis Acne Vulgaris

Acne vulgaris is a disease for which its occurrence and severity depend on various factors. These include, e.g., demographic, diet and lifestyle, and hormonal and genetic factors [47]. Current scientific reports on genes related to clinical symptoms and acne severity are scarce. Recent genome-wide studies have shown that genes associated with acne influence sebaceous gland functions or the development of an inflammatory immune response [48,49]. The *TNF* gene variants located on chromosome 6p21.33 are the most frequently studied genes in terms of the severity of acne lesions caused by pro-inflammatory immune responses [47]. The studies present that the crucial variants are variability in positions -308, -238, -863, -857, and -1031 TNF SNP in acne [50,51]. The polymorphism of genes for interleukins (IL) such as *IL1A*, *IL1B*, *IL4*, *IL6*, *IL8*, *IL10*, *IL17A*, *IL17F*, and related antagonists and receptors *IL1RN*, *IL4R*, *IL17RB*, and *IL23R* family genes are also responsible for the develop inflammation during acne vulgaris [47].

The groups of genes related to acne and a serious risk of acne can affect the function and activity of sebaceous glands. The families of the cytochrome P450 (CYP) gene and the 3-β HSD family (HSD3B) are two frequently examined families in analysis with respect to acne vulgaris [47,52,53].

5. Targeted Therapeutic Strategies in Acne Vulgaris

Targeted therapy for acne vulgaris is still under research and clinical trials. Recent studies report that agents that may be used to treat acne act by modulating the immune system.

One of these therapeutics include the inhibitors of interleukin-1β signaling, for example, Gevokizumab (XOMA 052) [54,55]. Gevokizumab is an anti-Il-1β humanized monoclonal immunoglobulin IgG2 antibody. Tle therapeutic role of Gevokizumab in acne vulgairs is actually studied in clinical trials (ClinicalTrial.gov Identifier: NCT01498874) [54,55]. IL-1β plays an important role in pathogenesis of acne vulgaris. The trial suggests that the inhibitors of interleukin-1β could be potentially used in acne treatment in the future.

6. Conclusions

Acne is a multifactorial immune-mediated chronic inflammatory disease of the pilosebaceous unit. *C. acnes*, which is present in sebaceous glands both in acne patients and in healthy individuals, plays a critical role in triggering host immune responses, which are considered crucial to the pathogenesis of acne vulgaris and are responsible for the clinical signs of acne vulgaris. There are at least four main pathways via which *C. acnes* interacts with the innate immune system to induce an inflammation: via TLRs, the activation of inflammasomes, the induction of the generation of matrix metalloproteinases (MMP), and the stimulation of antimicrobial peptides (AMP). Specific immune response cells, mainly Th1 and Th17 cells, also play a significant role in the pathogenesis of acne.

It is worth stressing that, in the future, the full understanding of the role of skin immune cells in acne pathogenesis might contribute to the development of state-of-the-art therapeutic strategies.

Author Contributions: Conceptualization, E.F. and W.K.; methodology, E.F., W.K., K.S., J.B. and J.R.; resources, E.F. and W.K.; data curation, W.K.; writing—original draft preparation, E.F, W.K. and J.B.; writing—review and editing, E.F., W.K. and J.R.; visualization, J.B.; supervision, J.B. and J.R.; project administration, E.F. All authors have read and agreed to the published version of the manuscript.

Funding: This research and APC was funded by Medical University of Lublin, grant number PBmb95.

Institutional Review Board Statement: Not applicable.

Informed Consent Statement: Not applicable.

Data Availability Statement: Not applicable.

Conflicts of Interest: The authors declare no conflict of interest.

References

1. Dréno, B.; Dagnelie, M.A.; Khammari, A.; Corvec, S. The Skin Microbiome: A New Actor in Inflammatory Acne. *Am. J. Clin. Dermatol.* **2020**, *21*, 18–24. [CrossRef] [PubMed]
2. Claudel, J.-P.; Auffret, N.; Leccia, M.-T.; Poli, F.; Corvec, S.; Dréno, B. Staphylococcus epidermidis: A Potential New Player in the Physiopathology of Acne? *Dermatology* **2019**, *235*, 287–294. [CrossRef] [PubMed]
3. Saurat, J.-H. Strategic Targets in Acne: The Comedone Switch in Question. *Dermatology* **2015**, *231*, 105–111. [CrossRef] [PubMed]
4. Veraldi, S.; Barbareschi, M. Comedone switch and reverse in acne pathogenesis and treatment. A role for silimarin? *AboutOpen* **2020**, *7*, 74–75. [CrossRef]
5. Manfredini, M.; Bettoli, V.; Sacripanti, G.; Farnetani, F.; Bigi, L.; Puviani, M.; Corazza, M.; Pellacani, G. The evolution of healthy skin to acne lesions: A longitudinal, in vivo evaluation with reflectance confocal microscopy and optical coherence tomography. *J. Eur. Acad. Dermatol. Venereol.* **2019**, *33*, 1768–1774. [CrossRef] [PubMed]
6. Harris, V.R.; Cooper, A.J. Modern management of acne. *Med. J. Aust.* **2017**, *206*, 41–45. [CrossRef] [PubMed]
7. Tanghetti, E.A. The role of inflammation in the pathology of acne. *J. Clin. Aesthet. Dermatol.* **2013**, *6*, 27–35.
8. Williams, H.C.; Dellavalle, R.; Garner, S. Acne vulgaris. *Lancet* **2011**, *379*, 361–372. [CrossRef]
9. Dreno, B.; Gollnick, H.; Kang, S.; Thiboutot, D.; Bettoli, V.; Torres, V.; Leyden, J.; The Global Alliance to Improve Outcomes in Acne. Understanding innate immunity and inflammation in acne: Implications for management. *J. Eur. Acad. Dermatol. Venereol.* **2015**, *29*, 3–11. [CrossRef]
10. Dréno, B.; Bettoli, V.; Araviiskaia, E.; Viera, M.S.; Bouloc, A. The influence of exposome on acne. *J. Eur. Acad. Dermatol. Venereol.* **2018**, *32*, 812–819. [CrossRef]
11. Kircik, L.H. Advances in the Understanding of the Pathogenesis of Inflammatory Acne. *J. Drugs Dermatol.* **2016**, *15*, 7–10.

12. Nguyen, A.V.; Soulika, A.M. The Dynamics of the Skin's Immune System. *Int. J. Mol. Sci.* **2019**, *20*, 1811. [CrossRef] [PubMed]
13. Nestle, F.O.; Di Meglio, P.; Qin, J.-Z.; Nickoloff, B.J. Skin immune sentinels in health and disease. *Nat. Rev. Immunol.* **2009**, *9*, 679–691. [CrossRef] [PubMed]
14. Szepietowski, J.; Kapińska-Mrowiecka, M.; Kaszuba, A.; Langner, A.; Placek, W.; Wolska, H.; Matusiak, Ł. Trądzik zwyczajny: Patogeneza i leczenie. Konsensus Polskiego Towarzystwa Dermatologicznego. *Przegl. Dermatol.* **2012**, *99*, 649–673.
15. Wilusz-Ludwiczak, K.; Kuchciak-Brancewicz, M.; Czyż, A.; Lesiak, A. Trądzik chorobą zapalną, a nie bakteryjną. *Forum Dermat.* **2019**, *5*, 92–95. [CrossRef]
16. Cao, H.; Yang, G.; Wang, Y.; Liu, J.P.; Smith, C.A.; Luo, H.; Liu, Y. Complementary therapies for acne vulgaris. *Cochrane Database Syst. Rev.* **2015**, *1*, CD009436. [CrossRef] [PubMed]
17. Zouboulis, C.C. Endocrinology and immunology of acne: Two sides of the same coin. *Exp. Dermatol.* **2020**, *29*, 840–859. [CrossRef]
18. Bergler-Czop, B. Trądzik odwrócony (acne inversa)—Najczęstsze błędy w postępowaniu diagnos-tyczno-terapeutycznym. *Diabetol. Dypl.* **2014**, *5*, 15–20.
19. Głowaczewska, A.; Reszke, R.; Szepietowski, J.C.; Matusiak, Ł. Indirect Self-Destructiveness in Hidradenitis Suppurativa Patients. *J. Clin. Med.* **2021**, *10*, 4194. [CrossRef]
20. Braun-Falco, M.; Kovnerystyy, O.; Lohse, P.; Ruzicka, T. Pyoderma gangrenosum, acne, and suppurative hidradenitis (PASH)? A new autoinflammatory syndrome distinct from PAPA syndrome. *J. Am. Acad. Dermatol.* **2012**, *66*, 409–415. [CrossRef]
21. Marzano, A.V.; Trevisan, V.; Gattorno, M.; Ceccherini, I.; De Simone, C.; Crosti, C. Pyogenic Arthritis, Pyoderma Gangrenosum, Acne, and Hidradenitis Suppurativa (PAPASH): A New Autoinflammatory Syndrome Associated with a Novel Mutation of the PSTPIP1 Gene. *JAMA Dermatol.* **2013**, *149*, 762–764. [CrossRef] [PubMed]
22. Bruzzese, V. Pyoderma Gangrenosum, Acne Conglobata, Suppurative Hidradenitis, and Axial Spondyloarthritis. *JCR J. Clin. Rheumatol.* **2012**, *18*, 413–415. [CrossRef] [PubMed]
23. Kumar, B.; Pathak, R.; Mary, P.B.; Jha, D.; Sardana, K.; Gautam, H.K. New insights into acne pathogenesis: Exploring the role of acne-associated microbial populations. *Dermatol. Sin.* **2016**, *34*, 67–73. [CrossRef]
24. Harder, J.; Tsuruta, D.; Murakami, M.; Kurokawa, I. What is the role of antimicrobial peptides (AMP) in acne vulgaris? *Exp. Dermatol.* **2013**, *22*, 386–391. [CrossRef] [PubMed]
25. Yang, L.; Shou, Y.-H.; Yang, Y.-S.; Xu, J.-H. Elucidating the immune infiltration in acne and its comparison with rosacea by integrated bioinformatics analysis. *PLoS ONE* **2021**, *16*, e0248650. [CrossRef] [PubMed]
26. Ozlu, E.; Karadag, A.S.; Ozkanli, S.; Oguztuzun, S.; Kilic, M.; Zemheri, E.; Akbulak, O.; Akdeniz, N. Comparison of TLR-2, TLR-4, and antimicrobial peptide levels in different lesions of acne vulgaris. *Cutan. Ocul. Toxicol.* **2015**, *35*, 300–309. [CrossRef] [PubMed]
27. Jugeau, S.; Tenaud, I.; Knol, A.C.; Jarrousse, V.; Quereux, G.; Khammari, A.; Dreno, B. Induction of toll-like receptors by Propionibacterium acnes. *Br. J. Dermatol.* **2005**, *153*, 1105–1113. [CrossRef] [PubMed]
28. Kutlubay, Z.; Kecici, A.S.; Engin, B.; Serdaroglu, S.; Tuzun, Y. Acne Vulgaris. In *Acne and Acneiform Eruptions*, 1st ed.; Kartal, S.P., Gönül, M., Eds.; IntechOpen: Rijeka, Croatia, 2017; pp. 7–30. [CrossRef]
29. Moreno-Arrones, O.; Boixeda, P. The Importance of Innate Immunity in Acne. *Actas Dermo-Sifiliográficas* **2016**, *107*, 801–805. [CrossRef] [PubMed]
30. Selway, J.L.; Kurczab, T.; Kealey, T.; Langlands, K. Toll-like receptor 2 activation and comedogenesis: Implications for the pathogenesis of acne. *BMC Dermatol.* **2013**, *13*, 10. [CrossRef]
31. Tenaud, I.; Khammari, A.; Dreno, B. In Vitro modulation of TLR-2, CD1d and IL-10 by adapalene on normal human skin and acne inflammatory lesions. *Exp. Dermatol.* **2007**, *16*, 500–506. [CrossRef] [PubMed]
32. Jarrousse, V.; Castex-Rizzi, N.; Khammari, A.; Charveron, M.; Dréno, B. Modulation of integrins and filaggrin expression by Propionibacterium acnes extracts on keratinocytes. *Arch. Dermatol. Res.* **2007**, *299*, 441–447. [CrossRef] [PubMed]
33. Jeong, E.; Hong, J.W.; Min, J.A.; Lee, D.W.; Sohn, M.Y.; Lee, W.J.; Lee, J.Y.; Park, Y.M. Topical ALA-Photodynamic Therapy for Acne Can Induce Apoptosis of Sebocytes and Down-regulate Their TLR-2 and TLR-4 Expression. *Ann. Dermatol.* **2011**, *23*, 23–32. [CrossRef] [PubMed]
34. Bakry, O.A.; Samaka, R.M.; Sebika, H.; Seleit, I. Toll-like receptor 2 and P. acnes: Do they trigger initial acne vulgaris lesions? *Anal. Quant. Cytopathol. Histpathol.* **2014**, *36*, 100–110. [PubMed]
35. Qin, M.; Pirouz, A.; Kim, M.-H.; Krutzik, S.R.; Garbán, H.J.; Kim, J. Propionibacterium acnes Induces IL-1β Secretion via the NLRP3 Inflammasome in Human Monocytes. *J. Investig. Dermatol.* **2014**, *134*, 381–388. [CrossRef] [PubMed]
36. Hammam, M.A.; Nesreen, G.A.; Mahmoud, S.N.H. Matrix metalloproteinase-9 in the blood of acne patients: The possible use of matrix metalloproteinase-9 as a biomarker of acne severity. *Menoufia Med. J.* **2020**, *33*, 1055–1058.
37. Nakatsuji, T.; Gallo, R.L. Antimicrobial Peptides: Old Molecules with New Ideas. *J. Investig. Dermatol.* **2012**, *132*, 887–895. [CrossRef] [PubMed]
38. Marcinkiewicz, M.; Majewski, S. The role of antimicrobial peptides in chronic inflammatory skin diseases. *Adv. Dermatol. Allergol.* **2016**, *1*, 6–12. [CrossRef] [PubMed]
39. Aksoy, B. Derinin dogal bagisiklik sistemi/Skin innate immune system. *Turk. Arch. Dermatol. Venereol.* **2013**, *47*, 2–11. [CrossRef]
40. Poiraud, C.; Quereux, G.; Knol, A.-C.; Zuliani, T.; Allix, R.; Khammari, A.; Dreno, B. Human β-defensin-2 and psoriasin, two new innate immunity targets of zinc gluconate. *Eur. J. Dermatol.* **2012**, *22*, 634–639. [CrossRef] [PubMed]
41. Borovaya, A.; Dombrowski, Y.; Zwicker, S.; Olisova, O.; Ruzicka, T.; Wolf, R.; Schauber, J.; Sárdy, M. Isotretinoin therapy changes the expression of antimicrobial peptides in acne vulgaris. *Arch. Dermatol. Res.* **2014**, *306*, 689. [CrossRef]

42. Kistowska, M.; Meier-Schiesser, B.; Proust, T.; Feldmeyer, L.; Cozzio, A.; Kuendig, T.; Contassot, E.; French, L.E. Propionibacterium acnes Promotes Th17 and Th17/Th1 Responses in Acne Patients. *J. Investig. Dermatol.* **2015**, *135*, 110–118. [CrossRef] [PubMed]
43. Verma, G.; Sardana, K. Propionibacterium acnes and the Th1/Th17 Axis, implications in acne pathogenesis and treatment. *Indian J. Dermatol.* **2017**, *62*, 392–394. [CrossRef] [PubMed]
44. Agak, G.W.; Kao, S.; Ouyang, K.; Qin, M.; Moon, D.; Butt, A.; Kim, J. Phenotype and Antimicrobial Activity of Th17 Cells Induced by Propionibacterium acnes Strains Associated with Healthy and Acne Skin. *J. Investig. Dermatol.* **2017**, *138*, 316–324. [CrossRef] [PubMed]
45. Kelhälä, H.-L.; Palatsi, R.; Fyhrquist, N.; Lehtimäki, S.; Väyrynen, J.; Kallioinen, M.; Kubin, M.E.; Greco, D.; Tasanen, K.; Alenius, H.; et al. IL-17/Th17 Pathway Is Activated in Acne Lesions. *PLoS ONE* **2014**, *9*, e105238. [CrossRef]
46. Antiga, E.; Verdelli, A.; Bonciani, D.; Bonciolini, V.; Caproni, M.; Fabbri, P. Acne: A new model of immune-mediated chronic inflammatory skin disease. *G. Ital. Dermatol. Venereol.* **2015**, *150*, 247–254. [PubMed]
47. Heng, A.H.S.; Say, Y.-H.; Sio, Y.Y.; Ng, Y.T.; Chew, F.T. Gene variants associated with acne vulgaris presentation and severity: A systematic review and meta-analysis. *BMC Med. Genom.* **2021**, *14*, 103. [CrossRef]
48. Navarini, A.A.; Simpson, M.A.; Weale, M.; Knight, J.; Carlavan, I.; Reiniche, P.; Burden, D.A.; Layton, A.; Bataille, V.; Allen, M.; et al. Genome-wide association study identifies three novel susceptibility loci for severe Acne vulgaris. *Nat. Commun.* **2014**, *5*, 4020. [CrossRef] [PubMed]
49. Petridis, C.; Navarini, A.A.; Dand, N.; Saklatvala, J.; Baudry, D.; Duckworth, M.; Allen, M.H.; Curtis, C.J.; Lee, S.H.; Burden, A.D.; et al. Genome-wide meta-analysis implicates mediators of hair follicle development and morphogenesis in risk for severe acne. *Nat. Commun.* **2018**, *9*, 5075. [CrossRef]
50. Grech, I.; Giatrakos, S.; Damoraki, G.; Kaldrimidis, P.; Rigopoulos, D.; Giamarellos-Bourboulis, E.J. Impact of TNF Haplotypes in the Physical Course of Acne Vulgaris. *Dermatology* **2013**, *228*, 152–157. [CrossRef]
51. Szabó, K.; Tax, G.; Teodorescu-Brinzeu, D.; Koreck, A.; Kemény, L. TNFα gene polymorphisms in the pathogenesis of acne vulgaris. *Arch. Dermatol. Res.* **2010**, *303*, 19–27. [CrossRef]
52. Chamaie-Nejad, F.; Saeidi, S.; Najafi, F.; Ebrahimi, A.; Rahimi, Z.; Shakiba, E. Association of the CYP17 MSP AI (T-34C) and CYP19 codon 39 (Trp/Arg) polymorphisms with susceptibility to acne vulgaris. *Clin. Exp. Dermatol.* **2017**, *43*, 183–186. [CrossRef] [PubMed]
53. Yang, X.-Y.; Wu, W.-J.; Yang, C.; Yang, T.; He, J.-D.; Yang, Z.; He, L. Association of HSD17B3 and HSD3B1 Polymorphisms with Acne Vulgaris in Southwestern Han Chinese. *Dermatology* **2013**, *227*, 202–208. [CrossRef] [PubMed]
54. Bhat, Y.; Latief, I.; Hassan, I. Update on etiopathogenesis and treatment of Acne. *Indian J. Dermatol. Venereol. Leprol.* **2017**, *83*, 298–306. [CrossRef] [PubMed]
55. Owyang, A.M.; Issafras, H.; Corbin, J.; Ahluwalia, K.; Larsen, P.; Pongo, E.; Handa, M.; Horwitz, A.H.; Roell, M.K.; Haak-Frendscho, M.; et al. XOMA 052, a potent, high-affinity monoclonal antibody for the treatment of IL-1β-mediated diseases. *mAbs* **2011**, *3*, 49–60. [CrossRef] [PubMed]

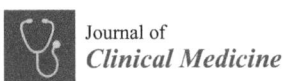

Review

Methods for the Improvement of Acne Scars Used in Dermatology and Cosmetology: A Review

Karolina Chilicka [1,*], Monika Rusztowicz [1], Renata Szyguła [1] and Danuta Nowicka [2]

[1] Department of Health Sciences, Institute of Health Sciences, University of Opole, 45-040 Opole, Poland; monika.rusztowicz@uni.opole.pl (M.R.); renata.szygula@uni.opole.pl (R.S.)

[2] Department of Dermatology, Venereology and Allergology, Wrocław Medical University, 50-368 Wrocław, Poland; danuta.nowicka@umed.wroc.pl

* Correspondence: karolina.chilicka@uni.opole.pl; Tel.: +48-665-43-94-43

Abstract: Acne vulgaris is a chronic skin disease that, depending on its course, is characterized by the occurrence of various skin eruptions such as open and closed comedones, pustules, papules, and cysts. Incorrectly selected treatment or the presence of severe acne vulgaris can lead to the formation of atrophic scars. In this review, we summarize current knowledge on acne scars and methods for their improvement. There are three types of atrophic scars: icepick, rolling, and boxcar. They are of different depths and widths and have different cross-sections. Scars can combine to form clusters. If acne scars are located on the face, they can reduce the patient's quality of life, leading to isolation and depression. There are multiple effective modalities to treat acne scars. Ablative lasers, radiofrequency, micro-needling, and pilings with trichloroacetic acid have very good treatment results. Contemporary dermatology and cosmetology use treatments that cause minimal side effects, so the patient can return to daily functioning shortly after treatment. Proper dermatological treatment and skincare, as well as the rapid implementation of cosmetological treatments, will certainly achieve satisfactory results in reducing atrophic scars.

Keywords: acne vulgaris; atrophic scars; dermatology; scar improvement

1. Introduction

Acne vulgaris is a chronic skin disease that, depending on its course, is characterized by the occurrence of skin eruptions such as open and closed comedones, pustules, and cysts [1,2]. It occurs in more than 80% of adolescents, 50–60% of women aged 20–25 years, and 12% of women over 25. Factors that cause the disease include abnormal keratinization of the pilosebaceous canal, increased sebum production, bacterial colonization, as well as inflammatory and hormonal disorders of the skin [3,4].

During the course of the disease, patients with acne experience itching and burning of the skin. Acne scars appear most often in people struggling with severe forms of acne, leading to a reduction in their quality of life. Patients often feel ashamed, embarrassed, anxious, and socially isolated, which can lead to depression and even suicidal thoughts [5–8].

A scar (also named cicatrix) is a skin lesion that results from the healing of wounds due to chemical, mechanical, or thermal injuries. Scars can develop after skin inflammation, for example, as a complication of acne. Scar formation is part of the wound healing process, which is divided into three phases: inflammatory, healing, and remodeling.

The inflammatory phase begins in the first 6 h after the skin is injured and continues for the next 48–72 h. During this phase, blood vessels dilate, and their permeability increases under the influence of kinins, histamine, prostaglandins, and leukotrienes. The skin is visibly swollen and red. The exudate starts to produce itself. Leukocytes migrate to the inflamed site under the influence of chemotaxins. The wound is debrided due to the dominance of white blood cells (neutrophils) and their phagocytic properties, as well as due to the release of proteolytic enzymes. The recruitment of monocytes, which replace neutrophilic granulocytes, increases on the second day after skin injury. Subsequently, after contact with the intercellular matrix, monocytes are transformed into macrophages, due to which microbial phagocytosis and wound debridement take place. A range of cytokines and a growth factor are produced due to macrophage activation, which stimulates fibroblasts and white blood cells. All those processes stimulate epithelialization and the formation of new blood vessels [9–11].

The second phase of wound healing is the proliferative phase. It begins 2–3 days after tissue damage and may continue for 3–6 weeks. It lasts from about 10 days to several weeks on average. In this phase, the number of fibroblasts stimulated by cytokines (PDGF, EGT, TGF beta, FGF) increases. The process of granulation tissue formation and collagen production begins. The skin defect is filled with granulation tissue containing a network of capillaries, fibroblasts, and white blood cells. This step begins between the third and fifth day after the injury and lasts up to several weeks. First, type III collagen is produced, and then it is replaced by type I collagen. Between the 14th and 28th days after the injury, collagen synthesis is most intense, and then it decreases due to the enzyme activity of the metalloproteinases of the extracellular matrix. During the production of granulation tissue in a wounded area, epithelization occurs, and new blood vessels are formed. During epithelialization, keratinocytes enter the wound from the periphery. This is followed by the proliferation of keratinocytes [12,13].

The last phase—the remodeling phase—is the rebuilding and maturation of the scar. This begins between the third and seventh day after the injury and lasts several months up to a year. Granulation is replaced by fibrous tissue. Approximately 5 days after the injury, the wound contracts, and this process continues for approximately 14 days. Microfibroblasts, present in a wound, have contractile properties due to active filaments that create gap junctions with fibronectin and collagen. As a result of their contraction, the edges of the wound are pulled together, and as a result, the wound gets smaller [14,15].

Types of the Acne Scars

Incorrect production and degradation of collagen during the healing process can lead to the development of various types of scars. Scars can be classified according to the cause and time of their formation and appearance. The last group of acne scars is divided into atrophic, hypertrophic, and discolored. Atrophic scars are below the surface of the skin and are recessed. On the other hand, hypertrophic scars are raised above the skin surface [16].

Atrophic scars can be divided into the following types: icepick, rolling, and boxcar. Icepick scars are deep, narrow, and can reach the border of the dermis with the subcutaneous tissue. They have sharp edges, a width of not more than 2 mm, and a V-shaped cross-section with a narrowing deep into the skin. The skin of a person with such scars looks like it has been pierced with a skewer or sharp instrument. Icepick scars account for 60% to 70% of atrophic scars. Boxcar scars are oval or round but quite wide and flat and resemble the letter U or a square. Their edges are well marked and have a demarcated edge. They are usually 0.1–0.5 mm deep and 1.5–4 mm wide. They can combine to form clusters. Boxcar scars have the cross-section of the letter M and account for 15 to 20% of atrophic scars. Rolling scars are the largest of all types and can reach a diameter of 5 mm. They comprise 15% to 25% of atrophic scars [16].

2. Methods of Acne Scars Management

Contemporary aesthetic medicine and cosmetology can offer a wide range of effective methods for reducing acne scars. Depending on the type of scar, its location, and the depth of the lesions, a dermatologist, in cooperation with a cosmetologist, can propose a series of treatments that will significantly flatten unwanted skin defects and improve the patient's quality of life.

2.1. Ablative Laser Resurfacing

Several traditional ablative lasers are used to treat acne scars, e.g., 10,600 nm carbon dioxide (CO_2) lasers and 2940 nm pulsed Er:YAG lasers [16]. Conventional 10,600 nm CO_2 lasers emit light in the far-infrared spectrum. Such a laser creates many microscopic treatment zones to activate new collagen formation and re-epithelialization [17]. The first application of the continuous CO_2 laser took place in the 1980s. Over the years, pulsed action lasers have started to be implemented, which has improved the precision of their action and depth of skin ablation and thus reduced the occurrence of side effects [18]. The CO_2 laser, either fully ablative or fractional mode, has been proposed to treat various conditions alone or combined with other devices [19–21].

The study by Fang et al. suggests that in treating atrophic acne scars in Asians using a fractional CO_2 laser, 3 treatment sessions led to better results as assessed after 3 months [22]. Several other studies indicate that combined treatments can give better results than single laser treatments alone. Li et al. also showed an improvement in skin texture in patients with atrophic scars after one treatment. In this study, fractional microplasma radiofrequency treatment combined with fractional ablative CO_2 laser treatment was performed in 45 patients, while a single procedure was performed in 19 patients. There were no statistically significant differences between the two groups; however, a greater number of combined treatments helped improve acne scars [23]. Gala et al. conducted a study on 30 patients using a fractional CO_2 laser on one side of the face and a fractional CO_2 laser followed by platelet-rich plasma (PRP) intradermal injections on the other half. In both groups, the effects were satisfactory; however, the synergy of the treatments contributed to a better improvement in atrophic scars, which was shown 3 months after completion of the treatments using the skin analysis camera [24]. Zhou et al. used a combination of the CO_2 laser with allogeneic stem cells. This treatment improved elasticity and skin hydration. A histological examination showed an increase in the density of dermal collagen and elastic fibers [25].

The traditional pulsed Er:YAG laser (2940 nm) was developed as a less aggressive alternative to the traditional CO_2 laser. The emitted wavelength is also in the infrared range; however, the thermal energy is more limited and precise at the same time, as the laser light closely approximates the absorption peak of water (3000 nm). For this reason, all energy is absorbed in the epidermis and superficial dermis. An Er:YAG laser at 5 J/cm vaporizes tissue at a depth of 20 to 25 µm with an additional 5 to 10 µm zone of thermal necrosis. This causes less damage to the skin than when a CO_2 laser is used [16,18,26].

Tidwell et al. compared the fractional Er:YAG laser with fully ablative Er:YAG in people with hypertrophic scars. Twenty patients with scars not younger than 8 weeks and not older than 1 year were enrolled in the study, but only 16 patients completed the entire series of treatments. A fractionated Er:YAG laser was used on one half of the face, while treatments with a fully ablative Er:YAG laser was applied on the other side. A series of 3 treatments were performed with a one-month interval between them. Follow-up visits were made 1 and 2 months after the final treatment. The study showed superior outcomes in the fractionated Er:YAG group over the fully ablative Er:YAG group [27]. Zgavec and Loca demonstrated using a histological examination that wound healing after Er:YAG treatment is shorter when compared to full beam ablative treatment with milder side effects [28]. Cenk et al. investigated the effectiveness of a series of 4 multifractional Er:YAG laser treatments in women and men with acne scars. At the end of the 4th session, the improvement rate was 26% to 50% in 14 of 24 patients and 51% to 75% in 10 patients [29]. Emam et al. treated 21 people with the fractional Er:YAG laser and radiofrequency micro-needling (MN). Er:YAG laser treatment was performed on one side of the face and radiofrequency MN on the other side. A series of 4 treatments were performed, each with a month-long break. To compare the effectiveness of the treatments, optical coherence tomography was used. After the end of the series of treatments, both sides of the face were compared, showing very good results and a scar improvement. There were no significant differences between these two devices. Optical coherence tomography showed a significant increase in epidermal and dermal thickness after 4 treatments compared to the baseline [30].

2.2. Non-Ablative Lasers

This group of lasers includes a pulsed dye laser (PDL) with a wavelength of 585 to 600 nm, ND:YAG with a wavelength of 1320 nm, and a diode laser with a wavelength of 1450 nm. This kind of laser is helpful in reducing scars classified as boxcar or atrophic. The chromophore in PDL is hemoglobin, and the laser supports the reduction of scars of various etiologies with the simultaneous elimination of blood vessels within the lesion. The adverse effect of using this device include persistent post-operative purpura for up to 14 days [31].

Rogachefsky et al. investigated the treatment of atrophic or a mixed pattern scarring with a 1320-nm Nd:YAG laser. Twelve patients with atrophic facial acne scars (N = 6) or a combination of atrophic and pitted, sclerotic, or boxcar scars (N = 6) underwent 3 laser sessions. The mean improvement in acne scars was 1.5 points on physician assessments ($p = 0.002$) and 2.2 points on patient assessments ($p = 0.01$). There were no complications at 6 months [32].

Sadick et al. used a 1320-nm Nd:YAG laser to check the efficacy of lasers for the treatment of acne scars. Eight probants with acne scars received 6 monthly treatments with a 1320-nm Nd:YAG laser with built-in cryogen cooling. The scar improvement was significant [33].

The 1450-nm diode laser was used by Tanzi et al. to compare it with the 1320-nm Nd:YAG laser. Twenty patients with mild-to-moderate atrophic facial acne scars randomly received 3 monthly treatments with a long-pulsed 1320-nm Nd:YAG laser on one half of the face and a long-pulsed 1450-nm diode laser on the other half of the face. The 1450-nm diode laser had a better clinical scar response [34].

Rathod et al. conducted a study on 48 probants with acne scars with a low-energy double-pass 1450-nm diode laser (5 treatment sessions). At the end of the 3rd month, 92.9% of the patients demonstrated >30% improvement. The diode laser treatment was efficient in facial acne scars when used with a double pass at low energy [35].

The studies conducted by Cannarozzo et al. deserve special attention. These two investigations showed the effect of a 675-nm laser on the skin. This device is recommended to treat hyperpigmentation, scars, and various types of wrinkles. In a case report of a 42-year-old man, after the laser treatment, skin biopsies showed the proliferation of new collagen fibers in the treated area. Histological analysis suggests that the 675-nm laser has a potential role in stimulating collagen remodeling, with a significant increase in thin and new collagen fibers. Another study by the same authors was conducted on 24 patients with acne scars. The patients had 3 sessions of the 675-nm laser. The efficacy of the treatment was evaluated using the Goodman and Baron grading scale before and 3 months after the last treatment. All patients had significant scar improvement and no side effects. This laser system is well tolerated with comfortable and easy posttreatment management for patients [36,37].

2.3. Trichloroacetic Acid

Trichloroacetic acid (TCA) is an organic compound of the class of carboxylic acids with the following chemical formula $C(Cl)_3COOH$. It is the most effective and one of the strongest acids. Its power (pKa) is 0.26 and, for comparison, the pKa of glycolic acid is 3.83. Depending on the effects to achieve, superficial peeling (10–30% TCA), medium-deep peeling (35% TCA), and deep peeling (50% TCA) can be used. This acid coagulates proteins and damages living cells of the epidermis, resulting in necrosis of the epidermis and the upper layer of the dermis, as well as exfoliation of the cells. In the long term, the treatment with TCA stimulates the production of new collagen fibers. The application of TCA to the skin causes protein denaturation (keratocoagulation), resulting in the appearance of white shedding on the patient's skin, the so-called frost [38,39].

Agarwal et al. evaluated the application of 70% TCA every 2 weeks in 53 patients with atrophic scars using the chemical reconstruction of skin scars (CROSS) technique. Good or very good improvement was seen in 66% of the patients. In total, 81.1% of the patients reported being satisfied or very satisfied [40]. Bhardwaj et al. used the same CROSS technique in 12 patients with atrophic scars but with 100% TCA every 2 weeks. Eight out of 10 patients reported an improvement in post-acne scars of more than 70%. No side effects were observed during treatment. One of the patients reported a lack of further improvement after 3 months after treatment [41]. Al-Hamamy et al. evaluated the effectiveness of 25% TCA combined with dermasanding. They reported a satisfactory improvement in acne scars. No significant complications were found except erythema and post-inflammatory hyperpigmentation, which disappeared after 3 months in affected patients [42]. Puri researched 25 patients who were divided into 2 groups. The first group had Jassner's peeling with 20% TCA, while the latter had only 20% TCA. In the first group, mild improvement in acne scars was observed in 8% of the patients, moderate improvement was observed in 32% of the patients, and marked improvement was observed in 60% of the patients. In the group treated with 20% TCA alone, mild improvement was seen in 32% of the patients, moderate improvement was observed in 40% of the patients, and marked improvement was observed in 25% of the patients. The results in both groups were similar. The group using the combination of Jessner's peel with 20% TCA did not show better results than the group treated with 20% TCA alone [43].

Concerning TCA, our research team is finishing researching its influence on acne scars. The results after only 2 treatments are very promising, and the skin structure is significantly improved. This study will be published soon.

2.4. Microneedling

MN is used in cosmetology as a treatment that rejuvenates the skin, improves its tension, and also improves stretch marks and scars. Due to the lack of post-inflammatory discoloration after MN, it is often used as an alternative to laser treatment in the case of skins with IV and V phototypes. The following MN devices can be used: rollers, stampers, and pens (electric or non-electric) [44]. Research has shown that after a series of treatments, there is increased expression of type I collagen, as well as glycosaminoglycans, vascular endothelial growth factor (VEGF), fibroblast growth factor (FGF)-7, epidermal growth factor (EGF), and transforming growth factor (TGF)-β, all important signaling molecules for collagen production and neovascularization [45,46].

In the study by El-Domyati et al., 10 patients were treated with skin MN in a series of 6 treatments performed every 2 weeks. Skin biopsies were obtained at baseline and after 3 months from the start of the treatment. The authors reported an improvement in acne scars and a significant increase in collagen types I, III, and VII [47]. Tirmizi et al. enrolled 50 patients with moderate to severe grade atrophic acne spars classified using the Goodman and Baron's Global Acne Scarring System. Three treatments were carried out every 4 weeks. The authors concluded that after MN, scars improved together with the improvement in scar grade, resulting in a greater number of patients classified as grade II after MN compared to the baseline. The study showed a beneficial effect of MN on the patient's skin [48]. Biesman et al. evaluated the effects of MN used in combination with Polymethylmethacrylate-Collagen Gel Dermal Filler (PMMA). In the study, 44 probants were enrolled and divided into 2 groups. The first group received 3 MN treatments and the second group received 3 MN treatments combined with PMMA. After 24 weeks, the group that had combined treatment showed better treatment effects. This fact confirmed the occurrence of synergies of treatments, so a combined treatment is advisable to achieve better results [49]. Finally, Schoenberg et al., in their study and a short review, described the effect of combined MN treatments with PRP in a group of 50 patients. The MN procedure was carried out on the entire face. Each half was treated with PRP or distilled water injected into the skin. After the end of the series of treatments, combined treatment showed better results [50].

Our experience shows that combining an MN treatment with, e.g., BioRePeel, gives much better results than performing separate treatments.

2.5. Fractional Radiofrequency

The use of microneedle radiofrequency is based on the ability to selectively heat the tissue at a specific depth. The device also uses micro-needles through which a beam of radio waves is emitted directly into the tissue. Additionally, the needles only heat up at their tips, which allows precise control of the depth at which the tissue is heated. Such a feature of this technique is unique and important for final effects. The puncture depth can be adjusted to 0.5 to 3.5 mm. Microneedle radiofrequency has gained great popularity in cosmetology due to improvement in scars.

Kim et al. used a fractional radiofrequency microneedle treatment in 52 patients with atrophic acne scars located on the face. Each of the patients received 4-treatment series. The Goodman and Baron's Global Acne Scarring System evaluated treatment results. Overall, 73.1% of patients improved according to the grading system. Five patients experienced post-inflammatory hyperpigmentation. The authors concluded that this method is effective with minimal risk of complications [51]. Chandrashekar et al. used microneedle radiofrequency to treat 31 patients with moderate and severe acne scars. The study protocol was based on 4 treatments conducted over 6 months every 6 weeks. After the treatments, the scars improved. Of grade 3 and 4 acne scars, 80.64% improved by 2 grades, and 19.35% improved by 1 grade, according to the Goodman and Baron's Global Acne Scarring System. The transient adverse effects reported by the patients were pain, erythema, edema, and hyperpigmentation [52]. Elawar et al. recruited 19 patients to evaluate the improvement in acne scars and skin, as well as the reduction of skin pores after 2 to 4 microneedle fractional radiofrequency treatments conducted at intervals of 1 month. The authors concluded that this method effectively treats acne scars, as it improves skin texture, reduces pore size, and increases patient satisfaction. Furthermore, none of the patients experienced hyper/hypopigmentation [53]. Kim et al. aimed to investigate the effectiveness of bipolar fractional radiofrequency in patients with acne scars and enlarged pores. The study protocol was based on 4 treatments conducted at 3-week intervals. The evaluation was carried out 3 months after completion of the protocol and showed clinical improvement. Objective measures confirmed improved elasticity and the melanin/erythema index, as well as more procollagen types I and III, and elastin. Furthermore, bipolar fractional radiofrequency appeared to be safe, as none of the patients reported side effects [54]. Similar observations were made by Qin et al. after a series of 4 treatments performed every month on a group of 23 Asian patients. The acne score improved significantly at 4 and 12 weeks after the first treatment. Side effects included transient pain, erythema, and dryness of the skin [55]. Chilicka et al. in their case reports showed that it is extremely important to continue research on the effects of glycolic acid and fractional mesotherapy to reduce acne scars. The needle radiofrequency with the application of active substances provided very good results for the shallowing of post-acne scars. This therapy changed the structure, visual appearance of the skin, and made the scars more shallow, as analyzed using the Goodman and Baron's scale. In addition, only needle radiofrequency gave good results in shallowing the scars [56,57]. It should also be remembered that to prevent acne scars it is extremely important to care for the skin of people who suffer from acne. This is evidence-based on numerous scientific studies [58–61]. Combination treatments are very useful in scars and improve scars much better than a single treatment (Table 1).

Table 1. Combination treatments for acne scars.

	Type of Treatment			
	Platelet-rich plasma	CO$_2$ laser	Acids	Subcision
Combination treatments	Fractional laser resurfacing [62]	Fractional microplasma radiofrequency [23]	Dermasanding [42]	Cross-linked hyaluronic acid or poly-l-lactic acid threads [63]
	Chemical reconstruction of skin scars technique [64]	Platelet-rich plasma [24]	Jessner's peeling [43]	Endolift (200-nm fiber) [65]
	Subcision and needling [62]	Allogeneic steam cell [25]	Fractional radiofrequency [57]	Platelet-rich plasma [66]
	Microneedling [67]			
	Transplantation of autologous fat, stromal vascular fraction cell [68]			

2.6. Platelet-Rich Plasma

Platelet-rich plasma (PRP) is an autologous blood-derived product enriched in platelets, growth factors, and chemo/cytokines delivered in a volume of plasma. PRP has the potential to deliver a high concentration of growth factors to the target tissues [69]. Lee et al. conducted a split-face study with 14 probants from Korea. They underwent fractional laser resurfacing, and the researchers randomly assigned them to receive normal saline or PRP. The improvement after 4 months was superior in the group with laser and PRP [62].

Mumtaz et al. compared the efficacy of PRP versus 50% TCA using the CROSS technique in treatment; PRP was significantly better than 50% TCA in reducing post-acne atrophic scars [64]. Bhargava et al. conducted a study using PRP as adjunctive therapy to a combined subcision and needling treatment in severe atrophic acne scarring. Thirty patients were randomly divided into 2 groups (15 patients for each group). Group A underwent 3 treatments-subcision and needling. Group B had 3 subcision, needling, and topical application treatments of PRP. Scar improvement ≥50% was better in group B than group A patients ($p = 0.025$) [70].

Ibrahim et al. used skin MN plus PRP versus skin MN alone to treat 35 patients with mild-to-severe acne scars. The patients received 4 sequential treatments of skin MN alone on the right side of the face and skin MN followed by topical application of PRP on the left side of the face. Treatment was conducted at intervals of 3 weeks. A significant improvement was observed on both sides of the face [67].

Nilforoushzadeh et al. used autologous fat, stromal vascular fraction cells, and PRP as cell therapy techniques in atrophic acne scars. Nine patients received autologous fat transplantation, PRP, and stromal vascular fraction cells. After 6 months, there was an improvement in skin lightness, skin elasticity, transepidermal water loss, spots, and skin pores. More than 66% of the patients were satisfied after these treatments [68].

Chawla S. used MN with PRP on one side of the face and MN with vitamin C on the other side. The treatments had an interval of 1 month. Overall, 27 out of 30 patients completed the study. The PRP group achieved a better response than the MN with the vitamin C group. The patients treated with MN and vitamin C were also more satisfied [71].

2.7. Subcision and Punch Techniques

2.7.1. Subcision

Subcision is based on inserting the needle under the scar to sever the fibrous tissue and binding down the scar. This method releases fibrous tissue and raises the scar so that it is effective in rolling and other tethered scars. Ebrahim et al. conducted a study to evaluate the efficacy of subcision versus its combination with cross-linked hyaluronic acid or poly-l-lactic acid threads in atrophic post-acne scars. Forty men and women took part in this study based on 3 sessions conducted at 1-month intervals. Subcision combined with hyaluronic acid or threads gave better clinical improvement than subcision alone [63].

Nilforoushzadeh et al. conducted a pilot study with 9 patients with acne scars. The probants underwent subcision with the Endolift (200-nm fiber). The study showed a 90% improvement. The number of lesions before the treatment was 25.5 ± 12.1, and after treatment, it was reduced to 11.4 ± 2.1 ($p < 0.05$) [65].

Deshmukh et al. used PRP and the subcision method in their study. Forty patients completed the split-face study. The right side of the face was treated with autologous PRP injected after subcision. The left side was the control side, where only subcision was performed. The right side, after treatment, showed better improvement in post-acne scars than subcision alone. This treatment performed better for rolling scars than for box scars. It shows that synergic treatments are better for treating scars [66].

2.7.2. Punch Elevation and Punch Excision

Punch elevation is the method developed for broad (3 mm) boxcar scars with sharp edges and normal bases. It is a technique where the scar is punched down to the subcutaneous tissue without being discarded. "The punched scar is then elevated and sutured in place at a level slightly higher than the surrounding skin to account for contraction during wound healing" [72].

Punch excision is suited for icepick and narrow (B 3 mm) boxcar scars. "The scar is excised down to the subcutaneous fat with the help of a punch instrument that is slightly larger than the scar, and the defect is closed with sutures along relaxed skin tension lines" [73].

3. Comparison of Methods

Notable is the comparison of various methods to reduce acne scars. Husein-El Ahmed et al. included 5 studies in their meta-analysis on non-ablative erbium versus CO_2 lasers for atrophic acne scars. The scar improvement was similar for both types of laser in terms of investigator-reported scar improvement. The ablative laser produced a slightly greater response compared to non-ablative lasers based on the physician's assessment [74].

Elsaie et al. conducted a study with 58 probants comparing these two methods. Each group included 29 patients, and each had 4 treatment sessions at 3-week intervals. The follow-up visit was after 3 months. Group A was treated with CO_2 lasers, and group B with a 1540-nm erbium glass laser. The improvement was higher in group A, but with a non-significant difference between both treatments. These two lasers were good for treating acne scars [75].

Reinholz et al. conducted a study with 14 patients with severe scars. Both cheeks were treated randomly 4 times with lasers. One side with Er:YAG, and the other side with CO_2 laser. The high-resolution, 3D small-field capture system, digital photography, and POSAS were used before and after the treatment sessions. The higher efficacy (better skin smoothing) was achieved in the group treated with the fractional CO_2 laser [76].

There is a lot of research on the use of TCA in the literature. Comparing the studies by Agarwal et al. in which they used 70% TCA CROSS, and the studies by Puri et al. with modified Jessner's Peel and 20% TCA versus 20% TCA peel alone, we can conclude that better results were obtained in the case of 70% TCA CROS [40,43].

Ahmed et al. used the CO_2 laser pinpoint irradiation technique versus CROSS technique for treating ice pick acne scars. Twenty-eight probants with acne scars were divided into 2 groups. Fourteen patients received pinpoint irradiation by CO_2 laser, and another 14 probants received TCA CROSS. Each patient had 4 sessions with 3-week intervals (3 months of follow-up). The researchers showed that clinical improvement was better with CO_2 laser [77].

Leheta et al. investigated the efficacy of combining a 1540-nm non-ablative fractional laser with percutaneous collagen induction (PCI) and 20% TCA) in treating atrophic acne scars. The results showed that the 1540-nm non-ablative fractional laser in alternation with PCI and 20%TCA effectively treats atrophic acne scars [78].

The study carried out by Nofal et al. included 45 patients with acne scars. Group A had intradermal injections of PRP, group B had a CROSS technique with 100% TCA, and group C had a combination of skin needling and PRP. Each group underwent 3 sessions (2-week intervals). The results showed that group C had the highest significant improvement [79].

El-Domyati et al. showed that combined treatment of a dermaroller and PRP or dermaroller and 15% TCA resulted in a better improvement when compared to a dermaroller. In addition, in the combined groups, the collagen bundles were better organized [80]. This study shows that combined treatments are much better than treatments conducted alone.

Fractional radiofrequency has also been used in scar reduction treatments. Currently, researchers are trying to combine treatments to increase their effectiveness. Rongsaard et al. used a 1550-nm fractional erbium-doped glass and a fractional bipolar radiofrequency to treat atrophic acne scars. Twenty patients participated in this study, and had 3 split-face monthly treatments. Fractional bipolar radiofrequency on one side of the face and 1550-nm fractional erbium-doped glass on the other side of the face was applied. This study concluded that fractional bipolar radiofrequency and fractional erbium-doped glass have similar effectiveness for scars. The pain was higher with fractional bipolar radiofrequency, while the duration of scab shedding was longer in erbium-doped glass [81].

Chae et al. conducted a study on the efficacy and safety of the 1550-nm Er:Glass fractional laser and fractional radiofrequency microneedle device. Each group (20 patients) received 3 treatments (4-week intervals) using the Er:Glass fractional laser or fractional radiofrequency microneedle device. Scars improved in both groups, but the laser was a more effective treatment than the radiofrequency microneedle [82].

Lan et al. in 2018 used micro-plasma radiofrequency to treat facial acne scars. Ninety-five patients participated in this study, and had 3 sessions of treatment at 2-month intervals. Eighty-six probants finished all sessions, 15 of 86 patients showed more than 75% improvement, 57 patients showed 50–75% improvement, and 14 patients showed 25–50%. The study confirmed that this treatment is safe and effective for acne scars [83].

Lan et al. in 2021 compared fractional micro-plasma radiofrequency and fractional microneedle radiofrequency for the treatment of scars in 60 patients. One treatment was conducted on the left part of the face, and another treatment, on the right part. The total sessions consisted of 3 treatments at 2-months intervals. Fractional micro-plasma radiofrequency was more effective for atrophic scars than fractional microneedle radiofrequency [84]. Zhang et al. compared fractional microplasma radiofrequency technology and CO_2 fractional laser in 33 Asian patients. This was a randomized split-face treatment. The patients received 3 sessions of treatment. There was no significant difference between these methods, but postinflammatory hyperpigmentation was observed with the CO_2 fractional laser. The microplasma radiofrequency might be better in patients with darker skin [85].

4. Conclusions

Acne scars are still an unpleasant complication for people who have suffered from acne vulgaris. They represent a real challenge for dermatologists and cosmetologists. Scientific research on improving acne scars is ongoing and shows multiple effective modalities to treat this type of scar. Ablative lasers and other modern devices that use, for example, radiofrequency or MN, as well as TCA, bring very good treatment results. However, it is worth noting that each scar reduction method has advantages and disadvantages. Nevertheless, research shows that the best results can be obtained through the synergy of treatments, for example: combining a 1540-nm non-ablative fractional laser with PCI and 20% TCA or combined treatment of dermaroller and PRP or dermaroller and 15% TCA. It should be remembered that each therapy should be selected individually for each patient. The best results in scar reduction are achieved with treatments using lasers, radiofrequency, MN, and PRP [24,32,47,55,78,80].

Contemporary dermatology and cosmetology use treatments that cause minimal side effects, so the patient can return to daily functioning shortly after treatment. Proper dermatological treatment and skincare, as well as the rapid implementation of cosmetological treatments, will certainly allow satisfactory results in reducing atrophic scars.

Author Contributions: Conceptualization, K.C. and D.N.; methodology, K.C.; writing—original draft preparation, K.C.; writing—review and editing, K.C., M.R., R.S. and D.N.; supervision, R.S. All authors have read and agreed to the published version of the manuscript.

Funding: This research received no external funding.

Institutional Review Board Statement: Not applicable.

Informed Consent Statement: Not applicable.

Data Availability Statement: No new data were created or analyzed in this study. Data sharing is not applicable to this article.

Conflicts of Interest: The authors declare no conflict of interest.

References

1. Chilicka, K.; Rogowska, A.M.; Szyguła, R.; Dzieńdziora-Urbińska, I.; Taradaj, J. A comparison of the effectiveness of azelaic and pyruvic acid peels in the treatment of female adult acne: A randomized controlled trial. *Sci. Rep.* **2020**, *10*, 12612. [CrossRef] [PubMed]
2. Leccia, M.; Auffret, N.; Poli, F.; Claudel, J.-P.; Corvec, S.; Dreno, B. Topical acne treatments in Europe and the issue of antimicrobial resistance. *J. Eur. Acad. Dermatol. Venereol.* **2015**, *29*, 1485–1492. [CrossRef] [PubMed]
3. Chilicka, K.; Rogowska, A.; Szyguła, R. Effects of Topical Hydrogen Purification on Skin Parameters and Acne Vulgaris in Adult Women. *Healthcare* **2021**, *9*, 144. [CrossRef] [PubMed]
4. Contassot, E.; French, L.E. New Insights into Acne Pathogenesis: Propionibacterium Acnes Activates the Inflammasome. *J. Investig. Dermatol.* **2014**, *134*, 310–313. [CrossRef] [PubMed]
5. Williams, H.C.; Dellavalle, R.; Garner, S. Acne vulgaris. *Lancet* **2012**, *379*, 361–372. [CrossRef]
6. Chilicka, K.; Rogowska, A.M.; Szyguła, R.; Taradaj, J. Examining Quality of Life after Treatment with Azelaic and Pyruvic Acid Peels in Women with Acne Vulgaris. *Clin. Cosmet. Investig. Dermatol.* **2020**, *13*, 469–477. [CrossRef]
7. Fabbrocini, G.; Cacciapuoti, S.; Monfrecola, G. A Qualitative Investigation of the Impact of Acne on Health-Related Quality of Life (HRQL): Development of a Conceptual Model. *Dermatol. Ther.* **2018**, *8*, 85–99. [CrossRef]
8. Gupta, M.A.; Gupta, A.K. A practical approach to the assessment of psychosocial and psychiatric comorbidity in the dermatology patient. *Clin. Dermatol.* **2013**, *31*, 57–61. [CrossRef]
9. Tredget, E.E.; Nedelec, B.; Scott, P.G.; Ghahary, A. Hypertrophic scars, keloids, and contractures: The cellular and molecular basis for therapy. *Surg. Clin. N. Am.* **1997**, *77*, 701–730. [CrossRef]
10. Imhof, B.A.; Jemelin, S.; Ballet, R.; Vesin, C.; Schapira, M.; Karaca, M.; Emre, Y. CCN1/CYR61-mediated meticulous patrolling by Ly6Clow monocytes fuels vascular inflammation. *Proc. Natl. Acad. Sci. USA* **2016**, *113*, E4847–E4856. [CrossRef]
11. Grose, R.; Werner, S. Wound-Healing Studies in Transgenic and Knockout Mice. *Mol. Biotechnol.* **2004**, *28*, 147–166. [CrossRef]
12. Werner, S.; Krieg, T.; Smola, H. Keratinocyte–Fibroblast Interactions in Wound Healing. *J. Investig. Dermatol.* **2007**, *127*, 998–1008. [CrossRef] [PubMed]
13. Zhu, Z.; Ding, J.; Tredget, E.E. The molecular basis of hypertrophic scars. *Burns Trauma* **2016**, *4*, 2. [CrossRef] [PubMed]
14. Lee, H.J.; Jang, Y.J. Recent Understandings of Biology, Prophylaxis and Treatment Strategies for Hypertrophic Scars and Keloids. *Int. J. Mol. Sci.* **2018**, *19*, 711. [CrossRef]
15. Stanirowski, P.; Sawicki, W. Modern methods of therapy of hard-to-heal post-operative wounds in obstetrics and gynecology—Analysis of applicability and effectiveness of use. *Postępy Nauk Medycznych* **2013**, *7*, 475–487.
16. Connolly, D.; Vu, H.L.; Mariwalla, K.; Saedi, N. Acne Scarring-Pathogenesis, Evaluation, and Treatment Options. *J. Clin. Aesthet. Dermatol.* **2017**, *10*, 12–23.
17. Magnani, L.R.; Schweiger, E.S. Fractional CO_2 lasers for the treatment of atrophic acne scars: A review of the literature. *J. Cosmet. Laser Ther.* **2014**, *16*, 48–56. [CrossRef]
18. Verma, N.; Yumeen, S.; Raggio, B.S. Ablative Laser Resurfacing. In *StatPearls*; StatPearls Publishing: Treasure Island, FL, USA, 2022.
19. Nistico, S.P.; Silvestri, M.; Zingoni, T.; Tamburi, F.; Bennardo, L.; Cannarozzo, G. Combination of Fractional CO_2 Laser and Rhodamine-Intense Pulsed Light in Facial Rejuvenation: A Randomized Controlled Trial. *Photobiomodul. Photomed. Laser Surg.* **2021**, *39*, 113–117. [CrossRef]
20. Sannino, M.; Ambrosio, A.G.; Lodi, G.; Cannarozzo, G.; Bennardo, L.; Nisticò, S.P. A giant epidermal nevus of the face treated with a CO_2 and dye laser combination: A case report and literature review. *J. Cosmet. Laser Ther.* **2021**, *23*, 59–64. [CrossRef]

21. Lodi, G.; Sannino, M.; Caterino, P.; Cannarozzo, G.; Bennardo, L.; Nisticò, S.P. Fractional CO_2 laser-assisted topical rifamycin drug delivery in the treatment of pediatric cutaneous leishmaniasis. *Pediatr. Dermatol.* **2021**, *38*, 717–720. [CrossRef]
22. Fang, F.; Yang, H.; Liu, X.; Ding, H.; Yang, Y.; Ge, Y.; Lin, T. Treatment of acne scars with fractional carbon dioxide laser in Asians: A retrospective study to search for predicting factors associated with efficacy. *Lasers Med. Sci.* **2022**, 1–5. [CrossRef] [PubMed]
23. Li, J.; Wang, D.; Wang, Y.; Du, Y.; Yu, S. Effectiveness and safety of fractional micro-plasma radio-frequency treatment combined with ablative fractional carbon dioxide laser treatment for hypertrophic scar: A retrospective study. *Ann. Palliat. Med.* **2021**, *10*, 9800–9809. [CrossRef] [PubMed]
24. Galal, O.; Tawfik, A.A.; Abdalla, N.; Soliman, M. Fractional CO_2 laser versus combined platelet-rich plasma and fractional CO_2 laser in treatment of acne scars: Image analysis system evaluation. *J. Cosmet. Dermatol.* **2019**, *18*, 1665–1671. [CrossRef] [PubMed]
25. Zhou, B.-R.; Zhang, T.; Bin Jameel, A.A.; Xu, Y.; Guo, S.-L.; Wang, Y.; Permatasari, F.; Luo, D.; Xu, Y. The efficacy of conditioned media of adipose-derived stem cells combined with ablative carbon dioxide fractional resurfacing for atrophic acne scars and skin rejuvenation. *J. Cosmet. Laser Ther.* **2016**, *18*, 138–148. [CrossRef] [PubMed]
26. Al Harithy, R.; Pon, K. Scar Treatment with Lasers: A Review and Update. *Curr. Dermatol. Rep.* **2012**, *1*, 69–75. [CrossRef]
27. Tidwell, W.J.; Owen, C.E.; Kulp-Shorten, C.; Maity, A.; McCall, M.; Brown, T.S. Fractionated Er:YAG laser versus fully ablative Er:YAG laser for scar revision: Results of a split scar, double blinded, prospective trial. *Lasers Surg. Med.* **2016**, *48*, 837–843. [CrossRef]
28. Zgavec, B.; Loka, S. Clinical and histological evaluation of Er:YAG Ablative fractional skin resurfacing. *Laser Health Acad.* **2014**, *1*, 1–6.
29. Cenk, H.; Sarac, G. Effectiveness and safety of 2940-nm multifractional Er: YAG laser on acne scars. *Dermatol. Ther.* **2020**, *33*, e14270. [CrossRef]
30. Emam, A.A.; Nada, H.A.; Atwa, M.A.; Tawfik, N.Z. Split-face comparative study of fractional Er:YAG laser versus microneedling radiofrequency in treatment of atrophic acne scars, using optical coherence tomography for assessment. *J. Cosmet. Dermatol.* **2022**, *21*, 227–236. [CrossRef]
31. Załęska, I.; Atta-Motte, M. Laser therapy applied to reduce scars of various etiology. *Kosm. Estet.* **2017**, *1*, 81–86.
32. Rogachefsky, A.S.; Hussain, M.; Goldberg, D.J. Atrophic and a Mixed Pattern of Acne Scars Improved with a 1320-nm Nd:YAG Laser. *Dermatol. Surg.* **2003**, *29*, 904–908. [CrossRef] [PubMed]
33. Sadick, N.; Schecter, A.K. A preliminary study of utilization of the 1320-nm Nd:YAG laser for the treatment of acne scarring. *Dermatol. Surg.* **2004**, *30*, 995–1000. [PubMed]
34. Tanzi, E.L.; Alster, T.S. Comparison of a 1450-nm Diode Laser and a 1320-nm Nd:YAG Laser in the Treatment of Atrophic Facial Scars: A Prospective Clinical and Histologic Study. *Dermatol. Surg.* **2004**, *30*, 152–157. [CrossRef]
35. Rathod, D.; Foroughi, A.; Mekokishvili, L.; Wollina, U.; Lotti, T.; Rajan, A.; Goldust, M. A cross-sectional, multi-center study on treatment of facial acne scars with low-energy double-pass 1450-nm diode laser. *Dermatol. Ther.* **2020**, *33*, e13326. [CrossRef] [PubMed]
36. Cannarozzo, G.; Bennardo, L.; Zingoni, T.; Pieri, L.; Del Duca, E.; Nisticò, S.P. Histological Skin Changes After Treatment with 675 nm Laser. *Photobiomodul. Photomed. Laser Surg.* **2021**, *39*, 617–621. [CrossRef] [PubMed]
37. Cannarozzo, G.; Silvestri, M.; Tamburi, F.; Sicilia, C.; Del Duca, E.; Scali, E.; Bennardo, L.; Nisticò, S.P. A new 675-nm laser device in the treatment of acne scars: An observational study. *Lasers Med. Sci.* **2021**, *36*, 227–231. [CrossRef] [PubMed]
38. Fischer, T.; Perosino, E.; Poli, F.; Viera, M.; Dreno, B. For the Cosmetic Dermatology European Expert Group Chemical peels in aesthetic dermatology: An update 2009. *J. Eur. Acad. Dermatol. Venereol.* **2010**, *24*, 281–292. [CrossRef]
39. O'Daniel, T.G. Multimodal Management of Atrophic Acne Scarring in the Aging Face. *Aesthet. Plast. Surg.* **2011**, *35*, 1143–1150. [CrossRef]
40. Agarwal, N.; Gupta, L.K.; Khare, A.K.; Kuldeep, C.M.; Mittal, A. Therapeutic Response of 70% Trichloroacetic Acid CROSS in Atrophic Acne Scars. *Dermatol. Surg.* **2015**, *41*, 597–604. [CrossRef]
41. Bhardwaj, D.; Khunger, N. An Assessment of the Efficacy and Safety of CROSS Technique with 100% TCA in the Management of Ice Pick Acne Scars. *J. Cutan. Aesthet. Surg.* **2010**, *3*, 93–96. [CrossRef]
42. Al-Hamamy, H.R.; Al-Dhalimi, M.A.; Abtan, A.F. Evaluation of treatment of acne scars with 25% trichloroacetic acid chemical peel followed by manual dermasanding. *J. Cosmet. Dermatol.* **2021**, *20*, 1750–1755. [CrossRef] [PubMed]
43. Puri, N. Efficacy of modified Jessner's peel and 20% TCA versus 20% TCA peel alone for the treatment of acne scars. *J. Cutan. Aesthet. Surg.* **2015**, *8*, 42–45. [CrossRef] [PubMed]
44. Juhasz, M.L.; Cohen, J.L. Microneedling for the Treatment of Scars: An Update for Clinicians. *Clin. Cosmet. Investig. Dermatol.* **2020**, *13*, 997–1003. [CrossRef] [PubMed]
45. Moftah, N.H.; El Khayyat, M.A.; Ragai, M.H.; Alaa, H. Carboxytherapy Versus Skin Microneedling in Treatment of Atrophic Postacne Scars: A Comparative Clinical, Histopathological, and Histometrical Study. *Dermatol. Surg.* **2018**, *44*, 1332–1341. [CrossRef]
46. Busch, K.-H.; Aliu, A.; Walezko, N.; Aust, M. Medical Needling: Effect on Skin Erythema of Hypertrophic Burn Scars. *Cureus* **2018**, *10*, e3260. [CrossRef]
47. El-Domyati, M.; Barakat, M.; Awad, S.; Medhat, W.; El-Fakahany, H.; Farag, H. Microneedling Therapy for Atrophic Acne Scars: An Objective Evaluation. *J. Clin. Aesthet. Dermatol.* **2015**, *8*, 36–42.

48. Tirmizi, S.S.; Iqbal, T.; Mansoor, M.; Farooq, N.; Ather, S.; Fatima, F.; Kapadia, N.; Anwar, A.; Hashmi, A.A. Role of Microneedling in Atrophic Post-Acne Scars: An Experience from a Tertiary Care Hospital. *Cureus* **2021**, *13*, e12578. [CrossRef]
49. Biesman, B.S.; Cohen, J.L.; Dibernardo, B.E.; Emer, J.J.; Geronemus, R.G.; Gold, M.H.; Lehman, A.S.; Pilcher, B.K.; Monheit, G.D.; Schlesinger, T.E.; et al. Treatment of Atrophic Facial Acne Scars with Microneedling Followed by Polymethylmethacrylate-Collagen Gel Dermal Filler. *Dermatol. Surg.* **2019**, *45*, 1570–1579. [CrossRef]
50. Schoenberg, E.; O'Connor, M.; Wang, J.V.; Yang, S.; Saedi, N. Microneedling and PRP for acne scars: A new tool in our arsenal. *J. Cosmet. Dermatol.* **2020**, *19*, 112–114. [CrossRef]
51. Kim, C.N.T.; Thi, L.P.; Van, T.N.; Minh, P.P.T.; Nguyet, M.V.; Le Thi, M.; Huu, N.D.; Hau, K.T.; Gandolfi, M.; Satolli, F.; et al. Successful Treatment of Facial Atrophic Acne Scars by Fractional Radiofrequency Microneedle in Vietnamese Patients. *Open Access Maced. J. Med. Sci.* **2019**, *7*, 192–194. [CrossRef]
52. Chandrashekar, B.S.; Sriram, R.; Mysore, R.; Bhaskar, S.; Shetty, A. Evaluation of microneedling fractional radiofrequency device for treatment of acne scars. *J. Cutan. Aesthet. Surg.* **2014**, *7*, 93–97. [CrossRef] [PubMed]
53. Elawar, A.; Dahan, S. Non-insulated Fractional Microneedle Radiofrequency Treatment with Smooth Motor Insertion for Reduction of Depressed Acne Scars, Pore Size, and Skin Texture Improvement: A Preliminary Study. *J. Clin. Aesthet. Dermatol.* **2018**, *11*, 41–44. [PubMed]
54. Kim, J.E.; Lee, H.W.; Kim, J.K.; Moon, S.H.; Ko, J.Y.; Lee, M.W.; Chang, S.E. Objective Evaluation of the Clinical Efficacy of Fractional Radiofrequency Treatment for Acne Scars and Enlarged Pores in Asian Skin. *Dermatol. Surg.* **2014**, *40*, 988–995. [CrossRef] [PubMed]
55. Qin, X.; Li, H.; Jian, X.; Yu, B. Evaluation of the efficacy and safety of fractional bipolar radiofrequency with high-energy strategy for treatment of acne scars in Chinese. *J. Cosmet. Laser Ther.* **2015**, *17*, 237–245. [CrossRef] [PubMed]
56. Pagacz, K.; Chilicka, K. The application of needle radiofrequency for the reduction of acne scars: A case report. *Med. Sci. Pulse* **2019**, *13*, 50–53. [CrossRef]
57. Chilicka, K.; Pagacz, K. The use of combination therapy with 20% glycolic acid and fractional mesotherapy to reduce acne scars: A case report. *Med. Sci. Pulse* **2019**, *13*, 49–51. [CrossRef]
58. Chilicka, K.; Rusztowicz, M.; Dzieńdziora, I. The effectiveness of alkaline water on oily and acne-prone skin: A case report. *Med. Sci. Pulse* **2021**, *15*, 50–54. [CrossRef]
59. Nowicka, D.; Chilicka, K.; Dzieńdziora-Urbińska, I. Host-Microbe Interaction on the Skin and Its Role in the Pathogenesis and Treatment of Atopic Dermatitis. *Pathogens* **2022**, *11*, 71. [CrossRef]
60. Chilicka, K.; Dzieńdziora-Urbińska, I.; Szyguła, R.; Asanova, B.; Nowicka, D. Microbiome and Probiotics in Acne Vulgaris—A Narrative Review. *Life* **2022**, *12*, 422. [CrossRef]
61. Chilicka, K.; Rogowska, A.M.; Rusztowicz, M.; Szyguła, R.; Yanakieva, A.; Asanova, B.; Wilczyński, S. The Effects of Green Tea (*Camellia sinensis*), Bamboo Extract (*Bambusa vulgaris*) and Lactic Acid on Sebum Production in Young Women with Acne Vulgaris Using Sonophoresis Treatment. *Healthcare* **2022**, *10*, 684. [CrossRef]
62. Lee, J.W.; Kim, B.J.; Kim, M.N.; Mun, S.K. The Efficacy of Autologous Platelet Rich Plasma Combined with Ablative Carbon Dioxide Fractional Resurfacing for Acne Scars: A Simultaneous Split-Face Trial. *Dermatol. Surg.* **2011**, *37*, 931–938. [CrossRef] [PubMed]
63. Ebrahim, H.M.; Nassar, A.; ElKashishy, K.; Artima, A.Y.M.; Morsi, H.M. A combined approach of subcision with either cross-linked hyaluronic acid or threads in the treatment of atrophic acne scars. *J. Cosmet. Dermatol.* **2021**. [CrossRef]
64. Mumtaz, M.; Hassan, T.; Shahzad, M.K.; Hanif, N.; Anwar, S.; Anjum, R. Comparing the Efficacy of Intra-dermal Platelet Rich Plasma (PRP) Versus 50% Trichloracetic Acid (TCA) using Cross Technique for Atrophic Acne Scars. *J. Coll. Physicians Surg. Pak.* **2021**, *31*, 55–59. [CrossRef]
65. Nilforoushzadeh, M.A.; Fakhim, T.; Heidari-Kharaji, M.; Hanifnia, A.R.; Hejazi, S.; Torkamaniha, E. Efficacy evaluation of Endolift-based Subcision on acne scar treatment. *J. Cosmet. Dermatol.* **2021**, *20*, 2579–2582. [CrossRef] [PubMed]
66. Deshmukh, N.S.; Belgaumkar, V.A. Platelet-Rich Plasma Augments Subcision in Atrophic Acne Scars: A Split-Face Comparative Study. *Dermatol. Surg.* **2019**, *45*, 90–98. [CrossRef] [PubMed]
67. Ibrahim, M.K.; Ibrahim, S.M.; Salem, A.M. Skin microneedling plus platelet-rich plasma versus skin microneedling alone in the treatment of atrophic post acne scars: A split face comparative study. *J. Dermatol. Treat.* **2018**, *29*, 281–286. [CrossRef]
68. Nilforoushzadeh, M.A.; Heidari-Kharaji, M.; Alavi, S.; Nouri, M.; Nikkhah, N.; Jahangiri, F.; Mahmoudbeyk, M.; Peyrovan, A.; Tork, B.B.; Torkamaniha, E.; et al. Transplantation of autologous fat, stromal vascular fraction (SVF) cell, and platelet-rich plasma (PRP) for cell therapy of atrophic acne scars: Clinical evaluation and biometric assessment. *J. Cosmet. Dermatol.* **2021**. [CrossRef]
69. Alser, O.H.; Goutos, I. The evidence behind the use of platelet-rich plasma (PRP) in scar management: A literature review. *Scars Burns Heal.* **2018**, *4*, 2059513118808773. [CrossRef]
70. Bhargava, S.; Kroumpouzos, G.; Varma, K.; Kumar, U. Combination therapy using subcision, needling, and platelet-rich plasma in the management of grade 4 atrophic acne scars: A pilot study. *J. Cosmet. Dermatol.* **2019**, *18*, 1092–1097. [CrossRef]
71. Chawla, S. Split face comparative study of microneedling with PRP versus microneedling with vitamin C in treating atrophic post acne scars. *J. Cutan. Aesthet. Surg.* **2014**, *7*, 209–212. [CrossRef]
72. Bhargava, S.; Cunha, P.R.; Lee, J.; Kroumpouzos, G. Acne Scarring Management: Systematic Review and Evaluation of the Evidence. *Am. J. Clin. Dermatol.* **2018**, *19*, 459–477. [CrossRef] [PubMed]

73. Gupta, A.; Kaur, M.; Patra, S.; Khunger, N.; Gupta, S. Evidence-based Surgical Management of Post-acne Scarring in Skin of Color. *J. Cutan. Aesthet. Surg.* **2020**, *13*, 124–141. [PubMed]
74. Husein-ElAhmed, H.; Steinhoff, M. Comparative appraisal with meta-analysis of erbium vs. CO_2 lasers for atrophic acne scars. *JDDG J. Dtsch. Dermatol. Ges.* **2021**, *19*, 1559–1568. [CrossRef] [PubMed]
75. Elsaie, M.L.; Ibrahim, S.; Saudi, W. Ablative Fractional 10,600 nm Carbon Dioxide Laser Versus Non-ablative Fractional 1540 nm Erbium-Glass Laser in Egyptian Post-acne Scar patients. *J. Lasers Med. Sci.* **2018**, *9*, 32–35. [CrossRef]
76. Reinholz, M.; Schwaiger, H.; Heppt, M.V.; Poetschke, J.; Tietze, J.; Epple, A.; Ruzicka, T.; Kaudewitz, P.; Gauglitz, G.G. Comparison of Two Kinds of Lasers in the Treatment of Acne Scars. *Facial Plast. Surg.* **2015**, *31*, 523–531. [CrossRef]
77. Ahmed, R.; Mohammed, G.; Ismail, N.; Elakhras, A. Randomized clinical trial of CO_2 LASER pinpoint irradiation technique versus chemical reconstruction of skin scars (CROSS) in treating ice pick acne scars. *J. Cosmet. Laser Ther.* **2014**, *16*, 8–13. [CrossRef]
78. Leheta, T.M.; Abdel Hay, R.M.; Hegazy, R.A.; El Garem, Y.F. Do combined alternating sessions of 1540 nm nonablative fractional laser and percutaneous collagen induction with trichloroacetic acid 20% show better results than each individual modality in the treatment of atrophic acne scars? A randomized controlled trial. *J. Dermatol. Treat.* **2014**, *25*, 137–141. [CrossRef]
79. Nofal, E.; Helmy, A.; Nofal, A.; Alakad, R.; Nasr, M. Platelet-rich plasma versus CROSS technique with 100% trichloroacetic acid versus combined skin needling and platelet rich plasma in the treatment of atrophic acne scars: A comparative study. *Dermatol. Surg.* **2014**, *40*, 864–873. [CrossRef]
80. El-Domyati, M.; Abdel-Wahab, H.; Hossam, A. Microneedling combined with platelet-rich plasma or trichloroacetic acid peeling for management of acne scarring: A split-face clinical and histologic comparison. *J. Cosmet. Dermatol.* **2018**, *17*, 73–83. [CrossRef]
81. Rongsaard, N.; Rummaneethorn, P. Comparison of a Fractional Bipolar Radiofrequency Device and a Fractional Erbium-Doped Glass 1,550-nm Device for the Treatment of Atrophic Acne Scars: A Randomized Split-Face Clinical Study. *Dermatol. Surg.* **2014**, *40*, 14–21. [CrossRef]
82. Chae, W.S.; Seong, J.Y.; Jung, H.N.; Kong, S.H.; Kim, M.H.; Suh, H.S.; Choi, Y.S. Comparative study on efficacy and safety of 1550 nm Er:Glass fractional laser and fractional radiofrequency microneedle device for facial atrophic acne scar. *J. Cosmet. Dermatol.* **2015**, *14*, 100–106. [CrossRef] [PubMed]
83. Lan, T.; Xiao, Y.; Tang, L.; Hamblin, M.R.; Yin, R. Treatment of atrophic acne scarring with fractional micro-plasma radio-frequency in Chinese patients: A prospective study. *Lasers Surg. Med.* **2018**, *50*, 844–850. [CrossRef] [PubMed]
84. Lan, T.; Tang, L.; Xia, A.; Hamblin, M.R.; Jian, D.; Yin, R. Comparison of Fractional Micro-Plasma Radiofrequency and Fractional Microneedle Radiofrequency for the Treatment of Atrophic Acne Scars: A Pilot Randomized Split-Face Clinical Study in China. *Lasers Surg. Med.* **2021**, *53*, 906–913. [CrossRef] [PubMed]
85. Zhang, Z.; Fei, Y.; Chen, X.; Lu, W.; Chen, J. Comparison of a Fractional Microplasma Radio Frequency Technology and Carbon Dioxide Fractional Laser for the Treatment of Atrophic Acne Scars: A Randomized Split-Face Clinical Study. *Dermatol. Surg.* **2013**, *39*, 559–566. [CrossRef]

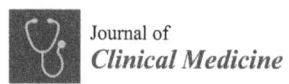

Review

Truncal Acne: An Overview

Yu Ri Woo and Hei Sung Kim *

Department of Dermatology, Incheon St. Mary's Hospital, The Catholic University of Korea, 222 Banpo-daero, Seocho-gu, Seoul 06591, Korea; w1206@naver.com
* Correspondence: hazelkimhoho@gmail.com

Abstract: Acne is a relatively common disease of the pilosebaceous units. Many aspects of facial acne have been studied. However, there is limited evidence regarding truncal acne. Truncal acne is also observed in a significant number of patients, but it is often ignored by patients and clinicians. Although the pathogenesis of facial and trunk acne is considered to be similar, the characteristics of the skin on the trunk and face are thought to be different. As truncal acne can cause scars on large areas of the body and adversely affect the quality of life of patients, more attention should be given to patients with truncal acne. Although only a few studies have been published to date, the epidemiology, etiology, severity assessment tool, assessments of the quality of life, and new treatments targeting truncal acne are currently being studied. Therefore, in this review, the latest knowledge on truncal acne will be discussed.

Keywords: acne; face; truncal acne

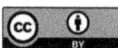

1. Introduction

Acne vulgaris is a common cutaneous disorder of the pilosebaceous unit with a high prevalence in the general population. A global burden of disease study in 2010 identified acne vulgaris as the eighth most common skin disease, with an estimated global prevalence of 9.38% [1]. A recent systematic review also estimated the prevalence of acne to range from 20% to 95% [2]. Of note, the global lifetime prevalence of acne is estimated to be 70–85% [3]. Despite its high prevalence, truncal acne has been neglected by many clinicians and patients. Although there has been a paucity of evidence on the epidemiology, pathogenesis, clinical features, and treatment of truncal acne, some recent studies are updating the evidence on truncal acne. Therefore, this review aimed to provide the evidence-based recent perspectives on truncal acne.

2. Epidemiology

The prevalence of truncal acne has not yet been well established to date. Previous studies report that about 48–52% of facial acne patients also have truncal acne [4–6]. In 2007, Del Rosso et al. [4] examined 696 patients aged 14 to 20 years with acne and found that 52.3% exhibited truncal involvement. Among them, 10.6% showed truncal acne scarring [4]. Isaacsson et al. [5] reported that 50% of Brazilian adolescents had acne on their chest or back. A large-scale international study of 2926 adult females found that 48.8% of the patients with facial acne also had truncal acne [6]. Recently, Dreno et al. reported that a family history of acne was associated with the extension of acne to the trunk [7].

With regards to sex, there is a slight male predominance of truncal acne (54%) over female (43%) [4]. Truncal acne is known to occur in adolescents as well as adults. Despite the results of the above-mentioned studies, few studies have studied only truncal acne, and additional research including large-scale and diverse ethnic groups is needed to identify the epidemiology of truncal acne.

3. Clinical Features of Truncal Acne

The clinical manifestations of truncal acne can range from noninflammatory comedones to inflammatory papules, pustules, and nodules located on the chest and/or back (Figure 1). When truncal acne is observed, it tends to be clustered near the midline of the trunk [8]. As the severe form of acne is usually accompanied by truncal involvement [9], truncal acne should always be considered by clinicians in cases of severe facial acne.

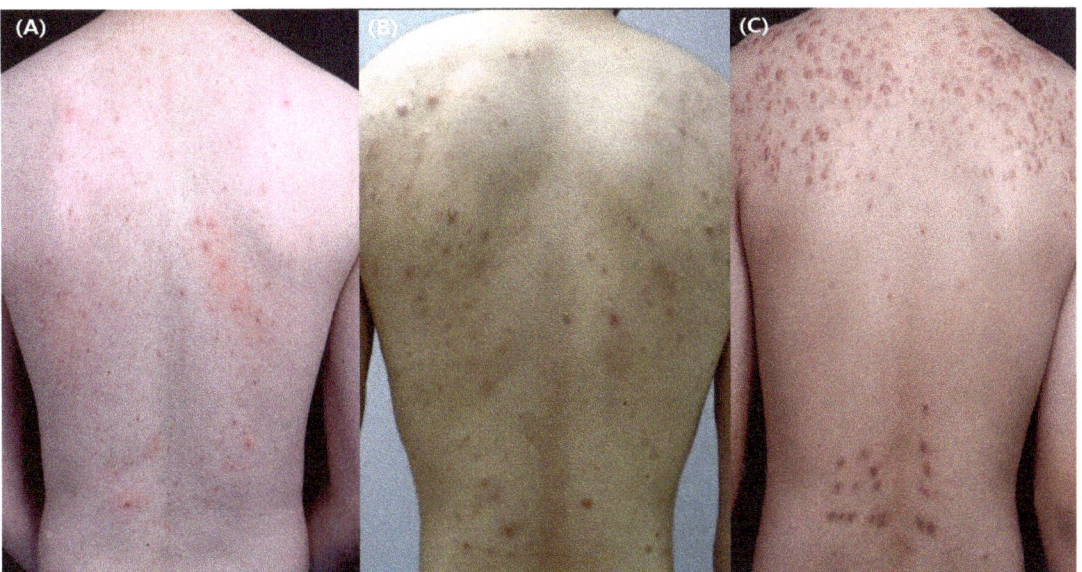

Figure 1. Clinical manifestations of truncal acne. (**A,B**) Truncal acne. (**C**) Truncal acne with severe scarring.

The most frequently involved anatomical site of truncal acne is the upper back (52%), followed by the upper chest (30%), lower back (22%), shoulders and upper extremities (16%), and neck (8%) [10]. A study conducted in East China also found that the back (25%) was the most frequently involved anatomical site, followed by the chest (16%), neck (7%), and arms (6%) [11]. A multicenter questionnaire-based study conducted in Korea found that the site most frequently affected with truncal acne in males was the back (19.4%), followed by the chest (18.1%) [12]. In females, the most frequently affected site was the back (13.9%), followed by the neck (12.7%) and chest (11.1%), which showed slight sex differences in the sites affected by acne [12]. Although there are some inconsistencies between the studies, most found that the back was the most frequently affected area in truncal acne. Scar formation from truncal acne is common and is mainly hypertrophic [9].

A severe form of acne, acne conglobata, usually presents with nodules, abscesses with sinus formation, and cysts on the chest, shoulders, back, and upper extremities [13]. As acne conglobata is characterized by suppurative severe inflammation, scar formation is common [13]. Acne fulminans is also known as acute febrile ulcerative acne and is the most severe type of acne [14]. It can be manifested with or without systemic symptoms and often heals with scarring [14]. The sudden appearance of tender inflammatory plaques with ulcers and hemorrhagic crusts on the chest and back, whilst sparing the neck, can be the characteristic signs of acne fulminans [14]. Nodules and polymorphous comedones are less frequently observed in acne fulminans than in acne vulgaris [14].

4. Pathophysiology of Truncal Acne

To date, the etiology of truncal acne is generally considered to be similar to that of facial acne. Follicular hyperkeratosis, the colonization of pilosebaceous units with *Cutibacterium acnes* (*C. acnes*), and inflammation are all considered major pathogenic factors in the development of facial and truncal acne [15,16]. Although facial and truncal acne have been considered to have shared pathogenesis, some differences between them have been reported. Kim et al. [17] found that sebum secretion was relatively lower in the trunk than in the face of patients with acne vulgaris. They suggested that hyperseborrhea might not play a major pathogenic role in the development of truncal acne [17].

Human hormones affect the biological functions of the pilosebaceous unit. The rise in androgen level during puberty is associated with the development of acne [18]. Among various hormones, receptors for androgens are also found in sebocytes and follicular keratinocytes [18]. Androgen can induce lipogenesis of the sebaceous gland, hyperproliferation of the follicular keratinocyte, proliferation of *C. acnes*, and follicular hypoxia, which could contribute to the development acne [18,19].

A variety of evidence has proved a link between the gut microbiota and acne. Previous studies found that patients with acne had dysbiosis of the gut microbiota [20–22]. However, to date, no study has analyzed the characteristics of gut microbiota in patients with truncal acne, and further studies are needed. In addition to the gut microbiota, alterations in the skin microbiota are also considered an important player in truncal acne. Dagnelie et al. [23] reported differences in the dominant bacterial families between facial acne and truncal acne. Colonization with *Enterococcaceae* was more frequently observed in truncal samples, whereas colonization with *Staphylococcaceae* and *Propionibacteriaceae* was frequently observed in facial samples [23]. Using the single-locus sequence typing method, Dagnelie et al. [24] found that phylotype IA1 was the most predominant type on the back of the acne patients compared to the healthy controls. Severe acne on the back was associated with a loss of *C. acnes* phylotype diversity [24]. Taken together, alterations in the composition of the skin bacterial microbiota might affect the inflammatory processes of the acne skin. In addition to the bacterial microbiota, the possible role of the fungal mycobiota in the development of truncal acne should be investigated further. Although little is known about the fungal mycobiota in truncal acne, a recent study found a negative interaction between *Malassezia globosa* and *C. acnes* among patients with facial acne [25]. Thus, we suppose that an interaction between the bacterial microbiota and fungal mycobiota, along with host factors, might be involved in the development of truncal acne, which remains to be elucidated in the future.

Endocrine abnormalities are also associated with acne [26]. Acne is a frequently observed clinical feature of polycystic ovarian syndrome (PCOS), congenital adrenal hyperplasia, Cushing syndrome, and androgen-secreting tumors [26,27]. Among patients with female acne, acne with hyperandrogenic signs was more strongly associated with truncal acne, longer disease duration, inappropriate diet, and PCOS than acne without hyperandrogenic signs [28].

As truncal acne is associated with post-acne scarring, some studies have investigated the mechanisms of scarring in truncal acne. A recent study found a difference in the profile of skin innate immunity in patients with acne by performing skin biopsies of the back [29]. The significant overexpression of pro-inflammatory markers such as Toll-like receptor-4 and interleukin-2 was observed both in the normal-appearing skin and inflammatory skin of acne patients with atrophic scars compared to acne patients without atrophic scars [29]. The authors suggested that the degree of activation of innate immunity was associated with the levels of acne inflammation and further scar formation [29].

Hypertrophic post-acne scarring was associated with the CC genotype of *MMP-2* [30]. Among patients with hypertrophic acne scars, 95.8% were shown to have the CC genotype of *MMP-2* [30]. Hypertrophic acne scarring patients with the CC genotype of *MMP-2* showed a 7.8-times increased risk of developing hypertrophic acne scars than acne patients without scar formation [30].

Although the etiology of truncal acne is generally considered to be similar to that of facial acne, there are differences between the skin on the face and the trunk in thickness, pH, and the distribution of sebaceous glands. Truncal skin is also more vulnerable to mechanical stimuli such as sweat, oils, pressure, friction, and occlusion than facial acne [31]. We hypothesize that these factors might be associated with the severity of truncal acne. Further large-scale clinical studies should be conducted to elucidate the relationship between these factors.

5. Assessment Tool for Truncal Acne

Previously, a tool for assessing the severity of truncal acne was used along with a tool for evaluating facial acne.

After Pillsbury et al. [32] proposed a tool for assessing truncal acne, Burke et al. [33] introduced the Leeds technique in 1984, which uses two simple scoring systems for evaluating the acne severity. In 1998, O'Brian et al. [34] proposed the Leeds Revised Acne Grading (LRAG) system based on the photographic templates for acne grading of the face, chest, and back. Tan et al. [35] introduced the comprehensive acne severity scale (CLASS) by modifying the investigator's global assessment of facial acne to evaluate truncal acne severity. The CLASS was strongly correlated with the Leeds grading system in a validation study [35]. In 2010, Tan et al. [36] developed a scale for assessing acne scar severity by developing a six-category global severity scale (SCAR-S) evaluating the severity of each region of the face, chest, and back.

Bernadis et al. [37] proposed a new acne global grading scale in 2021 for assessing acne severity by combining primary lesions and secondary changes. A very recent study provided the truncal acne severity scale (TRASS), which is very easy for dermatologists to use for assessing the severity of truncal acne. The TRASS evaluates the severity of truncal acne by utilizing a severity tool based on the global evaluation acne (GEA) and the Echelle de Cotation des Lesions d'Acne (ECLA) scales, and includes an assessment tool considering family history, clinical signs, and quality of life (QoL) [38]. In the TRASS, the xiphoid process is defined as the lower limit for the location of chest acne [38]. For back acne, the back is divided into two regions compromising the upper and lower backs, with the lower limit of the scapular defined as a line to separate them [38].

Despite the development of various assessment tools for truncal acne, the above-mentioned tools are mostly used as tools for clinical research (Table 1). In real-world clinical practice, the investigator's global assessment (IGA), the Leeds visual severity scale, ECLA scales, and the comprehensive acne severity scale are widely used for assessing the severity of truncal acne [39]. Given the anatomical variations in acne, there are unmet needs to properly evaluate the severity of truncal acne in real-world clinical practice. Therefore, more attention should be paid to develop more practical assessment tools for truncal acne in the future.

Table 1. Summary of recently developed assessment tool for truncal acne.

Tool	Sites	Grading	Descriptions of the Grading
LRAG	Each of face, chest, and back	Based on photographic templates Based on the number of inflamed lesions and their inflammatory intensity (Grade 1–12) Predominant noninflamed lesions (Grade 1–3)	Grade 1, least severe–Grade 3, most severe Grade 1, least severe–Grade 12, most severe
CLASS	Each of face, chest, and back	Clear (0) Almost clear (1) Mild (2) Moderate (3) Severe (4) Very severe (5)	No lesions to barely noticeable ones, very few scattered comedones and papules Hardly visible from 2.5 m away. A few scattered comedones, few small papules, and very few pustules Easily recognizable; less than half of the affected area is involved. Many comedones, papules, and pustules; 0–5 papules and pustules More than half of the affected area is involved; numerous comedones, papules and pustules; 6–20 papules and pustules The entire area is involved. Covered with comedones, numerous pustules, and papules, a few nodules and cyst; 21–50 papules and pustules Highly inflammatory acne covering the affected area, with nodules and cyst present; >50 inflammatory lesions
SCAR-S	Each of face, chest, and back	The overall scar score is the sum of scores from each of these three sites. Clear (0) Almost clear (1) Mild (2) Moderate (3) Severe (4) Very severe (5)	No visible scars from acne Hardly visible scars from 2.5 m away Easily recognizable; less than half the affected area (e.g., face, back, or chest) involved More than half the affected area (e.g., face, back, or chest) involved Entire area involved Entire area with prominent atrophic or hypertrophic scars
TRASS	Trunk (upper back, lower back, and chest)	Sum of the three sub-score items (ranging from 0–19) Sub-score 1: criteria of severity based on disease and family history (maximum score 6) Sub-score 2: Clinical marker of acne severity (maximum score 11) Sub-score 3: quality of life (maximum score 2)	Item 1: Duration of acne (0, 0–2 years; 1, 3–5 years; 2, ≥6 years) Item 2: Family history (0, none; 1, present) Item 3: Past systemic acne treatment (0, none; 1, oral systemics; 2, isotretinoin) Item 4: Areas on the trunk Upper back (0, no lesion; 1, lesion) Lower back (0, no lesion; 1, lesion) Chest (0, no lesion; 1, lesion) Item 5: Number of nodules (0, 0; 1, 1–5; 2, 6–9; 3, ≥10) Item 6: Scars (Hypertrophic/keloid: 0, no; 1, yes; atrophic: 0, no; 1, yes; elastosis: 0, no; 1, yes; hyperpigmentation/erythema: 0, no; 1, yes) Item 7: Facial acne (0, no; 1, yes) Item 8: Severity of impact on quality of life (0, none; 1, moderate; 2, important)

Abbreviation: CLASS, the comprehensive acne severity scale; LRAG, Leeds Revised Acne grading; SCAR-S, six-category global severity scale; TRASS, truncal acne severity scale.

6. Differential Diagnosis of Truncal Acne

A variety of papulopustular eruptions on the trunk should be differentiated from truncal acne.

Folliculitis is defined as an infection of the hair follicles by *Staphylococcus aureus* or other factors [40]. The clinical features of folliculitis are characterized by solitary or multiple inflammatory follicular erythematous papules and/or pustules without comedones on hair-bearing areas [40]. Pityrosporum folliculitis is the cutaneous disorder most frequently misdiagnosed as truncal acne. Clinically, pityrosporum folliculitis is manifested by pruritic monomorphic tiny follicular papules and pustules with or without perifollicular erythema on the upper portion of the trunk, neck, and upper arms [41]. Pityrosporum folliculitis can be differentiated from truncal acne by the absence of comedones, the lack of response to topical or oral antibiotics, and the presence of pruritic skin lesions [42].

In addition, acneiform eruptions, which are caused by several drugs including glucocorticoids, phenytoin, lithium, isoniazid, high-dose vitamin B complex, halogenated compounds, cyclosporine, epidermal growth factor receptor inhibitors, and BRAF inhibitors, are always considered when diagnosing truncal acne [43]. Usually, drug-induced acneiform eruptions present as diffuse monomorphic follicular papules on the trunk. Regarding steroid folliculitis, skin eruptions can generally be observed after two weeks of steroid use [43]. Unlike acne vulgaris, steroid folliculitis usually presents as inflammatory papules and pustules on the trunk, shoulders, and upper arms, with less involvement on the face. Comedones, cysts, and scarring are uncommonly observed, although post-inflammatory hyperpigmentation could be observed after improvement [43]. Recently, the term "bodybuilding acne" has been proposed for individuals who have been administered anabolic androgenic steroids such as methandrostenolone, nandrolone, testosterone, oxandrolone, stanozolol, or methenolone, which are usually taken by bodybuilders [18]. The clinical manifestations of bodybuilding acne vary from the occurrence of new-onset acne to the exacerbation of pre-existing acne, or the occurrence of acne conglobate or acne fulminans [18]. In addition to the above-mentioned medications, diverse drugs have recently been shown to cause acneiform eruptions. Therefore, for the correct diagnosis of drug-induced acneiform eruptions, it is necessary to properly evaluate the relationship between the drug intake history and the onset of the skin lesions through a detailed medical history [43].

7. Psychosocial Burden of Truncal Acne

The degree of the impact of acne on QoL is similar to that of other chronic general disorders such as diabetes, asthma, epilepsy, back pain, or arthritis [44]. Although the negative impact on QoL is correlated with the severity of acne, mild acne patients can also suffer from a significant negative impact on QoL, despite their mild signs [45].

To date, most previous studies determining the psychosocial burden of acne have been focused only on the impact of facial acne. As the face is the exposed area of the body, much attention is indeed paid to the facial regions. However, interest in truncal acne has increased recently, and studies on the effects of truncal acne on QoL are being conducted. A study by Papadopoulos et al. [46] found that the patients with facial and truncal acne had significantly lower self-esteem and body image than the controls. Compared to truncal acne patients, patients with facial acne exhibited lower self-esteem and body image [46]. A recent cross-sectional study identified that the negative impact on all health-related QoL was higher in patients with combined facial and truncal acne than in facial acne patients [47]. Among a variety of health-related QoL domains, having combined facial and truncal acne was associated with poorer emotional well-being, everyday life activities, participation in social activities and sports, and routine acne treatment than having facial acne alone [47].

The burden of truncal acne is obvious in many patients; however, it is thought that the degree of the impact of truncal acne could vary from patient to patient, and there is a difference in psychosocial burdens between patients with truncal acne and those with facial acne. As the truncal regions are usually exposed in summer, there might be a seasonal variation in the burden of truncal acne. The consensus of an expert panel suggested that the visual analog scale (VAS) could be a useful tool for assessing the factors associated with the impact of disease on patients, and thereby help to identify the treatment goal for each patient [39].

8. Management of Truncal Acne

In general, treatment-specific guidelines for acne have been established and updated in various countries [48–51]. However, the management guidelines for truncal acne are limited. In clinical practice, some clinicians are managing truncal acne based on the guidelines for facial acne. The recent consensus of an expert panel recommended managing truncal acne similar to facial acne [39]. Although the underlying pathogenic mechanisms between facial acne and truncal acne are similar, as there are some differences between the face and trunk, the management of truncal acne should be considered from a slightly different perspective. As the involved body surface area is broader in truncal acne than facial acne, and there is a difference in the characteristics of the skin between the trunk and face, these aspects should always be considered when choosing optimal treatment options for truncal acne. Although the clinical evidence for using topical and systemic agents for truncal acne is limited, some recent evidence confirmed the clinical efficacy of using these agents to treat truncal acne (Table 2).

Table 2. Summary of clinical trials for management of truncal acne.

Drug (Trade Name)	Company	Clinical Trial Number	Phase and Status	Study Design	Results
Topical management					
Dapsone 7.5 % gel (Aczone®)	Almirall	NCT02944461	Phase 4, completed	A 16-week open label pilot study ($n = 20$) with moderate truncal acne	At week 16, 46.7% showed at least two grade improvement and a rating of clear or almost clear on the investigator global assessment (IGA) scale.
Azelaic acid 20% cream (Skinoren®)	GSK	N/A	Phase 4, completed	A prospective, noninterventional multicenter study in adult female patients ($n = 251$) with mild to moderate acne	A significant improvement of acne on the face, chest, and back was observed after 12 weeks of the treatment.
Tazarotene foam and gel (Tazorac®)	GSK	NCT01019603	Phase 1, completed	A single-center, randomized, open-label, comparative bioavailability study in subjects with moderate to severe acne vulgaris ($n = 30$)	Mean concentration of tazarotene was higher for gel versus foam.
Trifarotene (Aklief®)	Galderma	NCT02189629	Phase 3, completed	An open-label, 52-week study with moderate facial and truncal acne ($n = 453$)	66.9% patients with truncal acne demonstrated treatment success by physician's global assessment rating (no or almost no acne).
		NCT02566369 NCT02556788	Phase 3, completed	Two double-blind, randomized, vehicle-controlled, 12-weeks studies of trifarotene cream versus vehicle in moderate facial and truncal acne	A highly significant difference in favor of trifarotene compared to the vehicle was observed based on physician's global assessment and the change in inflammatory and noninflammatory lesion counts.
Cortexolone 17a-propionate (CB-03-01) 1% cream (Clascoterone®)	Cassiopea S.p.A.	NCT02682264	Phase 3, completed	An open-label, long-term extension study ($n = 609$) to evaluate safety with acne	The 1% clascoterone cream showed a well-tolerable safety profile.

Table 2. Cont.

Drug (Trade Name)	Company	Clinical Trial Number	Phase and Status	Study Design	Results
Systemic management					
Sarecycline (Seysara®)	Almirall	NCT02322866	Phase 3, completed	Two double-blind, randomized, 12-week studies of sarecycline in the treatment of acne	The pooled analysis for truncal acne showed that chest and back IGA success rate was significantly greater with sarecycline than with the placebo at week 3, 6, and 12, respectively.
		NCT05010538	Phase 4, Active, not recruiting	A 12-week, single center open-label case series study for truncal acne ($n = 10$)	
Isotretinoin-Lidose (Absorica®)	Galephar	N/A	Phase 3, completed	A 20-week, multicenter, double-blind randomized study to evaluate the safety and efficacy of isotretinoin-lidose in patients with severe recalcitrant nodular facial and truncal acne ($n = 925$)	The mean change in facial and truncal nodular lesion counts from week 0 to week 20 was comparable between the isotretinoin-lidose group and the food-dependent generic isotretinoin group.
Drospirenone and Ethinyl Estradiol (YAZ®)	Bayer	NCT00722761	Phase 3, completed	A single center, randomized double-blind, parallel group study in moderate truncal acne vulgaris ($n = 30$)	The drospirenone/ethinyl estradiol showed treatment success among 53.3% of the patients based on IGA and 60% of the patients based on subject global assessment.

Abbreviation: N/A, not accessible.

8.1. Topical Management

Liu et al. [52] suggested that topical therapies could be the initial treatment options for mild-to-moderate truncal acne. Among a variety of topical agents used in acne, topical retinoids, benzoyl peroxide (BPO), azelaic acid, dapsone, and topical antibiotics can be used alone or in a combination of these for managing truncal acne.

BPO is a widely used topical agent for managing acne. BPO has a bactericidal efficacy against *C. acnes* and can reduce the inflammatory lesions of acne and the risk of antibiotic resistance. However, the previous use of BPO for treating the truncal area has been limited due to the bleaching effect of BPO on bed linens and clothing. Therefore, in the real-world, a wash-off cleanser formulation of BPO, including over-the-counter products, is commonly used for truncal acne. In 2010, Leyden et al. [53] designed a study examining the efficacy of 5.3% BPO emollient foam and 8% BPO wash in reducing *C. acnes* on the back of healthy individuals [53]. BPO 5.3% emollient foam decreased the total *C. acnes* count, whereas the 8% BPO wash did not significantly decrease *C. acnes* counts [53]. The authors suggested that the short contact time with the wash-off formulation was not enough for the sufficient penetration and deposition of BPO on the skin of the back. Therefore, the authors designed a further study which used a two-minute skin contact time with BPO wash. In that study, Leyden et al. [54] found that the application of 9.8% BPO foam to non-moistened skin during washing with a two-minute skin contact time in a once-daily application decreased the levels of *C. acnes* on the backs of healthy individuals. This suggests that the wash-off cleanser formulation of BPO could be used effectively for managing truncal acne.

Azelaic acid is a kind of natural compound that exerts its effect on acne through anti-keratinizing, anti-inflammatory, and antibacterial functions [55]. The topical application of azelaic acid is effective for both inflammatory acne and non-inflammatory acne lesions [55]. A prospective multicenter study in adult female patients with mild to moderate acne found that 12 weeks of treatment with twice-daily applications of 20% azelaic acid cream resulted in a significant improvement in acne on the face, chest, and back [56]. In addition, a significant decrease in the median dermatology life quality index (DLQI) was observed with very good or good tolerability of the treatment by both the patients and physicians [56].

A single center-pilot study found that 15% azelaic acid foam was effective in managing moderate truncal acne [57]. At week 16, 11 out of 16 patients with moderate truncal acne had clear or almost clear IGA scale scores after twice daily applications of 15% azelaic acid foam [57]. The authors suggested that this foam was effective in treating truncal acne due to its rapid skin penetration and spreadability [57]. A recent case series reported that the combination of 0.05% tretinoin lotion and 15% azelaic acid foam was effective in treating truncal acne in four female African-American patients [58].

The efficacy and safety of topical 7.5% dapsone gel were studied in patients with truncal acne [59]. Through 16 weeks of the treatment, 45% of the patients experienced clear/almost clear skin plus at least two-grade improvements in their truncal acne [59]. Topical 7.5% dapsone gel was relatively well-tolerated and safe for the patients throughout the study period [59].

Topical retinoids have been considered a potent treatment option for treatment of acne vulgaris. Several generations of topical retinoids have been developed. The binding affinity for several retinoid receptors and clinical considerations for use are summarized in Table 3. Among the diverse topical retinoids, Cunliffe et al. [60] reported that a 4-week treatment with topical isotretinoin was effective for facial and truncal acne without any clinically significant increase in plasma retinoid levels. A bioavailability study of 0.1% tazarotene foam compared to 0.1% tazarotene gel for moderate to severe acne was conducted [61]. Both agents were applied to the face, chest, shoulders, and upper back once daily. The authors concluded that both 0.1% tazarotene foam and 0.1% tazarotene gel were effective in managing moderate to severe acne with favorable safety and less potential for systemic exposure [61].

Recently, trifarotene, which selectively targets retinoic acid receptor gamma, was developed and shown to have potent anti-comedogenic, anti-inflammatory, and anti-pigmentary activities in an in vivo study [30]. The clinical effects of trifarotene on facial and truncal acne have been well demonstrated by clinical trials [62,63]. Two recent large-scale phase III clinical trials revealed that trifarotene cream was effective for both facial and truncal acne compared to the vehicle [62]. A long-term, open-label, 52-week study examining the safety and efficacy of trifarotene cream found that trifarotene was effective, safe, and well-tolerated by patients with moderate facial and truncal acne [63]. Of note, local irritation responses due to the application of trifarotene were less frequently observed in truncal acne than in facial acne [63], suggesting the tolerability of topical trifarotene in managing truncal acne.

The topical androgen receptor inhibitor clascoterone is a novel promising therapeutic option for acne. The mechanism of action of clascoterone on acne is supposed to be the inhibition of dihydrotestosterone-androgen receptor binding in sebocytes and the subsequent decrease in the downstream activation of androgen-driven lipid production and inflammation [64]. Two phase 3 clinical trials for clascoterone for facial acne were conducted from 2015 to 2018. The authors concluded that at week 12, 1% clascoterone cream significantly reduced the absolute noninflammatory lesion from baselines, with few and mild adverse events [65]. A nine-month, open-label extension trial to analyze the clinical safety and efficacy of clascoterone found that clascoterone could be used relatively safely and effectively for treating facial and truncal acne [64].

Table 3. Summary of topical retinoids for acne.

Retinoids	Trade Name (Formulations)	Binding Affinity to RARs	US FDA Pregnancy Category	Half-Life in Plasma
All-trans retinoic acid (Tretinoin)	Stieva-A®, Atralin®, Avita®, Retin-A®, Retin-A Micro®, Tretin-X® (Cream: 0.01%, 0.025%, 0.05%; gel: 0.01%, 0.025%, 0.04%, 0.05%, 0.1%)	RARα(++), RARβ(++), RARγ(++)	Category C	0.5–2 h
Adapalene	Differin® (Cream: 0.1%; gel: 0.1%, 0.3%; lotion: 0.1%)	RARβ(++), RARγ(++)	Category C	7–51 h
Tazarotene	Tazorac® (Cream: 0.05%, 0.1%; gel: 0.05%, 0.1%; foam: 0.1%)	RARα(+), RARβ(+++), RARγ(++)	Category X	18 h
Trifarotene	AKLIEF® (Cream: 0.005%)	RARγ(+++)	Not assigned	2–9 h

(+), Minimal binding affinity; (++) moderate binding affinity; (+++) strong binding affinity; Abbreviations: FDA, food and drug administration; RAR, retinoic acid receptor.

8.2. Systemic Management

Systemic management has been indicated for moderate to severe acne and inflammatory acne that are resistant to topical treatments. In moderate to severe acne, combined treatment with topical agents and systemic agents such as antibiotics, isotretinoin, oral contraceptives, or spironolactone can be applied [66].

The efficacy of tetracyclines and macrolides including tetracycline, doxycycline, minocycline, trimethoprim/sulfamethoxazole, trimethoprim, azithromycin, amoxicillin and cephalexin in treating acne has been well-documented [66]. Oral antibiotics are also effective options in managing truncal acne [67]. However, the use of trimethoprim-sulfamethoxazole and trimethoprim should be limited to patients who are unable to take tetracyclines or treatment-resistant patients. Systemic antibiotics should be used for the shortest possible duration of 3–4 months due to the potential for bacterial resistance [66]. Sarecycline is a third generation narrow-spectrum oral tetracycline that has been approved by the Food and Drug Administration (FDA) for treating acne [68]. Its unique structural characteristics enables it to exhibit anti-inflammatory and high anti-bacterial effects against *C. acnes*, *Staphylococci*, and *Streptococci* [69]. A phase 3 study of sarecycline for treating facial acne demonstrated that sarecycline was effective and well-tolerated [70]. A pooled analysis of two phase 3 studies on truncal acne was conducted [69]. Significant IGA success on the chest and back was, respectively, observed in the sarecycline group compared to the placebo group from three weeks to twelve weeks [69]. Thus, sarecycline could be a novel and effective option for managing moderate to severe truncal acne.

Isotretinoin is the treatment of choice for severe recalcitrant truncal acne [67]. The newer formulation of isotretinoin, isotretinoin-lidose, utilizes the lidose technique with micronized particles to increase the surface area of the drug. Therefore, isotretinoin-lidose can increase bioavailability by 50% compared to traditional isotretinoin. A double-blind, multicenter study of 925 patients with severe, recalcitrant nodular acne compared the clinical efficacy and safety of isotretinoin-lidose to standard isotretinoin for 20 weeks [71]. Both isotretinoin-lidose and traditional isotretinoin reduced the total number of nodules on the face and trunk to equivalent degrees, suggesting that both formulations had similar efficacy [71].

Hormone therapies such as oral contraceptives and spironolactone suppress the effect of androgens on the sebaceous glands, so they have been used for the treatment of acne.

Palli et al. [72] conducted a clinical trial to investigate the effects of 3 mg drospirenone/ 0.02 mg ethinyl estradiol on moderate truncal acne. Drospirenone has special antiandrogenic and anti-mineralocorticoid functions compared to other progestins. Due to these antiandrogenic properties, which can block male sex hormones associated with acne development, this hormone can be used to manage acne. In a single-center, double-blind, randomized study, 25 subjects, aged 18 to 45 years, with moderate truncal acne received 3 mg drospirenone/0.02 mg ethinyl estradiol or placebo for 24 weeks [72]. Treatment with 3 mg drospirenone/0.02 mg ethinyl estradiol showed treatment success among 53.3% of the patients based on IGA, and 60% of the patients based on subject global assessment (SGA) [72]. This regimen demonstrated significant clinical improvement with good tolerability by the patients [72].

8.3. Procedural Therapies

In general, truncal acne tends to have a slower response to treatment than facial acne, so it is likely to be approached with a more multidisciplinary treatment strategy. Among the variety of procedural therapies that can be applied to acne lesions such as lasers, light devices, chemical peels, and intralesional injections, there is a conspicuous absence of many randomized controlled trials evaluating the efficacy of these modalities in treating truncal acne. Regarding chemical peels, salicylic acid, glycolic acid, lactic acid, mandelic acid, retinoic acid, trichloroacetic acid, Jessner's solution, kojic acid, pyruvic acid, azelaic acid, and combination peels are used in management of acne [73]. Although most of the studies on chemical peels for acne studied facial acne, in general practice, most of the chemical peels are also applied to the trunk [73]. Among them, photodynamic therapy (PDT) has the greatest evidence for the management of truncal acne. A meta-analysis reported that PDT was effective in improving inflammatory acne vulgaris based on the analysis of 13 randomized controlled trials [74]. For truncal acne, the clinical efficacy of PDT with topical 5% 5-aminolevulinic acid was evaluated in Asian patients with truncal acne [75]. With a single treatment session with 5% 5-aminolevulinic acid PDT, a 64.2% reduction in inflammatory lesion counts and a 24.3% reduction in non-inflammatory lesion counts of truncal acne were observed at 12 weeks of follow-up among 15 patients [75].

For managing hypertrophic truncal scars, intralesional injections with corticosteroids, 5-fluorouracil, or bleomycin can be performed. In addition, cryotherapy and PDT can also be promising treatment modalities for managing hypertrophic truncal acne scars.

8.4. Future Directions

Although there is little clinical evidence on treatments to manage truncal acne, truncal acne is generally controlled in a similar way to that of facial acne. In the case of topical or oral formulations that have been recently developed, several clinical reports presented the effect of those agents in treating truncal acne. Although truncal acne occurs in covered areas, hypertrophic scars are common, calling for vigorous treatment as a scar preventive measure. Therefore, awareness should be established to actively treat body acne at an early stage.

9. Conclusions

Truncal acne is a condition that, despite being relatively common, is underreported by patients and underdiagnosed and undertreated by clinicians. More research on the epidemiology of truncal acne is needed, and in relation to treatment, evidence for effective therapeutic agents for truncal acne needs to be established independently of facial acne. Truncal acne can cause persistent scarring, such as macular atrophic scarring and keloids. Therefore, the early and prompt treatment of truncal acne patients is needed to prevent further scarring. In truncal acne patients who already have scars due to previous truncal acne, more attention and aggressive treatment should be conducted to normalize the condition.

Thus, there is an unmet need for treating truncal acne. As truncal acne occurs on an unexposed body part, more effort by the clinician to examine the lesions in detail is needed. In addition to multidisciplinary research for trunk acne to reveal its pathogenic characteristics and proper management options, significant effort should also be put into increasing the awareness of the importance of early and appropriate treatment for truncal acne.

Funding: This research received no external funding.

Conflicts of Interest: The authors declare no conflict of interest.

References

1. Vos, T.; Flaxman, A.D.; Naghavi, M.; Lozano, R.; Michaud, C.; Ezzati, M.; Shibuya, K.; Salomon, J.A.; Abdalla, S.; Aboyans, V. Years lived with disability (YLDs) for 1160 sequelae of 289 diseases and injuries 1990–2010: A systematic analysis for the Global Burden of Disease Study 2010. *Lancet* **2012**, *380*, 2163–2196. [CrossRef]
2. Heng, A.H.S.; Chew, F.T. Systematic review of the epidemiology of acne vulgaris. *Sci. Rep.* **2020**, *10*, 1–29. [CrossRef]
3. Marson, J.W.; Baldwin, H.E. Isotretinoin update. *Dermatol. Rev.* **2021**, *2*, 331–342. [CrossRef]
4. Del Rosso, J.Q.; Bikowski, J.B.; Baum, E.; Smith, J.; Hawkes, S.; Benes, V.; Bhatia, N. A closer look at truncal acne vulgaris: Prevalence, severity, and clinical significance. *J. Drugs Dermatol. JDD* **2007**, *6*, 597–600. [PubMed]
5. Isaacsson, V.C.S.; Almeida, H.L.D., Jr.; Duquia, R.P.; Breunig, J.D.A.; Souza, P.R.M.D. Dissatisfaction and acne vulgaris in male adolescents and associated factors. *An. Bras. De Dermatol.* **2014**, *89*, 576–579. [CrossRef]
6. Dreno, B.; Thiboutot, D.; Layton, A.; Berson, D.; Perez, M.; Kang, S. on behalf of the Global Alliance to Improve Outcomes in Acne. Large-scale international study enhances understanding of an emerging acne population: Adult females. *J. Eur. Acad. Dermatol. Venereol.* **2015**, *29*, 1096–1106. [CrossRef]
7. Dréno, B.; Jean-Decoster, C.; Georgescu, V. Profile of patients with mild-to-moderate acne in Europe: A survey. *Eur. J. Dermatol.* **2016**, *26*, 177–184. [CrossRef]
8. Barth, J.H.; Clark, S. Acne and hirsuties in teenagers. *Best Pract. Res. Clin. Obstet. Gynaecol.* **2003**, *17*, 131–148. [CrossRef]
9. Poli, F.; Auffret, N.; Leccia, M.T.; Claudel, J.P.; Dréno, B. Truncal acne, what do we know? *J. Eur. Acad. Dermatol. Venereol.* **2020**, *34*, 2241–2246. [CrossRef]
10. Nijsten, T.; Rombouts, S.; Lambert, J. Acne is prevalent but use of its treatments is infrequent among adolescents from the general population. *J. Eur. Acad. Dermatol. Venereol.* **2007**, *21*, 163–168. [CrossRef] [PubMed]
11. Wei, B.; Pang, Y.; Zhu, H.; Qu, L.; Xiao, T.; Wei, H.C.; Chen, H.D.; He, C.D. The epidemiology of adolescent acne in North East China. *J. Eur. Acad. Dermatol. Venereol.* **2010**, *24*, 953–957. [CrossRef] [PubMed]
12. Suh, D.H.; Kim, B.Y.; Min, S.U.; Lee, D.H.; Yoon, M.Y.; Kim, N.I.; Kye, Y.C.; Lee, E.S.; Ro, Y.S.; Kim, K.J. A multicenter epidemiological study of acne vulgaris in Korea. *Int. J. Dermatol.* **2011**, *50*, 673–681. [CrossRef] [PubMed]
13. Dessinioti, C.; Katsambas, A. Difficult and rare forms of acne. *Clin. Dermatol.* **2017**, *35*, 138–146. [CrossRef] [PubMed]
14. Zaba, R.; Schwartz, R.; Jarmuda, S.; Czarnecka-Operacz, M.; Silny, W. Acne fulminans: Explosive systemic form of acne. *J. Eur. Acad. Dermatol. Venereol.* **2011**, *25*, 501–507. [CrossRef]
15. Gollnick, H. From new findings in acne pathogenesis to new approaches in treatment. *J. Eur. Acad. Dermatol. Venereol.* **2015**, *29*, 1–7. [CrossRef]
16. Zouboulis, C.; Eady, A.; Philpott, M.; Goldsmith, L.; Orfanos, C.; Cunliffe, W.; Rosenfield, R. What is the pathogenesis of acne? *Exp. Dermatol.* **2005**, *14*, 143. [CrossRef]
17. Kim, B.R.; Chun, M.Y.; Kim, S.A.; Youn, S.W. Sebum secretion of the trunk and the development of truncal acne in women: Do truncal acne and sebum affect each other? *Dermatology* **2015**, *231*, 87–93. [CrossRef]
18. Melnik, B.; Jansen, T.; Grabbe, S. Abuse of anabolic-androgenic steroids and bodybuilding acne: An underestimated health problem. *JDDG J. Der Dtsch. Dermatol. Ges.* **2007**, *5*, 110–117. [CrossRef]
19. Zouboulis, C.C. Endocrinology and immunology of acne: Two sides of the same coin. *Exp. Dermatol.* **2020**, *29*, 840–859. [CrossRef]
20. Deng, Y.; Wang, H.; Zhou, J.; Mou, Y.; Wang, G.; Xiong, X. Patients with Acne Vulgaris Have a Distinct Gut Microbiota in Comparison with Healthy Controls. *Acta Derm. Venereol.* **2018**, *98*, 783–790. [CrossRef]
21. Yan, H.M.; Zhao, H.J.; Guo, D.Y.; Zhu, P.Q.; Zhang, C.L.; Jiang, W. Gut microbiota alterations in moderate to severe acne vulgaris patients. *J. Dermatol.* **2018**, *45*, 1166–1171. [CrossRef] [PubMed]
22. Huang, Y.; Liu, L.; Chen, L.; Zhou, L.; Xiong, X.; Deng, Y. Gender-Specific Differences in Gut Microbiota Composition Associated with Microbial Metabolites for Patients with Acne Vulgaris. *Ann. Dermatol.* **2021**, *33*, 531. [CrossRef] [PubMed]
23. Dagnelie, M.A.; Montassier, E.; Khammari, A.; Mounier, C.; Corvec, S.; Dréno, B. Inflammatory skin is associated with changes in the skin microbiota composition on the back of severe acne patients. *Exp. Dermatol.* **2019**, *28*, 961–967. [CrossRef] [PubMed]
24. Dagnelie, M.-A.; Corvec, S.; Saint-Jean, M.; Bourdès, V.; Nguyen, J.-M.; Khammari, A.; Dréno, B. Decrease in diversity of Propionibacterium acnes phylotypes in patients with severe acne on the back. *Acta Derm. Venereol.* **2018**, *98*, 262–267. [CrossRef]

25. Kim, J.; Park, T.; Kim, H.-J.; An, S.; Sul, W.J. Inferences in microbial structural signatures of acne microbiome and mycobiome. *J. Microbiol.* **2021**, *59*, 369–375. [CrossRef]
26. Nguyen, H.L.; Tollefson, M.M. Endocrine disorders and hormonal therapy for adolescent acne. *Curr. Opin. Pediatrics* **2017**, *29*, 455–465. [CrossRef]
27. Lolis, M.S.; Bowe, W.P.; Shalita, A.R. Acne and systemic disease. *Med. Clin.* **2009**, *93*, 1161–1181. [CrossRef]
28. Bansal, P.; Sardana, K.; Sharma, L.; Garga, U.C.; Vats, G. A prospective study examining isolated acne and acne with hyperandrogenic signs in adult females. *J. Dermatol. Treat.* **2021**, *32*, 752–755. [CrossRef]
29. Saint-Jean, M.; Khammari, A.; Jasson, F.; Nguyen, J.-M.; Dréno, B. Different cutaneous innate immunity profiles in acne patients with and without atrophic scars. *Eur. J. Dermatol.* **2016**, *26*, 68–74. [CrossRef]
30. Aubert, J.; Piwnica, D.; Bertino, B.; Blanchet-Réthoré, S.; Carlavan, I.; Déret, S.; Dreno, B.; Gamboa, B.; Jomard, A.; Luzy, A. Nonclinical and human pharmacology of the potent and selective topical retinoic acid receptor-γ agonist trifarotene. *Br. J. Dermatol.* **2018**, *179*, 442–456. [CrossRef]
31. Kim, S.A.; Kim, B.R.; Chun, M.Y.; Youn, S.W. Relation between pH in the trunk and face: Truncal pH can be easily predicted from facial pH. *Ann. Dermatol.* **2016**, *28*, 216–221. [CrossRef] [PubMed]
32. Pillsbury, D.M.; Shelley, W.B. Dermatology. *Annu. Rev. Med.* **1954**, *5*, 363–388. [CrossRef] [PubMed]
33. Burke, B.M.; Cunliffe, W. The assessment of acne vulgaris—The Leeds technique. *Br. J. Dermatol.* **1984**, *111*, 83–92. [CrossRef] [PubMed]
34. O'brien, S.; Lewis, J.; Cunliffe, W. The Leeds revised acne grading system. *J. Dermatol. Treat.* **1998**, *9*, 215–220. [CrossRef]
35. Tan, J.K.; Tang, J.; Fung, K.; Gupta, A.K.; Thomas, D.R.; Sapra, S.; Lynde, C.; Poulin, Y.; Gulliver, W.; Sebaldt, R.J. Development and validation of a comprehensive acne severity scale. *J. Cutan. Med. Surg.* **2007**, *11*, 211–216. [CrossRef]
36. Tan, J.K.; Tang, J.; Fung, K.; Gupta, A.K.; Thomas, D.R.; Sapra, S.; Lynde, C.; Poulin, Y.; Gulliver, W.; Sebaldt, R.J. Development and validation of a Scale for Acne Scar Severity (SCAR-S) of the face and trunk. *J. Cutan. Med. Surg.* **2010**, *14*, 156–160. [CrossRef]
37. Bernardis, E.; Shou, H.; Barbieri, J.S.; McMahon, P.J.; Perman, M.J.; Rola, L.A.; Streicher, J.L.; Treat, J.R.; Castelo-Soccio, L.; Yan, A.C. Development and initial validation of a multidimensional acne global grading system integrating primary lesions and secondary changes. *JAMA Dermatol.* **2020**, *156*, 296–302. [CrossRef]
38. Auffret, N.; Nguyen, J.; Leccia, M.T.; Claudel, J.; Dréno, B. TRASS: A global approach to assess the severity of truncal acne. *J. Eur. Acad. Dermatol. Venereol.* **2022**, *36*, 897–904. [CrossRef]
39. Tan, J.; Alexis, A.; Baldwin, H.; Beissert, S.; Bettoli, V.; Del Rosso, J.; Dréno, B.; Gold, L.S.; Harper, J.; Lynde, C. Gaps and recommendations for clinical management of truncal acne from the Personalising Acne: Consensus of Experts panel. *JAAD Int.* **2021**, *5*, 33–40. [CrossRef]
40. Sun, K.-L.; Chang, J.-M. Special types of folliculitis which should be differentiated from acne. *Derm. Endocrinol.* **2017**, *9*, e1356519. [CrossRef]
41. Prindaville, B.; Belazarian, L.; Levin, N.A.; Wiss, K. Pityrosporum folliculitis: A retrospective review of 110 cases. *J. Am. Acad. Dermatol.* **2018**, *78*, 511–514. [CrossRef] [PubMed]
42. Rubenstein, R.M.; Malerich, S.A. Malassezia (pityrosporum) folliculitis. *J. Clin. Aesthetic Dermatol.* **2014**, *7*, 37.
43. Kazandjieva, J.; Tsankov, N. Drug-induced acne. *Clin. Dermatol.* **2017**, *35*, 156–162. [CrossRef]
44. Mallon, E.; Newton, J.; Klassen, A.; Stewart-Brown, S.L.; Ryan, T.; Finlay, A. The quality of life in acne: A comparison with general medical conditions using generic questionnaires. *Br. J. Dermatol.* **1999**, *140*, 672–676. [CrossRef]
45. Rocha, M.A.; Bagatin, E. Adult-onset acne: Prevalence, impact, and management challenges. *Clin. Cosmet. Investig. Dermatol.* **2018**, *11*, 59. [CrossRef]
46. Papadopoulos, L.; Walker, C.; Aitken, D.; Bor, R. The relationship between body location and psychological morbidity in individuals with acne vulgaris. *Psychol. Health Med.* **2000**, *5*, 431–438. [CrossRef]
47. Tan, J.; Beissert, S.; Cook-Bolden, F.; Chavda, R.; Harper, J.; Hebert, A.; Lain, E.; Layton, A.; Rocha, M.; Weiss, J. Impact of facial and truncal acne on quality of life: A multi-country population-based survey. *JAAD Int.* **2021**, *3*, 102–110. [CrossRef]
48. Layton, A.; McDonald, B.; Mohd Mustapa, M.; Levell, N. National Institute for Health and Care Excellence (NICE) acne guideline: What's the latest for dermatologists? *Br. J. Dermatol.* **2022**, *186*, 426–428. [CrossRef]
49. Xu, Y.; Mavranezouli, I.; Kuznetsov, L.; Murphy, M.S.; Healy, E. Management of acne vulgaris: Summary of NICE guidance. *BMJ* **2021**, *374*, n1800. [CrossRef]
50. Harper, J.C. An update on the pathogenesis and management of acne vulgaris. *J. Am. Acad. Dermatol.* **2004**, *51*, 36–38. [CrossRef]
51. Conforti, C.; Chello, C.; Giuffrida, R.; di Meo, N.; Zalaudek, I.; Dianzani, C. An overview of treatment options for mild-to-moderate acne based on American Academy of Dermatology, European Academy of Dermatology and Venereology, and Italian Society of Dermatology and Venereology guidelines. *Dermatol. Ther.* **2020**, *33*, e13548. [CrossRef] [PubMed]
52. Liu, C.; Tan, J. Understanding truncal acne: A practical guide to diagnosis and management. *Skin Ther. Lett.* Available online: http://www.skintherapyletter.com/conditions/acne/truncal-diagnosis-management/ (accessed on 18 June 2022).
53. Leyden, J.J. Efficacy of benzoyl peroxide (5.3%) emollient foam and benzoyl peroxide (8%) wash in reducing Propionibacterium acnes on the back. *J. Drugs Dermatol. JDD* **2010**, *9*, 622–625. [PubMed]
54. Leyden, J.J.; Del Rosso, J.Q. The effect of benzoyl peroxide 9.8% emollient foam on reduction of Propionibacterium acnes on the back using a short contact therapy approach. *J. Drugs Dermatol. JDD* **2012**, *11*, 830–833. [PubMed]

55. Shemer, A.; Weiss, G.; Amichai, B.; Kaplan, B.; Trau, H. Azelaic acid (20%) cream in the treatment of acne vulgaris. *J. Eur. Acad. Dermatol. Venereol.* **2002**, *16*, 178–179. [CrossRef]
56. Kainz, J.T.; Berghammer, G.; Auer-Grumbach, P.; Lackner, V.; Perl-Convalexius, S.; Popa, R.; Wolfesberger, B. Azelaic acid 20% cream: Effects on quality of life and disease severity in adult female acne patients. *JDDG J. Der Dtsch. Dermatol. Ges.* **2016**, *14*, 1249–1259. [CrossRef]
57. Hoffman, L.K.; Del Rosso, J.Q.; Kircik, L.H. The Efficacy and Safety of Azelaic Acid 15% Foam in the Treatment of Truncal Acne Vulgaris. *J. Drugs Dermatol. JDD* **2017**, *16*, 534–538.
58. Surin-Lord, S.S.; Miller, J. Topical treatment of truncal acne with tretinoin lotion 0.05% and azelaic acid foam. *Case Rep. Dermatol. Med.* **2020**, *2020*, 5217567. [CrossRef]
59. Del Rosso, J.Q.; Kircik, L.; Tanghetti, E. Management of truncal acne vulgaris with topical dapsone 7.5% gel. *J. Clin. Aesthetic Dermatol.* **2018**, *11*, 45.
60. Cunliffe, W.J.; Glass, D.; Goode, K.; Stables, G.I.; Boorman, G.C. A double-blind investigation of the potential systemic absorption of isotretinoin, when combined with chemical sunscreens, following topical application to patients with widespread acne of the face and trunk. *Acta Derm. Venereol.* **2001**, *81*, 14–17. [CrossRef]
61. Jarratt, M.; Werner, C.P.; Alió Saenz, A.B. Tazarotene foam versus tazarotene gel: A randomized relative bioavailability study in acne vulgaris. *Clin. Drug Investig.* **2013**, *33*, 283–289. [CrossRef] [PubMed]
62. Tan, J.; Thiboutot, D.; Popp, G.; Gooderham, M.; Lynde, C.; Del Rosso, J.; Weiss, J.; Blume-Peytavi, U.; Weglovska, J.; Johnson, S. Randomized phase 3 evaluation of trifarotene 50 μg/g cream treatment of moderate facial and truncal acne. *J. Am. Acad. Dermatol.* **2019**, *80*, 1691–1699. [CrossRef] [PubMed]
63. Blume-Peytavi, U.; Fowler, J.; Kemény, L.; Draelos, Z.; Cook-Bolden, F.; Dirschka, T.; Eichenfield, L.; Graeber, M.; Ahmad, F.; Saenz, A.A. Long-term safety and efficacy of trifarotene 50 μg/g cream, a first-in-class RAR-γ selective topical retinoid, in patients with moderate facial and truncal acne. *J. Eur. Acad. Dermatol. Venereol.* **2020**, *34*, 166–173. [CrossRef] [PubMed]
64. Eichenfield, L.; Hebert, A.; Gold, L.S.; Cartwright, M.; Fragasso, E.; Moro, L.; Mazzetti, A. Open-label, long-term extension study to evaluate the safety of clascoterone (CB-03-01) cream, 1% twice daily, in patients with acne vulgaris. *J. Am. Acad. Dermatol.* **2020**, *83*, 477–485. [CrossRef]
65. Hebert, A.; Thiboutot, D.; Gold, L.S.; Cartwright, M.; Gerloni, M.; Fragasso, E.; Mazzetti, A. Efficacy and safety of topical clascoterone cream, 1%, for treatment in patients with facial acne: Two phase 3 randomized clinical trials. *JAMA Dermatol.* **2020**, *156*, 621–630. [CrossRef] [PubMed]
66. Zaenglein, A.L.; Pathy, A.L.; Schlosser, B.J.; Alikhan, A.; Baldwin, H.E.; Berson, D.S.; Bowe, W.P.; Graber, E.M.; Harper, J.C.; Kang, S. Guidelines of care for the management of acne vulgaris. *J. Am. Acad. Dermatol.* **2016**, *74*, 945–973.e933. [CrossRef]
67. Del Rosso, J.Q.; Stein-Gold, L.; Lynde, C.; Tanghetti, E.; Alexis, A.F. Truncal acne: A neglected entity. *J. Drugs Dermatol. JDD* **2019**, *18*, 205–1208.
68. Del Rosso, J.Q. Sarecycline and the Narrow-spectrum tetracycline concept: Currently Available Data and Potential Clinical Relevance in Dermatology. *J. Clin. Aesthetic Dermatol.* **2020**, *13*, 45.
69. Del Rosso, J.Q.; Baldwin, H.; Harper, J.; Zeichner, J.; Obagi, S.; Graber, E.; Jimenez, X.; Vicente, F.; Grada, A. Management of Truncal Acne With Oral Sarecycline: Pooled Results from Two Phase-3 Clinical Trials. *J. Drugs Dermatol. JDD* **2021**, *20*, 634–640.
70. Moore, A.; Green, L.J.; Bruce, S.; Sadick, N.; Tschen, E.; Werschler, P.; Cook-Bolden, F.E.; Dhawan, S.S.; Forsha, D.; Gold, M.H. Once-Daily Oral Sarecycline 1.5 mg/kg/day Is Effective for Moderate to Severe Acne Vulgaris: Results from Two Identically Designed, Phase 3, Randomized, Double-Blind Clinical Trials. *J. Drugs Dermatol. JDD* **2018**, *17*, 987–996. [CrossRef]
71. Webster, G.F.; Leyden, J.J.; Gross, J.A. Results of a Phase III, double-blind, randomized, parallel-group, non-inferiority study evaluating the safety and efficacy of isotretinoin-Lidose in patients with severe recalcitrant nodular acne. *J. Drugs Dermatol. JDD* **2014**, *13*, 665–670. [PubMed]
72. Palli, M.; Reyes-Habito, C.M.; Lima, X.T.; Kimball, A.B. A single-center, randomized double-blind, parallel-group study to examine the safety and efficacy of 3mg drospirenone/0.02 mg ethinyl estradiol compared with placebo in the treatment of moderate truncal acne vulgaris. *J. Drugs Dermatol. JDD* **2013**, *12*, 633–637. [PubMed]
73. Castillo, D.E.; Keri, J.E. Chemical peels in the treatment of acne: Patient selection and perspectives. *Clin. Cosmet. Investig. Dermatol.* **2018**, *11*, 365. [CrossRef] [PubMed]
74. Tang, X.; Li, C.; Ge, S.; Chen, Z.; Lu, L. Efficacy of photodynamic therapy for the treatment of inflammatory acne vulgaris: A systematic review and meta-analysis. *J. Cosmet. Dermatol.* **2020**, *19*, 10–21. [CrossRef]
75. Yew, Y.W.; Lai, Y.C.; Lim, Y.L.; Chong, W.-S.; Theng, C. Photodynamic Therapy With Topical 5% 5-Aminolevulinic Acid for the Treatment of Truncal Acne in Asian Patients. *J. Drugs Dermatol. JDD* **2016**, *15*, 727–732.

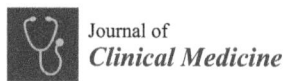

Article

Efficacy of Oxybrasion in the Treatment of Acne Vulgaris: A Preliminary Report

Karolina Chilicka [1,*], Aleksandra M. Rogowska [2], Renata Szyguła [1], Monika Rusztowicz [1] and Danuta Nowicka [3]

[1] Department of Health Sciences, Institute of Health Sciences, University of Opole, 45-040 Opole, Poland; renata.szygula@uni.opole.pl (R.S.); monika.rusztowicz@uni.opole.pl (M.R.)
[2] Institute of Psychology, University of Opole, 45-052 Opole, Poland; arogowska@uni.opole.pl
[3] Department of Dermatology, Venereology and Allergology, Wrocław Medical University, 50-368 Wrocław, Poland; danuta.nowicka@umed.wroc.pl
* Correspondence: karolina.chilicka@uni.opole.pl

Abstract: There are many cosmetic methods to reduce skin eruptions in people with acne vulgaris. As oxybrasion is a safe method of exfoliating dead epidermis, our objective was to investigate its effectiveness in young women with acne vulgaris. The Global Acne Grading System (GAGS) and Derma Unit SSC 3 device (Sebumeter SM 815, Corneometer CM 825) were used to assess acne vulgaris and skin properties. Twenty-four women aged 19–21 years ($M = 19.50$, $SD = 0.66$) with diagnosed mild acne vulgaris and a high level of sebum (more than 100 $\mu g/cm^2$) participated in the study. Women on any dermatological treatment within the last 12 months and/or hormonal contraception were excluded. Probands were randomly assigned to two equal groups. Group A (experimental) was oxybrased with 0.9% sodium chloride solution simultaneously with compressed oxygen. Group B (placebo) was the group treated with non-carbonated mineral water and oxygen from the device (not pure). A series of five treatments was performed at 10-day intervals. Skin parameters were measured before and 30 days after the end of treatment. As a result, in group A (experimental), skin hydration and GAGS improved, while sebum on the epidermis was reduced. No side effects were noted. We concluded that oxybrasion is effective in women with acne and safe, as it improved skin parameters; however, further research is needed.

Keywords: acne vulgaris; oxybrasion; sebumeter; corneometer

1. Introduction

Microdermabrasion is one of the methods of superficial controlled exfoliation of the stratum corneum. This treatment is safe and noninvasive, and as a result, patients can return to their daily activities without any recovery period [1–3]. Three types of microdermabrasion can be distinguished: diamond microdermabrasion, corundum microdermabrasion, and oxygen microdermabrasion oxybrasion. Diamond microdermabrasion uses the vacuum generated by a device and a tip covered with diamond crystals to exfoliate the surface of the epidermis. Corundum microdermabrasion uses corundum as an abrasive medium, while oxybrasion uses a stream of 0.9% sodium chloride solution ejected from an injector under pressure. In the case of corundum or diamond microdermabrasion, the friction causes skin redness and a feeling of warmth on the client's skin. During oxybrasion, the treatment area is cooled with the cold stream of saline, which reduces discomfort during exfoliation [4,5].

Oxybrasion is an exfoliating and cleansing treatment that stimulates and increases blood circulation. It stabilizes the functioning of the sebaceous glands, and also oxygenates and moisturizes the skin. This method can be combined with chemical exfoliation or intense pulsed light therapy. Oxybrasion exfoliates the stratum corneum and reduces seborrhea. The treatment is based on the use of a 0.9% sodium chloride solution and pure oxygen from a cylinder, which eliminates the environment of anaerobic bacteria, in turn contributing to better treatment effects and the reduction of skin inflammation.

Microdermabrasion treatments are recommended for people with acne scars, stretch marks, keratoconus, and excessive sebum secretion, as well as for those with mature skin and people suffering from acne [6–8].

Acne vulgaris is a chronic inflammatory skin disease, which is characterized by the appearance of skin eruptions such as comedones, papules, nodules, pustules, and seborrhea. In the course of this disease, there is also an excess of *Cutibacterium acnes* bacteria, which leads to inflammation. *C. acnes* is a gram-positive, polymorphic bacterium, which is mainly in a cylindrical form, and which does not produce spore forms. Additionally, it is devoid of motor organelles. *C. acnes* prefers anaerobic conditions, although it is partially oxygen tolerant. It produces large amounts of porphyrins, which may contribute to the destruction of keratinocytes [9].

Among the factors that make people predisposed to acne, apart from the presence of certain bacteria (*C. acnes*, *Staphylococcus aureus*, and *Staphylococcus epidermidis*), the following can be distinguished: increased sebum production, abnormal keratinization of the sebaceous canal, hormonal disorders, and genetic factors [10–12]. In people with severe acne, the first step is dermatological treatment, which is designed to reduce the number of nodules and cysts. If the acne is mild or moderate and the physician agrees to use cosmetology treatments, many different methods can be proposed to improve the quality of the patient's skin. The aim of the study was to check whether the oxybrasion treatment will have a positive effect on the reduction in skin eruptions.

2. Materials and Methods

2.1. Study Design

A single-blind placebo study with follow-up analysis was conducted at the Institute of Health Sciences of the University of Opole, Poland from February to April 2021. The research was approved by the Human Research Ethics Committee of the Opole Medical School (No. KB/57/NOZ/2019) and conducted according to the principles of the Declaration of Helsinki. The study was registered at https://www.isrctn.com (No. ISRCTN 28257448) and accessed on 7 May 2020. All patients signed a written informed consent prior to the research, and agreed to make photographic documentation. The photos were taken before the first treatment and 30 days after the end of the treatment series. The participants were informed that they may withdraw from the examination at any time and without giving any reason.

Initially, 40 people participated in the study, but only 16 met the exclusion criteria [oral supplementation with preparations that could reduce the amount of sebum produced was also forbidden (yeast tablets, sulfur tablets, herbal teas)—9 probants; claustrophobia—3 probants; skin irritation—4 probants]. The final study sample consisted of 24 women. The group was homogeneous due to the fact that no men entered the study. Twenty-four women, suffering from acne vulgaris, were divided into two groups. They were assigned to the groups on the basis of a random selection of envelopes containing a certain group designation (A or B). Group A (experimental) received the appropriate oxybrasion treatment using 0.9% sodium chloride solution and pure oxygen from a cylinder. Group B (placebo) had a "mock oxybrasion" procedure using still mineral water and oxygen from the compressor from the device (oxygen from the air). Patients from group B were not aware that they were a placebo group, and they were convinced that they were undergoing the procedure of oxybrasion. The process of inclusion of the patients is shown in Figure 1. All patients underwent a series of five treatments applied every 10 days. Any other cosmetic procedures, as well as the use of new cosmetics or sebum-regulating cosmetics, were forbidden during the study period. Only cosmetics such as micellar water and moisturizing creams were allowed.

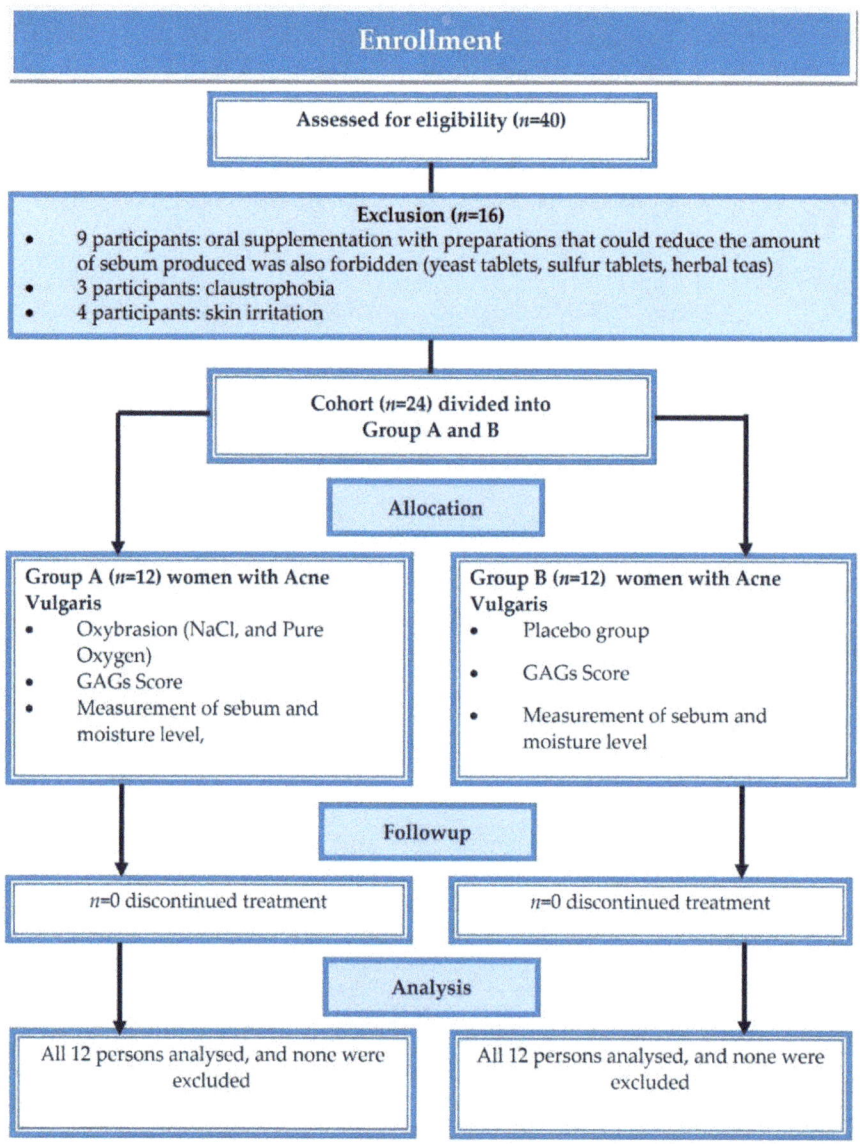

Figure 1. Patient follow in the study.

2.2. Participants

A group of 24 women aged 19–21 ($M = 19.50$, $SD = 0.66$) who suffered from acne vulgaris participated in the study. All the tested participants were diagnosed with mild acne (100%) by the same rater dermatologist using the GAGS before and after a series of treatments in group A (experimental) and group B (placebo).

The mean duration of acne was 6 years ($M = 5.79$, $SD = 0.83$), with a range between 5 and 7 years. Inclusion criteria for this study were no dermatological treatment within 12 months, no current hormonal contraception, age 19–23 years, and having mild acne which was measured by the Global Acne Grading System (GAGS). The study had contraindications that made it impossible for some people to participate. These included: pregnancy, breastfeeding, epilepsy, claustrophobia, skin damage, taking oral medications within the last 3 months, taking isotretinoin within the last year, taking contraceptives, sun exposure after the procedure, tanned skin, skin cancers, psoriasis, eczema, viral infections (including herpes), bacterial and fungal skin diseases, skin irritation, active inflammation, active rosacea, psoriasis, atopic dermatitis, general illness, and a tendency to having sinusitis. Oral supplementation with preparations that could reduce the amount of sebum produced was also forbidden (e.g., yeast tablets, sulfur tablets, and herbal teas).

Group A (n = 12) and B (n = 12) included young adult women with a higher sebum level (more than 100 µg/cm^2) and acne vulgaris. Acne, excessive seborrhea, blackheads, whiteheads, and papules were observed in the volunteers. Before and after the treatment series, the GAGS was used to determine the severity of acne and to check whether the treatments had a positive effect on the improvement of the skin condition of the patients.

2.3. Measures

2.3.1. Acne Vulgaris

The severity of acne vulgaris was assessed using the GAGS, which was developed in 1997 by Doshi, Zaheer, and Stiller [13]. Acne, excessive seborrhea, blackheads, whiteheads, and papules were observed in the volunteers. The GAGS scale, which is used to determine the degree of advancement of acne and also to check whether the treatments had a positive effect on the improvement of the skin of the patients, was used before and after the treatment series. The scale includes the following areas: nose, cheeks, forehead, chin, as well as the back and chest. Each of them is assigned a number based on size: nose = 1; left cheek = 2; right cheek = 2; forehead = 2; chin = 1; and back and chest = 3. Depending on the degree of severity, each lesion is given a grade: no cutaneous conditions—0, comedones—1, papules—2, pustules—3, and nodules—4. The local score calculated for each area has the following formula: Local score = factor × Grade (0–4). The global score is composed of the sum of the local results: 1–18—mild acne, 19–30—moderate acne, 31–38—severe acne, and above 39—acne with a very severe course [14].

2.3.2. Skin Parameters

Skin parameters were measured twice: before starting the tests (m0) and one month after the end of the last treatment (m1). The test subjects were asked to remove their face makeup the day before the measurements in the evening and not to apply any preparations to the face skin. The same applied to the morning care, with the difference that the patients could not remove make-up due to the fact that the parameters would be unreliable. Measurements were taken in the morning, with the test participants, after arriving in the room, acclimatizing for about 30 min. Room humidity was 40–50% and the temperature was 20–21 degrees C. The Derma Unit SCC 3 apparatus (Courge & Khazaka, Cologne, Germany) was used for the test. Skin hydration was tested with the Corneometer CM 825, while sebum was measured using the Sebumeter SM 815. The measurement points were as follows: forehead, nose, right and left cheeks, and chin.

2.4. Treatment Procedure (Intervention)

Before starting the treatment, in both groups A (experimental) and B (placebo), face makeup was removed using micellar fluid, and the skin was toned. The procedure was performed using a HEBE device. The patients' ears were covered with cotton wool, their eyes were protected with cotton pads and rubber glasses, and a cosmetic cap was put on their hair. The treatment in group A (experimental) was the actual treatment of oxybrasion. Saline was used for the treatment, and it was administered with a manipulator at the parameters of 5–5.5 bar. The treatment started from the forehead, and then progressed to the area between the eyebrows, cheeks, nose, and chin. The manipulator was located approximately 0.5–1 cm from the face. The exfoliation procedure was performed for a total of 5 min. Then, after this time, the face was toned, dried with wipes, and blown with pure oxygen from the cylinder for 5 min using a manipulator. The treatment in group B (placebo) was performed with the aid of an applicator with still mineral water at the pressure of 5–5.5 bar. The scheme was the same as in the case of group A, but at the same time, oxygen was supplied from the manipulator with the mineral water, which was taken from the air using a compressor. The mineral water contained 213.40 mg/L of minerals in total: bicarbonate 121.06 mg/L; fluorides 0.07 mg/L; magnesium 5.37 mg/L; calcium 36.39 mg/L; and sodium 7.79 mg/L. After the treatment, groups A and B had a tonic and moisturizing cream applied to their faces. Each group had a series of 5 treatments 10 days apart.

For home care, it was recommended to wash the face twice a day using Cetaphil MD Dermoprotector (aqua, glycerin, hydrogenated polyisobutene, cetearyl alcohol, macadamia ternifolia seed oil/macadamia ternifolia nut oil, ceteareth-20, tocopheryl acetate, dimethicone, acrylates/C10-30 alkyl acrylate crosspolymer, benzyl alcohol, citric acid, farnesol, panthenol, phenoxyethanol, sodium hydroxide, stearoxytrimethylsilane, stearyl alcohol, FIL 0133.V02). After using the above-mentioned preparation, the patients were meant to apply Alantan Plus cream (20 mg allantoin and 50 mg dexpanthenol) as a 50% solution of panthenol in propylene glycol, lanolin, liquid paraffin, cetostearyl alcohol, ethyl parahydroxybenzoate, methyl parahydroxybenzoate, propyl parahydroxybenzoate, propyl parahydroxybenzoate, purified water, and polawax.

The patients were instructed not to use the swimming pool, or sauna, and to avoid exposure to natural and artificial radiation. They were meant to use photoprotection every day and not use any preparations other than Cetaphil MD Dermoprotector and Alantan Plus cream. During the entire series of treatments, and a month after its completion, it was forbidden to use any other cosmetic and aesthetic medicine treatments. Dermatological procedures for the duration of the study were also prohibited.

2.5. Statistical Analysis

Several statistics were checked to examine the effect of oxybrasion treatment on the faces of young adult women with acne. Firstly, descriptive statistics were performed to check the normality assumptions for all variables in the study, including age, years of acne disease, the severity of acne before and after treatment, moisturizing, and lubrication after treatment. Next, a Student's *t*-test was conducted to examine differences between group A (experimental) and group B (placebo), for age, years of acne suffering, and severity of acne before and after the treatment with oxybrasion. Finally, the effect of oxybrasion on women's faces was tested using a repeated measure two-way ANOVA. A post hoc test with Bonferroni correction was used to check significant differences. All statistics were conducted using JASP software for Windows: JASP Team, Version 0.14.1 (Computer software; Amsterdam, The Netherlands: Department of Psychological Methods, University of Amsterdam; 2020).

3. Results

3.1. Changes in Acne Severity after Oxybrasion Treatment

The preliminary analysis regards the parametric properties of the variables, using median, mean (*M*), standard deviation (*SD*), skewness, and kurtosis. Skewness and kurtosis ranged between −1.5 and +1.5, therefore parametric statistics were performed in the next steps of statistical analysis. The Student's *t*-test was performed to examine differences between group A (experimental) and group B (placebo) in age, years of acne suffering, and acne severity diagnosis (Table 1). There were no group differences in age and diagnosis of acne before treatment. However, the groups differed slightly in years of acne suffering ($p < 0.05$), with a small effect size (Cohen's $d = -0.99$). In addition, group A demonstrated significantly lower scores in acne severity than group B after treatment of oxybrasion ($p < 0.001$), with a large effect size (Cohen's $d = -7.04$).

Table 1. Descriptive statistics.

Variable	Total Sample		Group A		Group B		$t(22)$	p	d
	M	SD	M	SD	M	SD			
Age	19.50	0.66	19.25	0.45	19.75	0.75	−1.97	0.062	−0.80
Years of acne	5.79	0.83	5.42	0.67	6.17	0.84	−2.43	0.024	−0.99
GAGS before	17.08	0.88	17.17	1.03	17.00	0.74	0.46	0.653	0.19
GAGS after	12.75	3.97	9.00	1.13	16.50	1.00	−17.23	<0.001	−7.04

Note. Group A = experimental, Group B = placebo, GAGS = Global Acne Grading System, M = mean, SD = standard deviation, t = Student's t-test, p = significance level, d = Cohen's d effect size.

A repeated measure two-way ANOVA was performed to examine the complex effect of oxybrasion on acne severity among women. The results indicated significant differences in acne severity (GAGS scores) before and after oxybrasion treatment, $F(1, 22) = 531.14$, $p < 0.001$, $\eta^2_p = 0.96$. The effect of group was also significant, $F(1, 22) = 106.48$, $p < 0.001$, $\eta^2_p = 0.83$, as well as the interaction effect between group and treatment, $F(1, 22) = 176.33$, $p < 0.001$, $\eta^2_p = 0.95$. The post hoc test with Bonferroni correction showed that groups A (experimental) and group B (placebo) did not differ significantly before treatment. Additionally, no differences were found between group A before treatment and group B after treatment. Acne severity was not changed significantly in group B before and after placebo treatment. However, a significant improvement was observed in group A regardless of acne severity before and after oxybrasion treatment. Figure 2 shows patients representing group A (experimental) while Figure 3 demonstrates participants from group B (placebo), both before and after treatment.

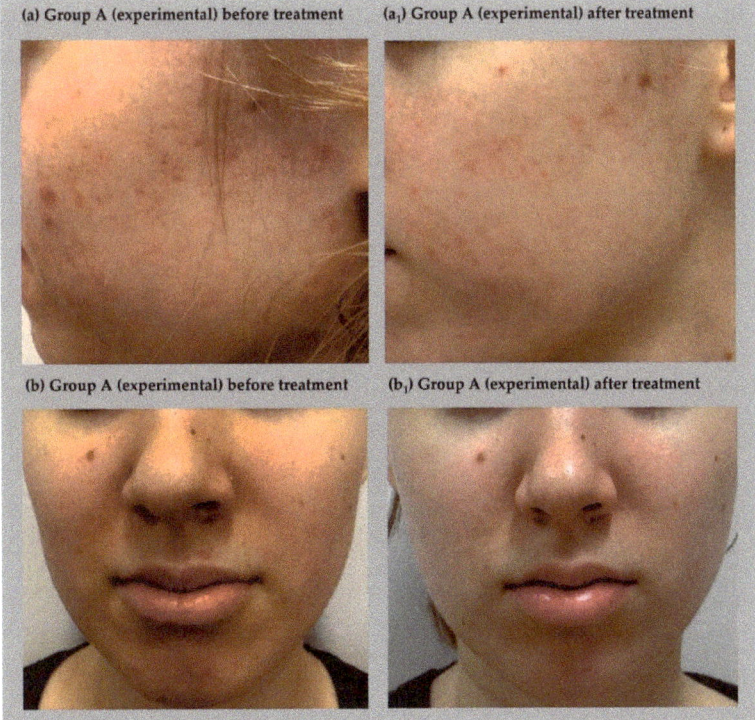

Figure 2. Effect of treatment on acne severity in two patients from group A (experimental) before (**a**,**b**) and after treatment (**a$_1$**,**b$_1$**).

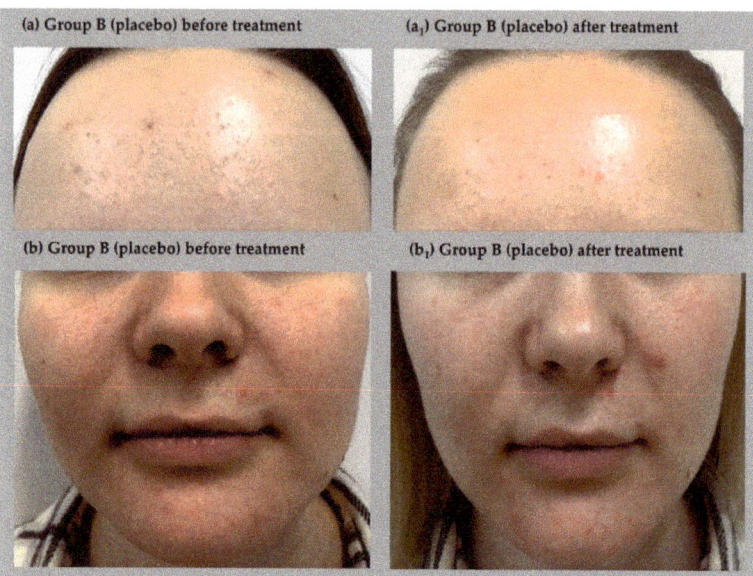

Figure 3. Effect of treatment on acne severity in two patients from group B (placebo) before (**a**,**b**) and after treatment (**a$_1$**,**b$_1$**).

3.2. Changes in Facial Skin Moisture after Oxybrasion Treatment

A series of repeated measures two-way ANOVAs were performed for the forehead, nose, right cheek, left cheek, and chin to examine the effect of oxybrasion on moisturizing faces of acne patients (Table 2). The group effect was not significant for moisturizing each part of the face. In contrast, a significant effect (with a medium effect size) of oxybrasion treatment and interaction between group and treatment was found for the forehead, nose, right cheek, and left cheek. In contrast, oxybrasion treatment did not have any significant effect on the chin. Furthermore, a very small interaction effect was presented for the chins of women with acne.

Table 2. The repeated measures one-way ANOVA for moisturizing using Corneometer CM825 (g/m^2).

Moisturizing	Group A		Group B		Effect	$F(1, 22)$	p	η^2_p
	M	SD	M	SD				
Forehead					G	2.61	0.120	0.11
Before	41.69	5.63	41.87	6.30	T	44.26	<0.001	0.67
After	49.81	5.44	42.18	6.01	T × G	37.86	<0.001	0.63
Nose					G	1.27	0.272	0.06
Before	41.93	6.92	43.58	6.45	T	30.87	<0.001	0.58
After	51.54	5.15	44.50	6.54	T × G	21.05	<0.001	0.49
Right Cheek					G	0.69	0.416	0.03
Before	41.61	8.54	41.97	8.07	T	43.92	<0.001	0.67
After	49.03	7.41	43.34	8.09	T × G	20.74	<0.001	0.49
Left Cheek					G	1.23	0.279	0.05
Before	43.72	8.03	43.63	7.89	T	20.57	<0.001	0.48
After	50.77	7.97	44.23	6.33	T × G	14.62	<0.001	0.40

Table 2. Cont.

Moisturizing	Group A		Group B		Effect	F(1, 22)	p	η^2_p
	M	SD	M	SD				
Chin					G	0.09	0.766	0.00
Before	38.98	4.62	40.84	5.58	T	3.61	0.071	0.14
After	41.30	4.57	40.71	6.34	T × G	4.54	0.045	0.17

Note. Group A = experimental, Group B = placebo, G = group, T = treatment. M = mean, SD = standard deviation, F = Fisher's F-test, p = significance level, η^2_p = partial eta-square effect size.

3.3. Changes in Facial Skin Greasing after Oxybrasion Treatment

Repeated measures of two-way ANOVAs were conducted to examine oxybrasion effect on greasing of various parts of women's faces (Table 3). The group effect was significant for the forehead, nose, right cheek, and left cheek, but insignificant for the chin. However, the effects of oxybrasion and interaction between treatment and group were significant for all parts of participants' faces, with a medium or strong effect size.

Table 3. The repeated measures one-way ANOVA for greasing using Sebumeter SM815 ($\mu g/cm^2$).

Greasing	Group A		Group B		Effect	F(1, 22)	p	η^2_p
	M	SD	M	SD				
Forehead					G	12.8	0.002	0.37
Before	187.08	30.73	191.08	28.86	T	146.8	<0.001	0.87
After	115.08	24.92	185.75	21.47	T × G	109.1	<0.001	0.83
Nose					G	9.1	0.006	0.29
Before	180.08	23.17	180.42	22.70	T	87.4	<0.001	0.80
After	124.42	16.42	174.67	24.93	T × G	57.7	<0.001	0.72
Right Cheek					G	7.4	0.013	0.25
Before	182.75	27.74	178.33	26.05	T	130.2	<0.001	0.86
After	112.83	18.91	170.83	28.27	T × G	84.6	<0.001	0.79
Left Cheek					G	9.1	0.006	0.29
Before	180.92	24.35	181.25	23.03	T	58.3	<0.001	0.73
After	125.00	13.12	171.42	24.37	T × G	28.6	<0.001	0.57
Chin					G	1.0	0.334	0.04
Before	180.17	19.63	165.92	25.34	T	78.0	<0.001	0.78
After	129.75	12.62	160.00	25.15	T × G	48.7	<0.001	0.69

Note. Group A = experimental, Group B = placebo, G = group, T = treatment. M = mean, SD = standard deviation, F = Fisher's F-test, p = significance level, η^2_p = partial eta-square effect size.

4. Discussion

Our study showed that the procedure performed in group A (experimental) contributed to a significant reduction in the number of skin eruptions (GAGS scale) and improved skin appearance in patients in this group. In addition, group A demonstrated significantly lower scores in acne severity than group B after treatment of oxybrasion ($p < 0.001$), with a large effect size (Cohen's $d = -7.04$) (Table 1). Table 3 shows how the oxybrasion affects greasing of various parts of women's faces. The group effect was significant for the forehead, nose, right cheek, and left cheek, but insignificant for the chin. However, the effects of oxybrasion and interaction between treatment and group were significant for all parts of participants' faces, with a medium or strong effect size. The study showed that a 0.9% sodium chloride solution exfoliated dead epidermis, and pure oxygen reduced skin eruptions in group A (experimental). C. acnes prefers anaerobic conditions, although it partially tolerates oxygen in temperatures of 36–37 °C.

Jarząbek et al. used oxybrasion on 27 healthy women; they examined sebum, skin hydration, pH, and transepidermal water loss (TEWL). Five treatments were performed every two weeks. The authors showed that the treatment had a positive effect on the reduction of the amount of sebum on the surface of the epidermis, in particular on the cheeks and nose. Oxybrasion increased skin hydration and decreased skin pH [4].

The most common method of microdermabrasion among researchers is diamond and corundum microdermabrasion. Chilicka et al. showed that treatments such as microdermabrasion and cavitation peeling had a positive effect on the condition of the skin in people with acne. There was a reduction in the number of skin eruptions, where as selected skin parameters, including sebum measurement, improved [15]. Fąk et al. performed the procedure for 16 women using aluminium oxide crystal microdermabrasion. The study examined whether the treatment would affect the level of hydration and lubrication of the epidermis. Statistically significant changes were observed on the cheeks and in the T-zone 30 min after the end of the procedure. There was a strong reduction of sebum all over the face; however, about an hour after the end of the treatment, this measurement began to return to the baseline. One hour after treatment, hydration started to gradually fall [16].

Kim et al. reported that diamond microdermabrasion was associated with an increase in TEWL immediately after the treatment, but after one day, it returned to the baseline value [17]. Abdel-Motaleb et al. showed morphological changes between the control group and the group treated using chemical peels and microdermabrasion. Salicylic acids and microdermabrasion significantly increased epidermal thickness, collagen fibres, and elastin thickness [18]. A study by El-Domyati et al. was conducted on 38 patients (four groups: acne scars, melasma, photoageing, and striae distensae). Eight microdermabrasion treatments were performed with a one-week interval. Punch biopsies were taken. Histometric analysis of epidermal thickness showed nonsignificant changes in all the groups. Collagen fibres with a more regular arrangement were detected in acne scars, and decreased melanization was also noted [19].

Kołodziejczak et al. used a combination of microdermabrasion and cavitation peeling in patients with seborrheic skin with acne punctata. Nine women had a series of six treatments with an interval of 10–14 days. Measurements such as skin hydration levels and sebumetric values were taken. In all patients, an improvement in skin sebum was observed. A significant improvement in skin hydration was seen in the chin area [19]. Scientists investigated 10 patients with a series of six microdermabrasion treatments with an interval of 14 days. One side of the face had two passes of microdermabrasion and the other side of the face had three passes. After the series of treatments, the sebum level was lower than baseline values. An increase in pH values was observed after finishing the series of microdermabrasion [20].

In the case of data concerning the effects of oxybrasion on acne-prone skin, there are no studies regarding this topic in the databases.

5. Study Limitations

This was a preliminary study, and therefore the research sample can be seen to be limited. In the future, we would like to increase the number of patients, as well as expand the group to include men, not only women.

6. Conclusions

Oxybrasion treatment using saline and pure oxygen from a cylinder significantly reduced the skin sebum level and increased the skin hydration level on the right part of the face. This method also reduced the number of skin eruptions in the study participants (group A). This was visible on the photographic documentation, and also due to the use of a dermatological scale for the determination of the degree of acne (GAGS). The oxybrasion treatment using 0.9% sodium chloride solutions and pure oxygen is a safe procedure with no side effects such as redness or skin irritation. It is a procedure that does not require the person undergoing it to be excluded from everyday functioning. However, it should be remembered that dermatological treatment cannot be replaced by cosmetological treatment.

Author Contributions: Conceptualization, K.C.; methodology, K.C.; software, K.C.; validation, K.C. and A.M.R.; formal analysis, A.M.R.; investigation, K.C.; resources, K.C. and R.S.; data curation, K.C. and A.M.R.; writing—original draft preparation, K.C., A.M.R., R.S., M.R. and D.N.; writing—review and editing, K.C. and A.M.R.; visualization, A.M.R.; supervision, R.S.; project administration, K.C. funding acquisition, R.S. All authors have read and agreed to the published version of the manuscript.

Funding: This research received no external funding.

Institutional Review Board Statement: The study was conducted according to the guidelines of the Declaration of Helsinki and approved by the Human Research Ethics Committee of the Opole Medical School No. KB/57/NOZ/2019.

Informed Consent Statement: Informed consent was obtained from all subjects involved in the study.

Data Availability Statement: Not applicable.

Conflicts of Interest: The authors declare no conflict of interest.

References

1. Kang, B.; Choi, J.H.; Jeong, K.H. A study of the effects of physical dermabrasion combined with chemical peeling in porcine skin. *J. Cosmet. Laser Ther.* **2015**, *17*, 24–30. [CrossRef] [PubMed]
2. Zapletalova, A.; Pata, V.; Stoklasek, P.; Janis, R.; Kejlova, K. Objective measurements of skin surface roughness after microdermabrasion treatment. *Skin Res. Technol.* **2017**, *23*, 346–353. [CrossRef] [PubMed]
3. El-Domyati, M.; Hosam, W.; Abdel-Azim, E.; Abdel-Wahab, H.; Mohamed, E. Microdermabrasion: A clinical, histometric, and histopathologic study. *J. Cosmet. Dermatol.* **2016**, *15*, 503–513. [CrossRef] [PubMed]
4. Jarząbek, S.; Rotsztejn, H. Effect of oxybrasion on selected skin parameters. *J. Cosmet. Dermatol.* **2021**, *20*, 657–663. [CrossRef] [PubMed]
5. Kordus, K.; Potempa, B.; Śpiewak, R. A survey of the motives for selecting the types of microdermabrasion and the opinion on their effectiveness in cosmetology practice. *Estetologia Med. Kosmetol.* **2011**, *1*, 21–26. [CrossRef]
6. Niewójt, K.E. Oxygen and salt in the main role- oxybrasion or oxydermabrasion. *Kosm. Estet.* **2016**, *2*, 136–139.
7. Nassar, A.; Ghomey, S.; Gohary, Y.; El-Desoky, F. Treatment of striae distensae with needling therapy versus microdermabrasion with sonophoresis. *J. Cosmet. Laser Ther.* **2016**, *18*, 330–334. [CrossRef] [PubMed]
8. Pallavi, R.V.; Seethalakshmi, G.V.; Kannan, G.; Nanjappachetty, G. A comparative study of the resurfacing effect of microdermabrasion versus glycolic acid peel in the management of acne scars. *J. Pak. Assoc. Dermatol.* **2018**, *28*, 224–232.
9. Perry, A.L.; Lambert, P.A. Propionibacterium acnes. *Lett. Appl. Microbiol.* **2006**, *42*, 185–188. [CrossRef] [PubMed]
10. Chilicka, K.; Rogowska, A.M.; Szyguła, R. Effects of Topical Hydrogen Purification on Skin Parameters and Acne Vulgaris in Adult Women. *Healthcare* **2021**, *9*, 144. [CrossRef] [PubMed]
11. Chilicka, K.; Rogowska, A.M.; Szyguła, R.; Dzieńdziora-Urbińska, I.; Taradaj, J. A comparison of the effectiveness of azelaic and pyruvic acid peels in the treatment of female adult acne: A randomized controlled trial. *Sci. Rep.* **2020**, *28*, 12612. [CrossRef] [PubMed]
12. Chilicka, K.; Rogowska, A.M.; Szyguła, R.; Taradaj, J. Examining Quality of Life after Treatment with Azelaic and Pyruvic Acid Peels in Women with Acne Vulgaris. *Clin. Cosmet. Investig. Dermatol.* **2020**, *27*, 469–477. [CrossRef] [PubMed]
13. Doshi, A.; Zaheer, A.; Stiller, M.J. A comparison of current acne trading systems and propos al of a novel system. *Int. J. Dermatol.* **1997**, *36*, 416–418. [CrossRef] [PubMed]
14. Adityan, B.; Kumari, R.; Thappa, D.M. Scoring systems in acne vulgaris. *Indian J. Dermatol. Venereol Leprol.* **2009**, *75*, 324–326.
15. Chilicka, K.; Maj, J.; Panaszek, B. General quality of life of patients with acne vulgaris before and after performing selected cosmetological treatments. *Patient Prefer. Adher.* **2017**, *4*, 1357–1361. [CrossRef] [PubMed]
16. Fąk, M.; Rotsztejn, H.; Erkiert-Polguj, A. The early effect of microdermabrasion on hydration and sebum level. *Skin Res. Technol.* **2018**, *24*, 650–655. [CrossRef] [PubMed]
17. Kim, H.S.; Lim, S.H.; Song, J.Y.; Kim, M.; Lee, J.H.; Park, J.G.; Kim, H.O.; Park, Y.M. Skin barrier function recovery after diamond microdermabrasion. *J. Dermatol.* **2009**, *36*, 529–533. [CrossRef] [PubMed]
18. Abdel-Motaleb, A.A.; Abu-Dief, E.E.; Hussein, M.R. Dermal morphological changes following salicylic acid peeling and microdermabrasion. *J. Cosmet. Dermatol.* **2017**, *16*, e9–e14. [CrossRef] [PubMed]
19. Kołodziejczak, A.; Wieczorek, A.; Rotsztejn, H. The assessment of the effects of the combination of microdermabrasion and cavitation peeling in the therapy of seborrhoeic skin with visible symptoms of acne punctata. *J. Cosmet. Laser Ther.* **2019**, *21*, 286–290. [CrossRef] [PubMed]
20. Davari, P.; Gorouhi, F.; Jafarian, S.; Dowlati, Y.; Firooz, A. A randomized investigator-blind trial of different passes of microdermabrasion therapy and their effects on skin biophysical characteristics. *Int. J. Dermatol.* **2008**, *47*, 508–513. [CrossRef] [PubMed]

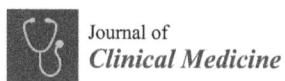

Article

A Split Face Comparative Study to Evaluate the Efficacy of 40% Pyruvic Acid vs. Microdermabrasion with 40% Pyruvic Acid on Biomechanical Skin Parameters in the Treatment of Acne Vulgaris

Monika Rusztowicz [1], Karolina Chilicka [1], Renata Szyguła [1], Wiktoria Odrzywołek [2], Antoniya Yanakieva [3], Binnaz Asanova [4] and Sławomir Wilczyński [2,*]

[1] Department of Health Sciences, Institute of Health Sciences, University of Opole, 45-040 Opole, Poland
[2] Department of Basic Biomedical Science, Faculty of Pharmaceutical Sciences in Sosnowiec, Medical University of Silesia in Katowice, 41-200 Sosnowiec, Poland
[3] Department of HTA, Faculty of Public Health, Medical University of Sofia, 1427 Sofia, Bulgaria
[4] Medical College Yordanka Filaretova, Medical University of Sofia, 1606 Sofia, Bulgaria
* Correspondence: swilczynski@sum.edu.pl; Tel.: +48-507-169-625

Abstract: The synergy of cosmetic acids, with their keratolytic and antibacterial properties, with the mechanical exfoliation of the epidermis brings faster and better treatment results. The aim of the study was to compare the effects of using only pyruvic acid and the synergy of microdermabrasion and chemical exfoliation. In total, 14 women diagnosed with acne took part in the study. Two areas were marked on the participants' faces: the right side (microdermabrasion treatment and a preparation containing pyruvic acid 40%) and the left side (preparation containing pyruvic acid 40%) without mechanical exfoliation. A series of four treatments was performed at 2-week intervals. Skin parameters such as stratum corneum hydration and sebum secretion were measured. Before the treatments, all patients had moderate acne according to GAGS (Min: 19, Max: 22, Md: 20), and after the treatments, it decreased to mild acne according to GAGS (Min: 13, Max: 17, Md: 140). On the right side of the face, there was a statistically significant reduction in sebum secretion in all the examined areas of the face and increase in the hydration of the stratum corneum. On the left side of the face, the differences were also observed in the decrease of sebum value and increase of hydration level; however, they were smaller than on the right side. The use of microdermabrasion in combination with pyruvic acid led to better results in the case of increased hydration and reduction of sebum secretion than using only pyruvic acid treatment.

Keywords: acne vulgaris; microdermabrasion; pyruvic acid; moisturizing; sebum

1. Introduction

Acne vulgaris is a dermatological disease that is characterized by whiteheads, blackheads, pustules, nodules, cysts or inflammatory papules [1]. The most common factors that can cause disease include: abnormal keratinization of the pilosebaceous canal, bacterial colonization (*Cutibacterium acnes*), hormonal disorders and excessive sebum production [2–4]. As a result of neglect or the acute course of the disease, scarring and discoloration of the skin may occur, which may be associated with a significantly reduced quality of life. Patients struggling with acne vulgaris often feel isolated, excluded from society and the disease limits their social life. An increased course of acne increases the risk of anxiety and depression [5–8].

Cosmetology offers many treatments, both with the use of chemicals and modern equipment that are able to alleviate the symptoms of acne. These include, among others, cosmetic acids, which cause coherence between keratinocytes and exfoliation of corneocytes. The advantages are also the reconstruction of the epidermis structure, as well as the reduction of sebum secretion onto the epidermis surface. The acids that are most often used in anti-acne treatments are: alpha hydroxy, beta hydroxy and alpha-keto acids [9–11].

Pyruvic acid is an alpha-keto acid that is found in apples, vinegar and fermented fruits, among others. It has good antibacterial and exfoliating properties, and also has a sebo-regulating effect. When it comes to acne scars, it also works well on this level, because it has the ability to stimulate the formation of new collagen and elastic fibers. Physiologically, PA converts to lactic acid, and it has a low risk of scarring. PA differs from lactic acid due to the presence of a ketone group in the alpha position instead of the hydroxyl group. PA is classified as a medium peeling agent that has a positive effect on acne vulgaris and greasy skin. It is also useful in photodamage of pigmentation in patients with light skin (tyrosinase inhibition properties) [12].

Microdermabrasion is classified as an apparatus treatment, which is a form of mechanical superficial exfoliation of the epidermis. It is a safe, non-invasive and effective method. This treatment is used for the reduction of acne, acne scars, photoaging, stretch marks and for superficial hyperpigmentation. Superficial exfoliation of the epidermis allows for better penetration of other substances that will be applied after the mechanical exfoliation treatment. As of today, there are three types of microdermabrasion: diamond microdermabrasion using diamond-coated heads, corundum microdermabrasion using corundum and oxybrasion using a stream of saline solution (0.9% NaCl). Thanks to special tips, diamond microdermabrasion can exfoliate the upper layers of the epidermis in a controlled way. The depth of exfoliation depends on the diamond-coated head used, the suction power set by the cosmetologist and the pressure of his hands on the skin of the person undergoing the procedure [13–15].

The aim of the study was to check whether the synergy of treatments would have a positive effect on the improvement of skin quality in people with acne vulgaris.

2. Materials and Methods

2.1. Patients

In total, 14 women with acne vulgaris were classified in this study. Full characteristics of the patients are summarized in Table 1. The Bioethicas Committee of the Opole Medical School agreed (KB/54/NOZ/2019) to conduct the project entitled: "Assessment of selected skin parameters and quality of life after cosmetics procedures in people with acne vulgaris and oily skin".

Table 1. Patient characteristics.

	N	Mean	SD	Min	Max
age (years)	14	19.6	0.7	19.0	21.0
duration of the disease (years)	14	5.4	1.7	2.0	8.0

2.1.1. Inclusion Criteria

Inclusion criteria for this study were no dermatological treatment within 12 months, no current hormonal contraception, age 19–22 and mild-to-moderate acne which was measured by the global acne severity scale (GAGS). GAGS is clinical tool for assessing the severity of acne vulgaris that was first proposed by Doshi et al., in 1997.

2.1.2. Exclusion Criteria

The study had contraindications that made it impossible for some people to participate. These included: taking oral medications within the last 3 months, taking isotretinoin within the last year, taking contraceptives, tendency to keloids, sun exposure weeks before and after procedure, telangiectasias, skin cancers, pregnancy and breastfeeding, viral, bacterial and fungal skin diseases, hypersensitivity to acids, skin irritation, active inflammation, active rosacea, psoriasis and atopic dermatitis.

Acne, excessive seborrhea, blackheads, whiteheads and papules were observed in the volunteers. Before and after the treatment series, the GAGS scale was used to determine the severity of acne and to check the effect of the treatments on the improvement of the skin condition of the patients. The scale includes the following areas: nose, cheeks, forehead, chin, as well as the back and chest. Each of them is assigned a number based on size: nose = 1; left cheek = 2; right cheek = 2; forehead = 2; chin = 1. Depending on the degree of severity, each lesion is given a grade: no cutaneous conditions—0, comedones—1, papules—2, pustules—3 and nodules—4. The local score calculated for each area has the formula: Local score = factor × Grade (0–4). The global score is composed of the sum of the local results: 1–18 = mild acne, 19–30 = moderate acne, 31–38 = severe acne, above 39 = acne with very severe course [16]. All volunteers underwent a series of four treatments applied every 2 weeks.

2.2. Procedure

The skin parameters were measured before and one month after the end of the treatment. The participants removed their face makeup the day before the measurements in the evening and did not apply any preparations to the face skin. Measurements were taken in the morning, and the test participants, after arriving in the room, acclimatized for about 30 minutes. The humidity in the room was 40–50%, while the temperature was 20–21 degrees C.

Corneometer CM 825 was used to measure stratum corneum hydration, while a Sebumeter SM 815 (Courage + Khazaka Electronic GmbH, Köln, Germany) was used to measure sebum. The measurement points were as follows: 1 cm above the brow, 1 cm from the lobe of the nose, cheek (5 cm from the lobe of the nose), 1 cm from the corner of the mouth. The measurements were made symmetrically.

Thermal camera FLIR T420 (FLIR Systems Company, Sweden) was used for thermal measurements. The thermal resolution was <0.045 °C; the wavelength range was 7.5–13 µm; the resolution of the obtained image was 320 × 240 pixels. FLIR ResearchIR software version 3.5 (FLIR®® Systems, Inc., Wilsonville, OR, USA) was used for analysis of the data.

The study was conducted from March 2021 to April 2021.

Before starting the treatment procedure, the face was cleansed with micellar fluid. The treatment was divided into two parts: the right and the left side of the face. The entire face was first degreased with alcohol. On the right side of the patients' face, microdermabrasion was performed for a period of 5 minutes (tip gradation 200, negative pressure 15 mmHg). Then, after the end of the treatment, the face was washed with hydrogen peroxide solution and a preparation containing 40% pyruvic acid (Perfarma Pyruvic Peeling 40 strong) was applied. The preparation was applied to the right surface of the face with a brush for 2 minutes and then washed off with water. No microdermabrasion was performed on the left side of the patients' face. After degreasing the face, 40% pyruvic acid was applied with a brush to the left part of the face for 2 minutes and washed off with water. Then, a post-treatment cream with a 50+ filter (Dives Global Protection) was applied to the entire treatment area.

For home care, it was recommended to wash the face twice a day with the preparation Cetaphil MD Dermoprotector (Aqua, Glycerin, Hydrogenated Polyisobutene, Cetearyl Alcohol, Macadamia Ternifolia Seed Oil/Macadamia Ternifolia Nut Oil, Ceteareth-20, Tocopheryl Acetate, Dimethicone, Acrylates/C10-30 Alkyl Acrylate Crosspolymer, Benzyl Alcohol, Citric Acid, Farnesol, Panthenol, Phenoxyethanol, Sodium Hydroxide, Stearoxytrimethylsilane, Stearyl Alcohol, FIL 0133.V02.). After applying the above-mentioned preparation, the subjects were to apply Alantan Plus cream (20 mg allantoin and 50 mg dexpanthenol as a 50% solution of panthenol in propylene glycol, lanolin, liquid paraffin, cetostearyl alkohol, etyl parahydroxybenzoate, metyl parahydroxybenzoate, propyl parahydroxybenzoate, purified water, polawax).

The patients were instructed not to use a swimming pool or sauna, to avoid exposure to natural and artificial radiation, and to use photoprotection every day and not to use any preparations other than Cetaphil MD Dermoprotector and Alantan Plus cream.

During the entire series of treatments and a month after its treatment, it was forbidden to use any other cosmetic and aesthetic medicine treatments. Oral supplementation with preparations that could reduce the amount of sebum produced was also forbidden.

2.3. Statistical Analysis

Statistica 13.3 software was used for the statistical analysis of the results. Wilcoxon test was used to compare the effects before and after the treatments. The results at the level of $p < 0.05$ were considered statistically significant.

3. Results

The use of the treatments had a statistically significant effect on the severity of acne in each of the patients ($p < 0.001$) (Figure 1). Before the treatments, all patients had moderate acne according to GAGS (Min: 19, Max: 22, Md: 20), and after the treatments, it decreased to mild acne according to GAGS (Min: 13, Max: 17, Md: 14) (Table 2).

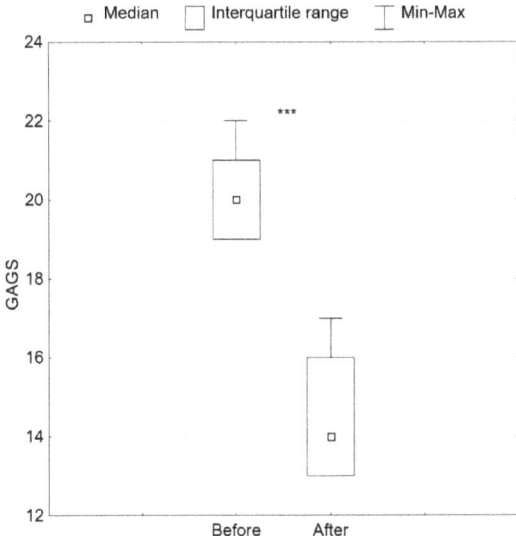

Figure 1. Advancement of acne according to GAGS before and after treatments, *** $p < 0.001$.

Table 2. Advancement of acne according to GAGS before and after treatments, *** $p < 0.001$, Md—Median, Q1—1st quartile, Q3—3rd quartile, Min—Minimum, Max—Maximum.

	GAGS ***	
	Before	After
Md	20	14
Q1	19	13
Q3	21	16
Min	19	13
Max	22	17

On the right side of the face, where treatments using both microdermabrasion and 40% pyruvic acid were applied, there was a statistically significant reduction in sebum secretion in all the examined areas of the face ($p < 0.001$) (Figure 2, Table 3). The reduction in sebum secretion on the right side of the face occurred in all patients, and the median sebum value decreased from 77.5 ug/cm^2 on the cheek to 113.0 ug/cm^2 on the forehead.

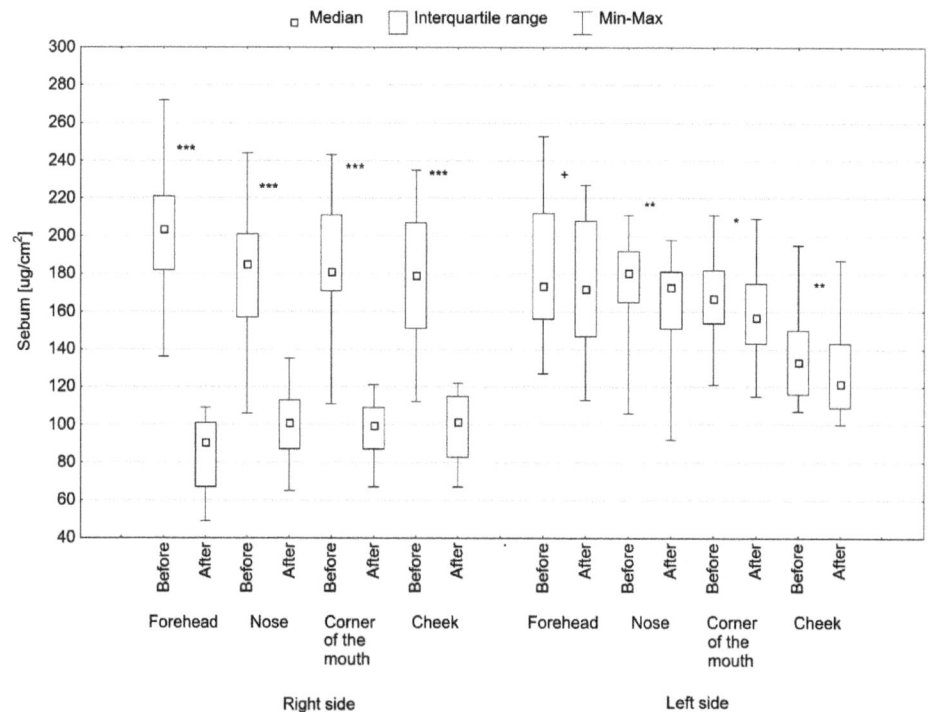

Figure 2. Sebum value in various areas of the face on the right side, treated with microdermabrasion and pyruvic acid, and on the left side, treated only with acid before and after treatments, + $p = 0.055$, * $p < 0.05$, ** $p < 0.01$, *** $p < 0.001$.

Table 3. Sebum value in various areas of the face on the right side, treated with microdermabrasion and pyruvic acid, and on the left side, treated only with acid before and after treatments, + $p = 0.055$, * $p < 0.05$, ** $p < 0.01$, *** $p < 0.001$, Md—Median, Q1—1st quartile, Q3—3rd quartile, Min—Minimum, Max—Maximum.

	Right Side								Left Side							
	Forehead ***		Nose ***		Corner of the Mouth ***		Cheek ***		Forehead +		Nose **		Corner of the Mouth *		Cheek **	
	Before	After	Before	After	Before	After	Before	After	Before	After	Before	After	Before	After	Before	After
Md	203.5	90.5	185.0	101.0	181.0	99.5	179.0	101.5	173.5	172.0	180.5	173.0	167.0	157.0	133.0	121.5
Q1	182.0	67.0	157.0	87.0	171.0	87.0	151.0	83.0	156.0	147.0	165.0	151.0	154.0	143.0	116.0	109.0
Q3	221.0	101.0	201.0	113.0	211.0	109.0	207.0	115.0	212.0	208.0	192.0	181.0	182.0	175.0	150.0	143.0
Min	136.0	49.0	106.0	65.0	111.0	67.0	112.0	67.0	127.0	113.0	106.0	92.0	121.0	115.0	107.0	100.0
Max	272.0	109.0	244.0	135.0	243.0	121.0	235.0	122.0	253.0	227.0	211.0	198.0	211.0	209.0	195.0	187.0

On the left side of the face, where only the 40% pyruvic acid procedure was performed, a reduction in sebum secretion was also achieved, but the effects were smaller than on the right side (Figure 2, Table 3). On the left side of the face, near the forehead, the reduction in sebum secretion did not fully reach the level of statistical significance ($p = 0.055$); in the remaining areas, the differences were statistically significant, and the median sebum secretion value decreased by o 7.5 ug/cm², respectively, ($p < 0.01$) on the nose, by 10 μg/cm² ($p < 0.05$) around the corner of the mouth and by 11.5 ug/cm² ($p < 0.01$) on the cheek.

The microdermabrasion procedure and the application of 40% pyruvic acid on the right side of the face resulted in a statistically significant increase in the hydration of the stratum corneum in the forehead ($p < 0.01$), the corner of the mouth ($p < 0.01$) and the cheek ($p < 0.05$) (Figure 3, Table 4). The median value of skin hydration increased by 7.2 in the forehead area, 2.3 in the nasal lobe, 3.2 in the corner of the mouth and 4.9 in the cheek area.

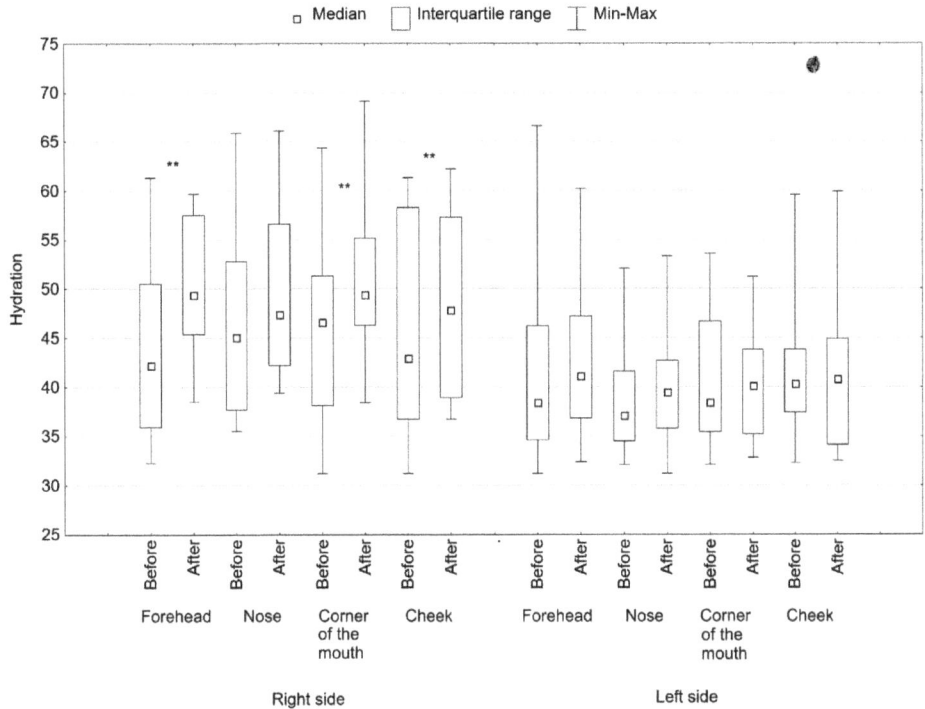

Figure 3. Moisturizing the skin in various areas of the face on the right side, treated with microdermabrasion and pyruvic acid, and on the left side, treated only with acid before and after treatments, ** $p < 0.01$.

Table 4. Moisturizing the skin in various areas of the face on the right side, treated with microdermabrasion and pyruvic acid, and on the left side, treated only with acid before and after treatments, ** $p < 0.01$, Md—Median, Q1—1st quartile, Q3—3rd quartile, Min—Minimum, Max—Maximum.

	Right Side								Left Side							
	Forehead **		Nose		Corner of ** the Mouth		Cheek **		Forehead		Nose		Corner of the Mouth		Cheek	
	Before	After	Before	After	Before	After	Before	After	Before	After	Before	After	Before	After	Before	After
Md	42.2	49.4	45.1	47.4	46.6	49.4	42.9	47.8	38.4	41.2	37.1	39.5	38.4	40.1	40.3	40.8
Q1	35.9	45.4	37.7	42.2	38.1	46.3	36.7	38.9	34.6	36.8	34.5	35.8	35.4	35.2	37.4	34.1
Q3	50.5	57.5	52.8	56.6	51.3	55.2	58.3	57.3	46.2	47.2	41.6	42.7	46.7	43.8	43.8	44.9
Min	32.3	38.5	35.5	39.4	31.2	38.4	31.2	36.7	31.2	32.4	32.1	31.2	32.1	32.8	32.3	32.5
Max	61.3	59.7	65.9	66.1	64.4	69.2	61.3	62.2	66.6	60.2	52.1	53.4	53.6	51.2	59.6	59.9

On the left side of the face, after the treatment with 40% pyruvic acid, improvement in skin hydration could also be observed, but it did not reach statistical significance in any of the examined areas of the face (Figure 3, Table 4).

The left and right side of the face were compared in the thermography assessment (Figure 4). Thermographic images of the face were recorded before and after treatment. The analysis of the patient's face temperature (Region of Interest) before and after procedure did not show statistically significant differences both on the right and on the left side of the face.

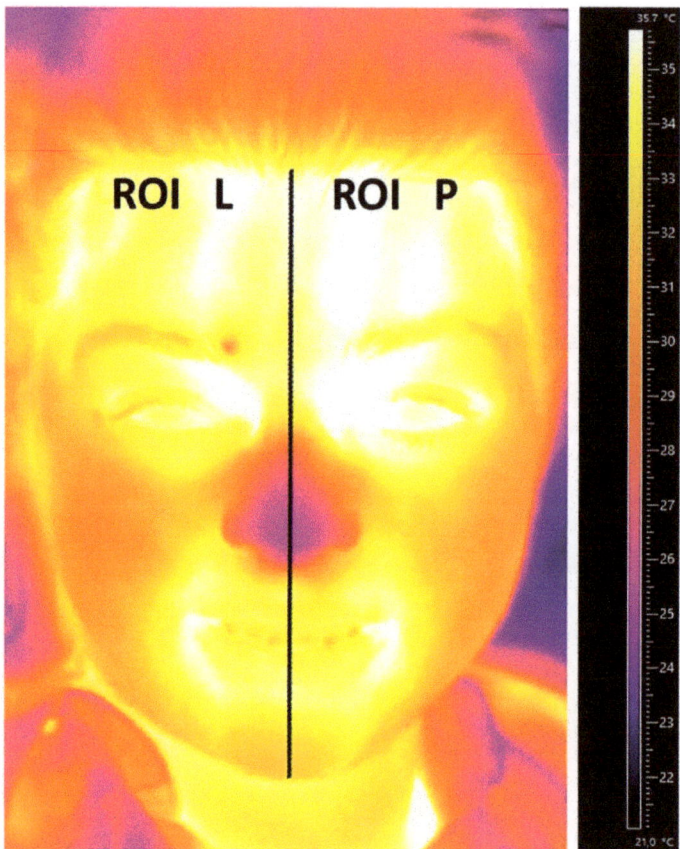

Figure 4. A thermogram of a sample patient with the left and right treatment area marked. The mean temperature difference in the ROI L and ROI R areas for all the studied patients was not statistically significant.

4. Discussion

Acne vulgaris therapy should lead to reduced skin lesions, inflammation and sebum secretion as well as to improved appearance [17]. Various treatments, e.g., topical therapies, oral antibiotic treatment, isotretinoin and hormonal therapies can cause side effects. Chemical peeling is one of the most popular non-invasive cosmetic treatments [18,19]. The use of chemical peels in combination with microdermabrasion for the reduction of acne lesion can be a response to the search for effective and safe methods of acne treatment [20].

The effectiveness of pyruvic acid has been confirmed in numerous studies. In the study by Jaffary et al., patients underwent four treatments with 50% hydroalcoholic solution of pyruvic acid for 2-week intervals. Patients showed a statistically significant reduction in the number of comedones, papules and ASI [21]. Marczyk et al. observed a statistically significant decrease in the level of secreted sebum after the third application (out of six) of 50% pyruvic peel [22]. The findings of Chilicka et al.'s research indicate a significant reduction of acne lesion after the PA six peeling sessions at 2-week intervals. An effect of reducing skin greasiness was also observed [12].

Microdermabrasion removes the superficial epidermal layer, which may contribute to the changes of the hydrolipid barrier. Fąk et al. examine the changes in hydration and sebum level on the skin after microdermabrasion. Thirty minutes after treatment on the cheeks and immediately after on the T-zone, significant differences in stratum corneum hydration have been observed. The reduction of sebum secretion level was observed immediately after the treatment [23].

The above studies show the effectiveness of pyruvic acid and microdermabrasion in reducing sebum secretion and increasing the hydration of the epidermis. The improvement of these skin parameters can reduce acne lesions, and the combination of these two methods may lead to better results than their individual action.

In our study, the use of microdermabrasion in combination with 40% pyruvic acid contributed to the reduction of sebum secretion in each of the measured areas. The differences were greater than when using the pyruvic acid procedure without microdermabrasion. The value of hydration of the stratum corneum increased after a series of treatments with pyruvic acid and microdermabrasion than in the case of treatments without microdermabrasion. Higher hydration of the stratum corneum and greater reduction of sebum secretion after the use of a series of microdermabrasion treatments in combination with pyruvic acid may be the result of the synergic effect of the combination of these treatments on acne-prone skin. Microdermabrasion can lead to exfoliation of epidermal cells and can accelerate and increase the penetration of pyruvic acid. Pyruvic acid has the ability to transform into a component of NMF (Natural Moisturizing Factor) lactic acid which leads to better hydration of the epidermis.

5. Study Limitations

The research sample can be seen to be limited. In the future, we would like to increase the number of patients, as well as expand the group to include men, not only women.

6. Conclusions

In conclusion, after the four peeling sessions using pyruvic acid and pyruvic acid with microdermabrasion, all patients showed better skin parameters in terms of reduced sebum secretion and increased stratum corneum hydration. However, the use of microdermabrasion in combination with pyruvic acid led to better results with increased hydration and reduction of sebum secretion than using only the pyruvic acid treatment. It should be remembered that dermatological treatment cannot be replaced by cosmetological treatment.

Author Contributions: Conceptualization, M.R. and K.C.; methodology, M.R. and R.S.; software, W.O.; validation, A.Y., B.A. and W.O.; formal analysis, M.R.; investigation, M.R. and K.C.; resources, R.S., B.A. and S.W.; data curation, R.S.; writing—original draft preparation, M.R.; writing—review and editing, K.C. and S.W.; visualization, W.O.; supervision, S.W. and R.S.; project administration, M.R.; funding acquisition, M.R., K.C. and R.S. All authors have read and agreed to the published version of the manuscript.

Funding: This research was funded by the University of Opole.

Institutional Review Board Statement: The study was conducted in accordance with the Declaration of Helsinki, and approved by the Bioethics Committee of the Opole Medical School (KB/54/NOZ/2019).

Informed Consent Statement: Informed consent was obtained from all subjects involved in the study.

Data Availability Statement: The data presented in this study are available on request from the corresponding author.

Conflicts of Interest: The authors declare no conflict of interest.

References

1. Chilicka, K.; Rogowska, A.M.; Szyguła, R. Effects of Topical Hydrogen Purification on Skin Parameters and Acne Vulgaris in Adult Women. *Healthcare* **2021**, *9*, 144. [CrossRef]
2. Mazzarello, V.; Donadu, M.G.; Ferrari, M.; Piga, G.; Usai, D.; Zanetti, S.; Sotgiu, M.A. Treatment of acne with a combination of propolis, tea tree oil, and Aloe vera compared to erythromycin cream: Two double-blind investigations. *Clin. Pharmacol. Adv. Appl.* **2018**, *10*, 175–181. [CrossRef] [PubMed]
3. Contassot, E.; French, L.E. New insights into acne pathogenesis: Propionibacterium Acnes activates the inflammasome. *J. Investig. Dermatol.* **2014**, *134*, 310–313. [CrossRef]
4. Oge, L.K.; Broussard, A.; Marshall, M.E. Acne vulgaris: Diagnosis and Treatment. *Am. Fam. Physician* **2019**, *100*, 475–484.
5. Chilicka, K.; Rogowska, A.M.; Szyguła, R.; Adamczyk, E. Association between Satisfaction with Life and Personality Types A and D in Young Women with Acne Vulgaris. *Int. J. Environ. Res. Public Health* **2020**, *17*, 8524. [CrossRef] [PubMed]
6. Chilicka, K.; Maj, J.; Panaszek, B. General quality of life of patients with acne vulgaris before and after performing selected cosmetological treatments. *Patient Prefer. Adherence* **2017**, *11*, 1357–1361. [CrossRef] [PubMed]
7. Chilicka, K.; Rogowska, A.M.; Szyguła, R.; Taradaj, J. Examining Quality of Life after Treatment with Azelaic and Pyruvic Acid Peels in Women with Acne Vulgaris. *Clin. Cosmet. Investig. Dermatol.* **2020**, *13*, 469–477. [CrossRef] [PubMed]
8. Vilar, G.N.; Santos, L.A.; Sobral Filho, J.F. Quality of life, self-esteem and psychosocial factors in adolescents with acne vulgaris. *An. Bras. Dermatol.* **2015**, *90*, 622–629. [CrossRef]
9. Liu, H.; Yu, H.; Xia, J.; Liu, L.; Liu, G.J.; Sang, H.; Peinemann, F. Topical azelaic acid, salicylic acid, nicotinamide, sulphur, zinc and fruit acid (alpha-hydroxy acid) for acne. *Cochrane Database Syst. Rev.* **2020**, *5*, CD011368.
10. Jeong, I.J.; Hyun, D.J.; Kim, D.H.; Moon, S.Y.; Hee, J.L. Comparative study of buffered 50% glycolic acid (pH 3.0) + 0.5% salicylic acid solution vs. Jessner's solution in patients with acne vulgaris. *J. Cosmet. Dermatol.* **2017**, *17*, 797–801.
11. Zdrada, J.; Odrzywołek, W.; Deda, A.; Wilczyński, S. A split-face comparative study to evaluate the efficacy of 50% pyruvic acid against a mixture of glycolic and salicylic acids in the treatment of acne vulgaris. *J. Cosmet. Dermatol.* **2020**, *19*, 2352–2358. [CrossRef]
12. Chilicka, K.; Rogowska, A.M.; Szyguła, R.; Dzieńdziora-Urbińska, I.; Taradaj, J. A comparison of the effectiveness of azelaic and pyruvic acid peels in the treatment of female adult acne: A randomized controlled trial. *Sci. Rep.* **2020**, *10*, 12612. [CrossRef]
13. Abdel-Motaleb, A.A.; Bakr, R.M. Microdermabrasion assisted delivery of glycolic acid 70% peel for the treatment of melasma in dark-skinned patients. *Dermatol. Ther.* **2021**, *34*, e15025. [CrossRef]
14. Jarząbek, S.; Rotsztejn, H. Effect of oxybrasion on selected skin parameters. *J. Cosmet. Dermatol.* **2021**, *20*, 657–663. [CrossRef]
15. Adamski, Z.; Gornowicz-Porowska, J.; Sobkowska, D.; Kaszuba, K.; Czajkowski, R. Acne—Therapeutic challenges to the cooperation between a dermatologist and a cosmetologist. *Postepy Dermatol. Alergol.* **2021**, *38*, 21–31. [CrossRef]
16. Chilicka, K.; Rusztowicz, M.; Dzieńdziora, I. The effectiveness of alkaline water on oily and acne-prone skin: A case report. *Med. Sci. Pulse* **2021**, *15*, 50–54. [CrossRef]
17. Chilicka, K.; Rogowska, A.M.; Rusztowicz, M.; Szyguła, R.; Yanakieva, A.; Asanova, B.; Wilczyński, S. The Effects of Green Tea (*Camellia sinensis*), Bamboo Extract (*Bambusa vulgaris*) and Lactic Acid on Sebum Production in Young Women with Acne Vulgaris Using Sonophoresis Treatment. *Healthcare* **2022**, *10*, 684. [CrossRef]
18. Castillo, D.E.; Keri, J.E. Chemical peels in the treatment of acne: Patient selection and perspectives. *Clin. Cosmet. Investig. Dermatol.* **2018**, *16*, 365–372. [CrossRef]
19. Zdrada, J.; Odrzywołek, W.; Deda, A.; Wilczyński, S.; Błońska-Fajfrowska, B. Analysis of the effectiveness of chemical peelings in the treatment of acne vulgaris assessed using high-frequency ultrasound—A comparative study. *J. Cosmet. Dermatol.* **2021**, *20*, 2810–2815. [CrossRef]
20. Kempiak, S.J.; Uebelhoer, N. Superficial chemical peels and microdermabrasion for acne vulgaris. *Semin. Cutan. Med. Surg* **2008**, *27*, 212–220. [CrossRef] [PubMed]
21. Jaffary, F.; Faghihi, G.; Saraeian, S.; Hosseini, S.M. Comparison the effectiveness of pyruvic acid 50% and salicylic acid 30% in the treatment of acne. *J. Res. Med. Sci.* **2016**, *9*, 21–31. [CrossRef]
22. Marczyk, B.; Mucha, P.; Budzisz, E.; Rotsztejn, H. Comparative study of the effect of 50% pyruvic and 30% salicylic peels on the skin lipid film in patients with acne vulgaris. *J. Cosmet. Dermatol.* **2014**, *13*, 15–21. [CrossRef] [PubMed]
23. Fąk, M.; Rotsztejn, H.; Erkiert-Polguj, A. The early effect of microdermabrasion on hydration and sebum level. *Skin. Res. Technol.* **2018**, *24*, 650–655. [CrossRef]

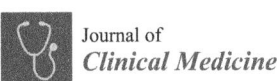

Article

Efficacy of Hydrogen Purification and Cosmetic Acids in the Treatment of Acne Vulgaris: A Preliminary Report

Karolina Chilicka [1,*], Monika Rusztowicz [1], Aleksandra M. Rogowska [2], Renata Szyguła [1], Binnaz Asanova [3] and Danuta Nowicka [4]

1. Department of Health Sciences, Institute of Health Sciences, University of Opole, 45-040 Opole, Poland
2. Department of Social Sciences, Institute of Psychology, University of Opole, 45-052 Opole, Poland
3. Medical College Yordanka Filaretova, Medical University of Sofia, 1606 Sofia, Bulgaria
4. Department of Dermatology, Venereology and Allergology, Wrocław Medical University, 50-368 Wrocław, Poland
* Correspondence: karolina.chilicka@uni.opole.pl

Abstract: Acne and skin lesions that appear in its course deteriorate the quality of life of patients, cause depression and the emergence of suicidal thoughts. Cosmetic treatments can have a positive effect on improving skin condition by cleaning up skin eruptions, thus improving the well-being of affected people. Hydrogen purification is a treatment that uses alkaline water generated by a device, which reduces sebum from the surface of the epidermis. This is a novel treatment that has recently been introduced to beauty salons. On the other hand, cosmetic acids have been used for many years for treating people with acne vulgaris and give spectacular results in terms of improving the skin condition. In this study, skin condition was evaluated with a Derma Unit SSC 3 device. The Global Acne Grading System (GAGS) was used to check acne severity. Twenty-four women aged 19–21 years ($M = 20.13$, $SD = 0.80$) diagnosed with mild acne vulgaris and a high sebum level participated in the study. Group A underwent a hydrogen purification treatment using an H2jet manipulator, which ejected alkaline water from the manipulator under pressure. Group B underwent a hydrogen purification treatment with the use of a phytic, pyruvic, lactic and ferulic acids at 40% mixture (pH 1.4). A series of four treatments was performed at 14-day intervals in both groups. Skin parameters were measured before and 30 days after the series of treatment. Very good results were obtained in both groups. The skin eruptions in patients were reduced and we also observed lower amounts of sebum on the surface of the epidermis, and an improvement in skin hydration. However, in group B, the results were better than in group A. The study showed that the synergy of the treatments produced much better effects than those obtained by completing the hydrogen purification treatment alone.

Keywords: acne vulgaris; hydrogen purification; chemical peels; Sebumeter; Corneometer; cosmetology

1. Introduction

Acne vulgaris is a chronic disease. Several types of lesions can occur during acne, including non-inflammatory and inflammatory lesions, scars, rush, and discolorations. Comedones are classified as non-inflammatory lesions. They can be microscopic (microblackheads) and serve as precursors of open or closed blackheads visible on the skin. The causes of acne revolve around the interplay of several factors, including increased sebum production, follicular hyperkeratosis, inflammation, and the action of anaerobic *Cutibacterium acnes* in the hair follicles [1–4].

Acne vulgaris is a common skin disease that affects teenagers and young adults. It is estimated that 80% to 90% of adolescents experience varying degrees of acne symptoms, which may continue into adulthood. Exacerbation of acne may depend on premenstrual flares, diet, and body mass index (BMI) [5,6]. Long-term treatment of acne, the constant appearance of skin eruptions, and acne scars can negatively affect mental and physical health. The presence of this disease causes discomfort that can lead to emotional disorders, reduced quality of life, and depression [7–10]. However, despite many years of research, the pathogenesis of acne vulgaris has not yet been fully elucidated, and effective treatments have not yet been developed.

Hydrogen is formed by two hydrogen atoms, and it is an odorless and colorless gas that dissolves in water. It builds most of the organic molecules and takes third place in terms of the number of elements found in the human body. Hydrogen is 1000 times smaller than bacteria and cells in the human body with a molecule size of 0.24 nm. Furthermore, it diffuses quickly, so it easily penetrates the structures of the human body and the skin barrier.

Alkaline water has recently begun to be used in cosmetology. In the hydrogen purification treatment, alkaline water, namely electrochemically reduced water (ERW), is used. Such water is rare in nature, but it can be produced by an instant chemical process called electrolysis; the pH of such water is 8–10. During the electrolysis process, by which a direct current is passed between two electrodes (anode and cathode) separated by a semi-permeable membrane, the elements contained in the water are broken down into hydrogen ions (H^+) that are gathered around the cathode and hydroxyl ions (OH^-) that are gathered around the anode. H^+ ions form ionized alkaline water. Negative OH^- ions form acidic water. Active molecular hydrogen that is present in alkaline water serves as the main factor in building the ORP. Its level is related to the concentration of alkaline water and falls within the range of 0.3–0.6 mg/L. Water with hydrogen ions is a natural antioxidant and can be produced solely during electrolysis (water ionizers) and hydrogen saturation (hydrogen generators). Recently, hydrogen cleansing has become one of the most popular treatments in cosmetology, which is used to reduce free radicals, and thus has an anti-aging effect. Once introduced into cells, the hydrogen atoms donate their electrons to free radicals, which are converted into water molecules. In this way, the activity of free radicals is neutralized [11].

In 2007, Ohsawa et al. [12] demonstrated that molecular hydrogen can selectively reduce reactive forms of oxygen in vitro and exert antioxidant, anti-inflammatory, and anti-apoptotic effects. For many years, scientists have been researching the internal effects of alkaline water in people with problems such as pyrosis, dysphoria, tympanites, and diarrhea. The research results confirm that drinking alkaline water significantly improves health conditions [13–16].

Cosmetic acids have been the basis for proper care of acne-prone skin, among others, for years. They cause exfoliation of the dead epidermis, thanks to which the skin pores are cleansed, the incidence of inflammatory skin eruptions is reduced, and the secreted sebum is reduced on the surface of the epidermis. Cosmetic acid treatments can complement dermatological therapies. The acids most commonly used for acne skin include ferulic, azelaic, mandelic, glycolic, salicylic, pyruvic, lactic, and phytic acids. However, combining different topical therapies may produce more beneficial results in treating problematic skin. An extremely important point is also the close cooperation between dermatologists and cosmetologists. Knowledge and shared experience will certainly bring the expected positive results of therapy [17]. For those reasons, the aim of this study was to investigate the efficacy of hydrogen purification in the treatment of acne vulgaris alone and in combination with cosmetic acids.

2. Materials and Methods

2.1. Study Design

A single-blind placebo study with follow-up analysis was conducted at the Institute of Health Sciences of the University of Opole, Poland, from January to March 2021 and at Medical College Yordanka Filaretova, Medical University of Sofia, Sofia, Bulgaria, from June to July 2021. The research was approved by the Human Research Ethics Committee of the Opole Medical School (No. KB/57/NOZ/2019) and conducted according to the principles of the Declaration of Helsinki. The study was registered at https://www.isrctn.com (No.

ISRCTN 28257448) and accessed on 7 May 2020. The patients signed informed consent forms and agreed to take photos before and after the series of treatments. The participants knew that they could withdraw from the examination at any time. They did not have to give any reason of withdrawing.

The G*Power ver. 3.1.9.6 software was used to determine a priori the appropriate sample size for the study. Considering 80% power and $\alpha = 0.05$ (two-tail) for the repeated measures ANOVA with the interaction of within- and between-factors (2 groups, 2 time-points) the total sample size should equal $N = 22$. Initially, 44 people participated in the study, but 20 met the exclusion criteria (Figure 1). The final study sample consisted of 24 women. The power for the final sample size $N = 24$ was $(1 - \beta) = 0.87$ for the ANOVA.

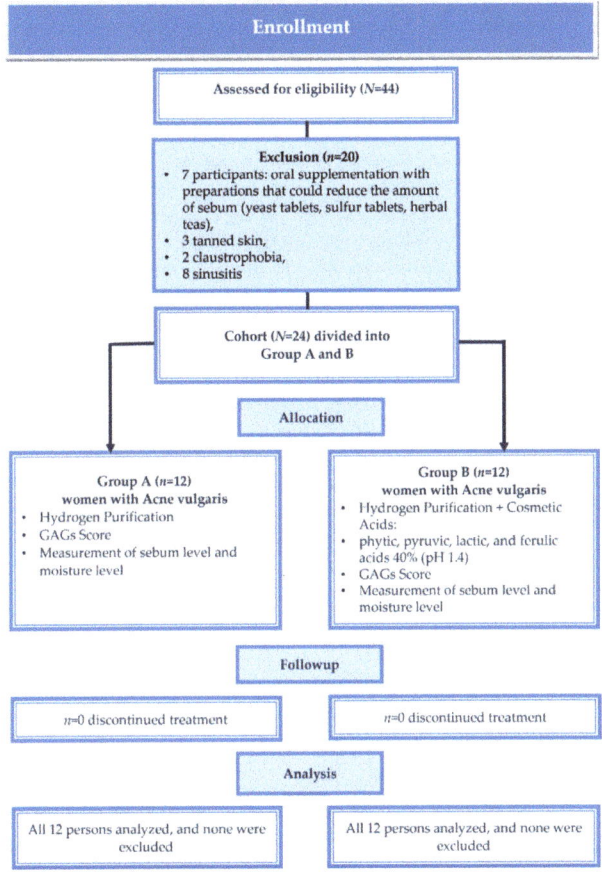

Figure 1. Patients follow in the study.

No men participated in the study. Twenty-four women suffering from acne vulgaris were divided into two groups. They were assigned to the groups of a random selection of envelopes containing groups A or B. Group A underwent hydrogen purification using the H2Jet manipulator, which ejects alkaline water prepared by the device's generator under pressure. Group B underwent hydrogen purification using the H2Jet manipulator with the subsequent use of a mixture of cosmetic acids (of phytic, pyruvic, lactic, and ferulic acids 40% (pH 1.4)).

All patients underwent a series of four treatments applied every 14 days. They could not have other cosmetic procedures. New cosmetics or sebum-regulating creams were forbidden during the entirety of the study period. Only cosmetics such as Cetaphil MD Dermoprotector, micellar water, SPF 50 cream, and Alantan Plus cream were approved to use.

2.2. Participants

A group of 24 women aged 19–21 ($M = 20.13$, $SD = 0.80$) who suffered from acne vulgaris were enrolled in the study. All participants were diagnosed with mild acne by the same rater dermatologist using the GAGS before and after a series of treatments.

The mean duration of acne was 6 years ($M = 5.67$, $SD = 0.76$), ranging between 5 and 7 years. Inclusion criteria for this study were: mild acne, no hormonal contraception, age 19–23 years, and no dermatological treatment within 12 months. The study had contraindications that made it impossible for some people to participate. For Group A it was: pregnancy, breastfeeding, claustrophobia, epilepsy, taking oral medications within the last 3 months, taking isotretinoin within the last year, active inflammation of the skin, fungal, viral, bacterial, allergic skin diseases, taking contraceptives, tanned skin, sun exposure after the procedure, psoriasis, eczema, skin cancers, numerous melanocytic nevi, atopic dermatitis, general illness, and a tendency to having sinusitis, numerous telangiectasias, recently having surgery (up to 2 months). For Group B it was: pregnancy, breastfeeding, claustrophobia, epilepsy, active inflammation of the skin, bacterial, viral, allergic, and fungal relapsing skin diseases, skin cancers, eczema, psoriasis, taking oral medications within the last 3 months, taking isotretinoin within the last year, taking contraceptives, sun exposure after the procedure, tanned skin, atopic dermatitis, general illness, and a tendency to having sinusitis, numerous telangiectasias, recently having surgery (up to 2 months), numerous melanocytic nevi, active herpes, reduced immunity, allergy to peeling ingredients, active rosacea, tanned skin, autoimmune diseases (pemphigus, collagenosis), having cryotherapy (up to 6 months), severe acne and propensity to keloids. Oral supplementation with yeast tablets, sulfur tablets, and herbal was forbidden.

Group A ($n = 12$) and B ($n = 12$) included young adult women with a higher sebum level (more than 100 µg/cm^2) and acne vulgaris. Acne, excessive seborrhea, blackheads, whiteheads, and papules were observed in the volunteers. Before and after the treatment series, the GAGS was used to determine the severity of acne and to check whether the treatments had a positive effect on the improvement of the skin condition of the patients.

2.3. Measures
2.3.1. Acne Vulgaris

The severity of acne vulgaris was assessed using the GAGS. Acne, excessive seborrhea, blackheads, whiteheads, and papules were observed. The GAGS scale is used to determine the degree of acne and to also check whether the treatments had a positive effect on the improvement of the skin [18].

2.3.2. Skin Parameters

Before starting the tests and one month after the end of the last treatment, the skin parameters were measured. The participants were asked to remove face makeup the day before the measurements in the evening and not to apply any preparations to the face skin. In the morning the patients could not use any micellar fluid or cosmetics due to the fact that the parameters would be unreliable. Measurements were taken in the morning, with the test participants, after arriving in the room, acclimatizing for about 30 min. Room humidity was 40–50%, and the temperature was 20–21 degrees C. The Derma Unit SCC 3 apparatus (Courge & Khazaka, Cologne, Germany) was used for the test. Skin hydration was tested with the Corneometer CM 825, and sebum was measured using the Sebumeter SM 815. The measurement points were as follows: forehead, nose, right and left cheeks, and chin. The reliability of measurement was Cronbach's $\alpha = 0.72$ for moisturizing and Cronbach's $\alpha = 0.73$ for greasing in the study sample.

2.4. Treatment Procedure

Face makeup was removed in both groups (micellar fluid) before starting the treatments and also the skin was toned. Group A underwent a hydrogen purification treatment using specialized equipment generating water with an alkaline pH. After putting the subject on a cosmetic bed, the hair was covered with a cosmetic cap, cotton pads, and rubber goggles were put on the eyes, and the ears were covered and secured with cotton wool. Then, when the device was turned on, the vacuum was set to 2 bar, and alkaline water was ejected under pressure from the H2jet manipulator. The manipulator was held approximately 2–3 cm away from the subject's skin, making epidermis exfoliation more precise. The exfoliation was carried out for about 5 min. The face was then dried with cosmetic wipes, and a sunscreen cream was applied to the treated skin. Treatment in group A was repeated in a series of 4 treatments every 2 weeks. Group B also underwent a hydrogen purification treatment, and the treatment algorithm was the same as that for group A. However, after drying the skin with a tissue, the skin was prepared with pre-peel cleanser and pre-peel lotion. Delicate areas such as the corners of the eyes, the area around the lobes of the nose, and the red lip were protected with petroleum jelly. Moistened cotton swabs were put on the eyes to protect against the penetration of acids into the eyeball. The acid was then applied to the entire treatment area of the face using a cotton baguette and left for 2 min during the first treatment. Each subsequent treatment had a longer exposure time to acid by 25 s. After treatment with acid, the neutralizer was applied to the skin for 1 min and then washed with cotton pads and cold water several times. Finally, the skin was dried, and a 50+ UV filter was applied to the face.

For home care, it was recommended to wash the face using Cetaphil MD Dermoprotector. After using the above-mentioned preparation, also, micellar fluid was allowed during the skin care. The patients were asked to use the Cetaphil MD Dermoprotector and micellar fluid twice a day for all periods of the study: in the morning and in the evening.

The patients were meant to apply Alantan Plus cream. Each patient used a thin layer of the cream in the morning and evening hours, after removing makeup.

The patients were instructed not to use the swimming pool and sauna and to avoid exposure to natural and artificial radiation. They were meant to use photoprotection every day and not use any preparations other than Cetaphil MD Dermoprotector, micellar fluid, and Alantan Plus cream. During the entire series of treatments, and a month after its completion, it was forbidden to use any other cosmetic and aesthetic medicine treatments. Dermatological procedures for the duration of the study were also prohibited.

2.5. Statistical Analysis

Initially, descriptive statistics (mean, standard deviation, median, skewness, kurtosis, and Shapiro–Wilk normality test) were performed to check the parametric properties of demographic variables, such as age and years of acne disease, and all dependent variables, such as the severity of acne (GAGS), face moisturizing and greasing, in both conditions before and after hydrogen purification treatment. Since the demographic variables did not meet the assumption of normal distribution of the data, the no-parametric Mann–Whitney U-test was conducted to check whether groups A and B of participants differed from each other. The effect of hydrogen purification treatment on the severity of acne and two parameters of face skin: moisturizing and greasing were examined using the repeated measures of one-way ANOVA. The Bonferroni post-hoc tests were performed to check the simultaneous statistically significant differences between the groups (A and B) and the conditions (before and after treatment). The effect size was assessed using $\eta^2{}_p$ (with a 0.01 value interpreted as small, 0.06 as a medium, and above 0.14 as a large effect size). All statistics were performed using JASP software for Windows: JASP Team, Version 0.14.1 (Computer software; Amsterdam, The Netherlands: Department of Psychological Methods, University of Amsterdam; 2020).

3. Results

3.1. Changes in Acne Severity after Hydrogen Purification and Cosmetic Acids

Initially, the A and B groups were compared to each other to examine differences in age and acne years. Because age and acne years did not meet normality criteria, the Mann–Whitney U-test was performed for this purpose. Group A (Range 19–21, M = 20.00, SD = 0.85, Mdn = 20) did not differ significantly from group B (Range 19–21, M = 20.25, SD = 0.75, Mdn = 20) in age, U = 60, Z = −0.66, p = 0.51. No significant differences in years of acne were found between group A (Range 5–7, M = 5.75, SD = 0.75, Mdn = 6) and group B (Range 5–7, M = 5.58, SD = 0.79, Mdn = 5), U = 62, Z = 0.55, p = 0.58. So, both groups A and B did not differ in age and years of acne.

Acne severity before and after treatment was measured in groups A and B, before and after treatment, respectively (Table 1). The repeated measures one-way ANOVA showed that groups A and B differed significantly (p < 0.01) in acne severity with a large effect size. Statistically significant differences in acne severity were also found between conditions before and after hydrogen purification treatment (p < 0.001), with a large effect size. The interaction effect between the group and treatment was significant (p < 0.001) with a large effect size. A Bonferroni post-hoc test showed that Group A and B did not differ from each other in acne severity before treatment (p > 0.05). However, all groups differed significantly (p < 0.001) between conditions before and after treatment (with higher severity before than after treatment) and between groups A and B after treatment (with lower acne severity in group B than A), which is presented in Figure 2.

Table 1. Repeated measures of one-way ANOVA for acne severity in groups A and B, before and after treatment, using the Global Acne Grading System (GAGS).

GAGS	Group A		Group B		Effect	F(1, 22)	p	η^2_p
	M	SD	M	SD				
Before treatment	16.42	1.00	16.50	1.00	G	12.32	0.002	0.359
After treatment	11.58	1.51	9.00	0.95	T	430.26	<0.001	0.951
					T × G	20.11	<0.001	0.478

Note. Group A = hydrogen purification, Group B = hydrogen purification and cosmetic acid, GAGS = Global Acne Grading System, M = mean, SD = standard deviation, F = Fisher's test, p = significance level, η^2_p = partial eta-square effect size, G = group effect, T = treatment effect, T × G = interaction between group and treatment effect.

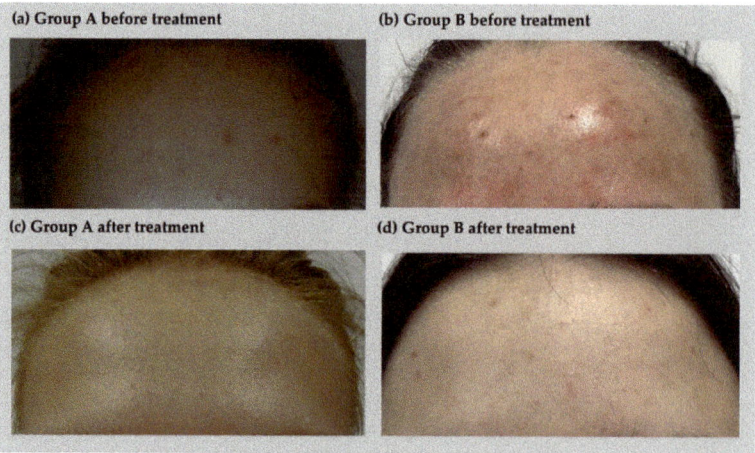

Figure 2. Effect of treatment on acne severity in a patient from group A before (**a**) and after treatment (**c**), group B before (**b**) and after treatment (**d**).

3.2. Changes in Facial Skin Moisture after Hydrogen Purification and Cosmetic Acids

The repeated measures one-way ANOVA was performed to examine the effect of hydrogen purification treatment on facial skin moisture in samples A and B. The results are presented in Table 2, separately for the forehead, nose, right and left cheek, and chin. The ANOVA showed no group, treatment, or interaction effect on forehead moisturizing in the women sample ($p < 0.05$).

Table 2. Repeated measures of one-way ANOVA for face moisturizing in groups A and B, before and after treatment, using Corneometer CM825 (g/m^2).

Face Moisturizing	Group A		Group B		Effect	$F(1, 22)$	p	η^2_p
	M	SD	M	SD				
Forehead					G	2.01	0.170	0.08
Before	39.83	3.53	41.09	3.20	T	0.00	0.991	0.00
After	39.91	2.32	41.03	1.63	T × G	0.01	0.922	0.00
Nose					G	5.30	0.031	0.19
Before	39.91	2.32	41.03	1.63	T	39.89	<0.001	0.65
After	42.08	3.53	45.53	3.14	T × G	4.91	0.037	0.18
Right Cheek					G	8.72	0.007	0.28
Before	38.78	3.49	42.96	2.87	T	15.20	<0.001	0.41
After	44.50	4.00	46.48	4.82	T × G	0.86	0.363	0.04
Left Cheek					G	13.63	0.001	0.38
Before	40.85	3.21	41.64	2.40	T	94.92	<0.001	0.81
After	45.73	3.66	51.53	1.89	T × G	10.96	0.003	0.33
Chin					G	14.97	<0.001	0.41
Before	38.90	3.41	40.93	2.18	T	111.46	<0.001	0.84
After	43.64	3.27	49.58	2.83	T × G	9.52	0.005	0.30

Note. Group A = hydrogen purification, Group B = hydrogen purification and cosmetic acid, M = mean, SD = standard deviation, F = Fisher's test, p = significance level, η^2_p = partial eta-square effect size, G = group effect, T = treatment effect, T × G = interaction between group and treatment effect.

The group effect was significant for nose moisturizing ($p < 0.05$), with a large effect size, indicating higher moisturizing in group B than A (Table 2). The treatment effect was significant ($p < 0.001$), with a large effect size, showing that the level of nose moisturizing was higher after treatment than before. In addition, the interaction effect between group and treatment was significant ($p < 0.05$), with a large effect size. The Bonferroni post-hoc test demonstrated that group B before treatment did not differ significantly from group A both before and after treatment ($p > 0.05$). The other differences between groups A and B before and after treatments were significant ($p < 0.05$), showing better nose moisturizing after treatment than before, with a greater effect in group B than A.

Regarding right check moisturizing (Table 2), ANOVA showed the significant effect of group ($p < 0.01$, large effect size) and treatment ($p < 0.001$, large effect size), but no interaction effect ($p > 0.05$, small effect size). Group A before treatment showed significantly lower right cheek moisturizing than groups A ($p < 0.05$) and B ($p < 0.001$) after treatment, as the Bonferroni post-hoc tests showed. The other differences between groups A and B before and after treatment were insignificant.

When the left check was examined using ANOVA (Table 2), all effects were significant, including group ($p < 0.01$, large effect size), treatment ($p < 0.001$, large effect size) and interaction ($p < 0.01$, large effect size) effects. Although group A did not differ from group B in left check moisturizing before the experiment ($p > 0.05$), the other differences between groups A and B before and after treatment were statistically significant ($p < 0.001$), showing a higher left check moisturizing after treatment than before, in particular among women from group B.

The ANOVA found significant group ($p < 0.001$, large effect size), treatment ($p < 0.001$, large effect size), and interaction ($p < 0.01$, large effect size) effects for check moisturizing among participants. The post-hoc test indicated that group B before treatment did not differ from group A before and after treatment, while the other differences between groups A and B before and after treatment were significant ($p < 0.001$), indicating higher check moisturizing after treatment, especially in the B group.

3.3. Changes in Facial Skin Greasing after Hydrogen Purification and Cosmetic Acids

The effect of hydrogen purification treatment on facial skin greasing was tested in samples A and B using repeated measures of one-way ANOVA (Table 3). The effects of group ($p < 0.05$, large effect size), treatment ($p < 0.001$, large effect size), and interaction ($p < 0.01$, large effect size) were significant for the forehead greasing. The post-hoc Bonferroni test showed that although groups A and B did not differ in forehead greasing before treatment ($p > 0.05$), all other differences between groups A and B before and after treatment were significant ($p < 0.001$), indicating lower forehead greasing after treatment than before, especially in the B group (Table 3).

Table 3. Repeated measures one-way ANOVA for face greasing in groups A and B, before and after treatment, using Sebumeter SM815 ($\mu g/cm^2$).

Face Greasing	Group A		Group B		Effect	$F(1, 22)$	p	η^2_p
	M	SD	M	SD				
Forehead					G	7.68	0.011	0.26
Before	191.58	17.55	189.58	14.58	T	454.62	<0.001	0.95
After	127.25	15.16	103.08	9.23	T × G	9.82	0.005	0.31
Nose					G	7.96	0.010	0.27
Before	185.33	19.42	189.08	17.43	T	366.86	<0.001	0.94
After	130.67	8.13	100.50	10.72	T × G	20.57	<0.001	0.48
Right Cheek					G	0.49	0.490	0.02
Before	191.42	20.22	191.33	16.82	T	0.49	0.491	0.02
After	194.33	19.34	184.25	20.10	T × G	2.82	0.107	0.11
Left Cheek					G	8.23	0.009	0.27
Before	194.33	19.34	184.25	20.10	T	351.12	<0.001	0.94
After	134.17	16.79	108.92	12.81	T × G	4.40	0.048	0.17
Chin					G	8.32	0.009	0.27
Before	191.83	15.95	186.17	17.79	T	177.16	<0.001	0.89
After	135.25	13.84	117.75	12.40	T × G	1.59	0.221	0.07

Note. Group A = hydrogen purification, Group B = hydrogen purification and cosmetic acid, M = mean, SD = standard deviation, F = Fisher's test, p = significance level, η^2_p = partial eta-square effect size, G = group effect, T = treatment effect, T × G = interaction between group and treatment effect.

Next, the nose greasing was examined before and after treatment in groups A and B, using ANOVA (Table 3). All effects were significant, including group ($p < 0.01$, large effect size), treatment ($p < 0.001$, large effect size), and interaction ($p < 0.001$, large effect size) effects. The Bonferroni post-hoc tests indicate that groups A and B before treatment did not differ from each other significantly ($p > 0.05$), but the other differences between samples A and B before and after treatment were significant ($p < 0.001$). The levels of nose greasing were significantly lower after treatment than before in both samples, but this effect was statistically stronger in group B compared to group A.

The ANOVA did not show any significant effect of group (A vs. B), treatment (before vs. after), and interaction between group and treatment on the greasing of the right cheek ($p > 0.05$). In contrast, significant effects of group ($p < 0.01$, large effect size), treatment ($p < 0.001$, large effect size), and interaction ($p < 0.05$, large effect size) were found on the left cheek greasing. Although no differences were demonstrated between groups A and B before treatment, the other differences between samples A and B, considering conditions before and after treatment, were significant ($p < 0.001$). More specifically, the level of left cheek greasing decreased after treatment, particularly among women in group B (see Table 3 for more details).

The significant effects of group ($p < 0.01$, large effect size) and treatment ($p < 0.001$, large effect size), but no interaction between group and treatment ($p > 0.05$), were shown for chin greasing in the A and B samples (Table 3). Apart from no differences between samples A and B before treatment, all other significant differences were found between groups (A and B) and conditions (before and after treatments) in the study ($p < 0.001$). Compared to the condition before the experiment, lower chin greasing was presented after treatment in both A and B samples, with a greater difference in group B than A.

4. Discussion

The results of the research presented in this article show that cosmetological treatments have a positive effect on improving basic skin parameters and reducing skin eruptions that occur in people struggling with acne. Furthermore, the synergy of two treatments is definitely a better solution and gives better results than the use of single cosmetic methods. The research conducted first by Chilicka et al. in 2021 on the use of hydrogen purification in people suffering from acne showed that the procedure is safe and improves the skin condition of the study participants [11]. To the best of our knowledge, there are no other reports in the literature on the influence of alkaline water on the skin of people with acne.

Much more is known about the use of cosmetic acids, as treatments with their use have been known in dermatology and cosmetology for many years. Cosmetic acids provide very good results in terms of reducing skin eruptions and restoring proper skin parameters. Sarkar et al. conducted a series of treatments involving 45 patients with acne. Group A underwent biweekly peeling sessions with 35% glycolic acid, group B underwent treatment with 20% salicylic–10% mandelic acid treatment, and group C received phytic acid peels for a total of six sessions. After 12 weeks of treatment, there was a significant reduction in the number of inflammatory and non-inflammatory eruptions in all groups. The reduction in the acne scores in the three study groups were 70.55%, 74.14%, and 69.7%, respectively [19].

Chilicka et al. conducted research on a group of 120 young women. Group A ($n = 60$) underwent Azelaic Peeling treatment (6 sessions, every 2 weeks), and group B ($n = 60$) underwent Pyruvic Peeling treatment (6 sessions, every 2 weeks). Both Azelaic Peeling and Pyruvic Peeling produced a significantly lower desquamation level. However, significant differences between these two agents were shown in the extent of the oily skin level [20].

Kamm et al. compared the effect of ferulic acid and the use of d'Arsonwal's high-frequency currents on acne-prone skin. Group A ($n = 30$) had a series of 5 treatments with ferulic acid performed every 7 days. The acid was applied to the face for 6 min. Group B ($n = 30$) had the same series of treatments but with the use of d'Arsonwal's high-frequency currents. With probants in the ferulic acid group, the number of inflammatory exanthema after the end of the treatment was significantly lowered. In d'Arsonwal's current group, the number of inflammatory exanthema also significantly reduced [21].

An interesting study was conducted by Marczyk et al. who compared the effect of the application of 50% pyruvic and 30% salicylic peels on the skin in patients with acne vulgaris. Ten patients were treated with 50% pyruvic acid and 10 patients with 30% salicylic acid. The series of the treatment included five treatments performed every two weeks. To measure the amount of sebum on the surface of the epidermis the Sebumeter SM 815 device was used. Better results in terms of sebum reduction were obtained in the group in which salicylic peel was used [22].

Jaffary et al. conducted a study with the use of the same acids at the same concentrations. The study group consisted of 86 patients randomly divided into two groups. Routine acne treatment (4% topical solution of erythromycin, triclocarban soap, and sunscreen) was used twice a day for 8 weeks. Additionally, 30% salicylic acid was used for the control group and 50% pyruvic acid for the study group. The reduction in the number of comedones, papules, and acne severity index was statistically significant ($p < 0.001$) in the course of treatment in both groups [23].

In another study by Zdrada et al. 50% pyruvic acid and preparation containing glycolic and salicylic acids were used. Fourteen women with a diagnosis of acne underwent a series of four treatments at 2-week intervals. Pyruvic acid was applied to the right side of the patient's face, and glycolic and salicylic acids were applied to the left side. Basic skin parameters such as hydration, sebum secretion, and skin color were evaluated. The increase in skin hydration on the left side of the chin and nose was not statistically significant. Treatment with a mixture of acids resulted in fewer side effects than a single acid used in high concentrations, but therapeutic effects were comparable [24].

In cosmetology, many treatments for acne-prone skin benefit from using modern devices, including those that are based on cosmetic acids. One of them is microdermabrasion. It is safe and effective without excluding the patient from his/her everyday life. The above-mentioned treatments have a positive effect on the reduction of acne lesions, reduction of the level of sebum on the surface of the epidermis, and improvement of skin hydration [25,26]. We hope that our research results and the treatments that we have proposed, can be used by other researchers to apply them to another disease, for example hidradenitis suppurativa [27–29].

5. Study Limitations

In the future, larger study samples should be carried out that include both genders and a wider age range. We would like to include additional measurements, such as pH. We could also compare the effectiveness of other cosmetic treatments or other types of cosmetic acids.

6. Conclusions

Hydrogen purification is a procedure that is increasingly used in cosmetology. Our research shows that it produces very good results in terms of reducing skin eruptions and improving skin parameters. The synergy of the treatments, namely hydrogen purification and cosmetic acids, indicates that they provide better results than their use as individual treatments. These procedures do not require patients to abandon their daily activities. Finally, they do not cause side effects such as redness or skin irritation. However, it should be remembered that dermatological treatment cannot be replaced by cosmetological treatment.

Author Contributions: Conceptualization, K.C.; methodology, K.C. and M.R.; software, K.C.; validation, K.C. and A.M.R.; formal analysis, A.M.R.; investigation, K.C. and B.A.; resources, K.C. and M.R.; data curation, K.C. and A.M.R.; writing—original draft preparation, K.C., A.M.R. and D.N.; writing—review and editing, K.C., A.M.R. and D.N.; visualization, A.M.R.; supervision, R.S.; project administration, K.C.; funding acquisition, R.S. All authors have read and agreed to the published version of the manuscript.

Funding: This research received no external funding.

Institutional Review Board Statement: The study was conducted according to the guidelines of the Declaration of Helsinki and approved by the Human Research Ethics Committee of the Opole Medical School No. KB/57/NOZ/2019.

Informed Consent Statement: Informed consent was obtained from all subjects involved in the study.

Data Availability Statement: Not applicable.

Conflicts of Interest: The authors declare no conflict of interest.

References

1. Zhu, W.; Wang, H.L.; Bu, X.L.; Zhang, J.B.; Lu, Y.G. A narrative review of research progress on the role of NLRP3 inflammasome in acne vulgaris. *Ann. Transl. Med.* **2022**, *10*, 645. [CrossRef] [PubMed]
2. Tuchayi, S.M.; Makrantonaki, E.; Ganceviciene, R.; Dessinioti, C.; Feldman, S.R.; Zouboulis, C.C. Acne vulgaris. *Nat. Rev. Dis. Primers* **2015**, *1*, 15029. [CrossRef] [PubMed]
3. Ogé, L.K.; Broussard, A.; Marshall, M.D. Acne Vulgaris: Diagnosis and Treatment. *Am. Fam. Physician* **2019**, *100*, 475–484.
4. Bernales Salinas, A. Acne vulgaris: Role of the immune system. *Int. J. Dermatol.* **2021**, *60*, 1076–1081. [CrossRef] [PubMed]

5. O'Neill, A.M.; Gallo, R.L. Host-microbiome interactions and recent progress into understanding the biology of acne vulgaris. *Microbiome* **2018**, *6*, 177. [CrossRef] [PubMed]
6. Anaba, E.L.; Oaku, R.I. Adult female acne: A cross-sectional study of diet, family history, body mass index, and premenstrual flare as risk factors and contributors to severity. *Int. J. Women Dermatol.* **2020**, *7*, 265–269. [CrossRef] [PubMed]
7. Chilicka, K.; Rogowska, A.M.; Szyguła, R.; Taradaj, J. Examining Quality of Life After Treatment with Azelaic and Pyruvic Acid Peels in Women with Acne Vulgaris. *Clin. Cosmet. Investig. Dermatol.* **2020**, *13*, 469–477. [CrossRef]
8. Fabbrocini, G.; Cacciapuoti, S.; Monfrecola, G. A qualitative investigation of the impact of acne on Health-Related Quality of Life (HRQL): Development of a conceptual model. *Dermatol. Ther.* **2018**, *8*, 85–99. [CrossRef]
9. Chilicka, K.; Maj, J.; Panaszek, B. General quality of life of patients with acne vulgaris before and after performing selected cosmetological treatments. *Patient Prefer. Adherence* **2017**, *11*, 1357–1361. [CrossRef]
10. Öztekin, C.; Öztekin, A. The association of depression, loneliness and internet addiction levels in patients with acne vulgaris. *Biopsychosoc. Med.* **2020**, *14*, 17. [CrossRef]
11. Chilicka, K.; Rogowska, A.M.; Szyguła, R. Effects of Topical Hydrogen Purification on Skin Parameters and Acne Vulgaris in Adult Women. *Healthcare* **2021**, *9*, 144. [CrossRef] [PubMed]
12. Ohsawa, I.; Ishikawa, M.; Takahashi, K.; Watanabe, M.; Nishimaki, K.; Yamagata, K.; Katsura, K.I.; Katayama, Y.; Asoh, S.; Ohta, S. Hydrogen acts as a therapeutic antioxidant by selectively reducing cytotoxic oxygen radicals. *Nat. Med.* **2007**, *13*, 688–694. [CrossRef] [PubMed]
13. Zeng, K.; Zhang, D.K. Recent progress in alkaline water electrolysis for hydrogen production and applications. *Prog. Energ. Combust. Sci.* **2010**, *36*, 307–326. [CrossRef]
14. Harris, D.C. *Quantitative Chemical Analysis*, 9th ed.; Macmillan: New York, NY, USA, 2010.
15. Shirahata, S.; Hamasaki, T.; Teruya, K. Advanced research on the health benefit of reduced water. *Trends Food Sci. Technol.* **2012**, *23*, 124–131. [CrossRef]
16. Hong, Y.; Chen, S.; Zhang, J.M. Hydrogen as a selective antioxidant: A review of clinical and experimental studies. *J. Int. Med. Res.* **2010**, *38*, 1893–1903. [CrossRef]
17. Adamski, Z.; Gornowicz-Porowska, J.; Sobkowska, D.; Kaszuba, K.; Czajkowski, R. Acne–therapeutic challenges to the cooperation between a dermatologist and a cosmetologist. *Postep. Dermatol. Alergol.* **2021**, *38*, 21–31. [CrossRef]
18. Chilicka, K.; Rogowska, A.M.; Szyguła, R.; Rusztowicz, M.; Nowicka, D. Efficacy of Oxybrasion in the Treatment of Acne Vulgaris: A Preliminary Report. *J. Clin. Med.* **2022**, *11*, 3824. [CrossRef]
19. Sarkar, R.; Ghunawat, S.; Garg, V.K. Comparative Study of 35% Glycolic Acid, 20% Salicylic-10% Mandelic Acid, and Phytic Acid Combination Peels in the Treatment of Active Acne and Postacne Pigmentation. *J. Cutan. Aesthet. Surg.* **2019**, *12*, 158–163.
20. Chilicka, K.; Rogowska, A.M.; Szyguła, R.; Dzieńdziora-Urbińska, I.; Taradaj, J. A comparison of the effectiveness of azelaic and pyruvic acid peels in the treatment of female adult acne: A randomized controlled trial. *Sci. Rep.* **2020**, *10*, 12612. [CrossRef]
21. Kamm, A.; Załęska, I. The Effect of Ferulic Acid and D'Arsonwal's High Frequency Currents Activity over the Number of Exanthema among Adult Women. *J. Med.-Cin. Res. Rev.* **2018**, *2*, 1–7.
22. Marczyk, B.; Mucha, P.; Budzisz, E.; Rotsztejn, H. Comparative study of the effect of 50% pyruvic and 30% salicylic peels on the skin lipid film in patients with acne vulgaris. *J. Cosmet. Dermatol.* **2014**, *13*, 15–21. [CrossRef] [PubMed]
23. Jaffary, F.; Faghihi, G.; Saraeian, S.; Hosseini, S.M. Comparison the effectiveness of pyruvic acid 50% and salicylic acid 30% in the treatment of acne. *J. Res. Med. Sci.* **2016**, *21*, 31. [PubMed]
24. Zdrada, J.; Odrzywołek, W.; Deda, A.; Wilczyński, S. A split-face comparative study to evaluate the efficacy of 50% pyruvic acid against a mixture of glycolic and salicylic acids in the treatment of acne vulgaris. *J. Cosmet. Dermatol.* **2020**, *19*, 2352–2358. [CrossRef] [PubMed]
25. Briden, E.; Jacobsen, E.; Johnson, C. Combining superficial glycolic acid (alpha-hydroxy acid) peels with microdermabrasion to maximize treatment results and patient satisfaction. *Cutis* **2007**, *79* (Suppl. 1), 13–16. [PubMed]
26. Kempiak, S.; Uebelhoer, N. Superficial chemical peels and microdermabrasion for acne vulgaris. *Semin. Cutan. Med. Surg.* **2008**, *27*, 212–220. [CrossRef]
27. Ruggiero, A.; Martora, F.; Picone, V.; Marano, L.; Fabbrocini, G.; Marasca, C. Paradoxical Hidradenitis Suppurativa during Biologic Therapy, an Emerging Challenge: A Systematic Review. *Biomedicines* **2022**, *10*, 455. [CrossRef]
28. Napolitano, M.; Fabbrocini, G.; Martora, F.; Picone, V.; Morelli, P.; Patruno, C. Role of Aryl Hydrocarbon Receptor Activation in Inflammatory Chronic Skin Diseases. *Cells* **2021**, *10*, 3559. [CrossRef]
29. Martora, F.; Marasca, C.; Fabbrocini, G.; Ruggiero, A. Strategies adopted in a southern Italian referral centre to reduce adalimumab discontinuation: Comment on 'Can we increase the drug survival time of biologic therapies in hidradenitis suppurativa?'. *Clin. Exp. Dermatol.* **2022**, *47*, 1864–1865. [CrossRef]

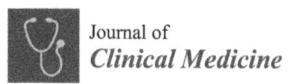

Review

Current Medical and Surgical Treatment of Hidradenitis Suppurativa—A Comprehensive Review

Lennart Ocker *, Nessr Abu Rached, Caroline Seifert, Christina Scheel and Falk G. Bechara *

International Centre for Hidradenitis Suppurativa/Acne Inversa (ICH), Department of Dermatology, Venereology and Allergology, Ruhr-University Bochum, 44791 Bochum, Germany
* Correspondence: lennart.ocker@kklbo.de (L.O.); falk.bechara@kklbo.de (F.G.B.); Tel.: +49-234-509-3420 (L.O.)

Abstract: Hidradenitis suppurativa (HS) is a chronic inflammatory skin disease presenting with recurrent inflammatory lesions in intertriginous body regions. HS has a pronounced impact on patients' quality of life and is associated with a variety of comorbidities. Treatment of HS is often complex, requiring an individual approach with medical and surgical treatments available. However, especially in moderate-to-severe HS, there is an urgent need for new treatment approaches. In recent years, increased research has led to the identification of new potential therapeutic targets. This review aims to give a comprehensive and practical overview of current treatment options for HS. Furthermore, the clinically most advanced novel treatment approaches will be discussed.

Keywords: hidradenitis suppurativa; acne inversa; dermatology; inflammation; treatment; adalimumab; targeted therapy; small molecules

1. Introduction

Hidradenitis suppurativa (HS) is a chronic inflammatory skin disease, presenting with recurrent inflammatory nodules, abscess formation and subsequently formation of subcutaneous sinus tracts and scars during disease progression.

Epidemiologic studies reported varying HS prevalence rates from 0.1% in the US to 1.8% in a Danish population, based on heterogeneous measurement methods [1,2]. A recent meta-analysis came to an overall prevalence of 0.4% [3]. The highest prevalence rates of around 4% are found in young adults between 20 and 40 years, while rates decline in older patients [4].

HS is associated with a high burden of disease, impairing the social and economic situation of affected patients [5]. The occurrence of inflammatory skin lesions and pus discharge in intertriginous areas compromises the sexual life, and causes chronic and exacerbating pain [6–8]. HS patients are more often absent from work with subsequent increasing risk of unemployment and loss of social status [9]. Diagnosis is often delayed with a European study reporting a delay of 7.2 years and a recent German cross-sectional study showing more than 10 years and consultation of more than three physicians before correct diagnosis [10,11].

Additionally, HS can be associated with multiple comorbidities [12]. Studies found strong associations with metabolic syndrome, obesity, cardiovascular disease, chronic inflammatory bowel disease, spondylarthritis and depression, underlining the need for a multi-professional treatment approach [12–20]. Physicians involved in the treatment of HS patients should be aware of potential comorbidities and further diagnostics should be performed in suspected cases. However, in contrast to other inflammatory skin conditions like psoriasis vulgaris, with adalimumab there is currently only one biologic agent available and the individual selection of treatment modalities is based on multiple factors, like inflammatory activity, objective disease severity and patients' preferences.

The pathophysiology of HS is complex and has gradually been elucidated in recent years due to increased research interest in inflammatory skin diseases [21,22]. However,

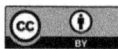

Citation: Ocker, L.; Abu Rached, N.; Seifert, C.; Scheel, C.; Bechara, F.G. Current Medical and Surgical Treatment of Hidradenitis Suppurativa—A Comprehensive Review. *J. Clin. Med.* **2022**, *11*, 7240. https://doi.org/10.3390/jcm11237240

Academic Editor: Dennis Paul Orgill

Received: 14 November 2022
Accepted: 2 December 2022
Published: 6 December 2022

Copyright: © 2022 by the authors. Licensee MDPI, Basel, Switzerland. This article is an open access article distributed under the terms and conditions of the Creative Commons Attribution (CC BY) license (https://creativecommons.org/licenses/by/4.0/).

we have still recognized only parts of the complex inflammatory mosaic, which is reflected in the lack of efficacy of various treatment approaches in recent trials. Possibly, due to the complex pathophysiology and high inflammatory load, combination therapies might be necessary to control HS on a sufficient level. However, data on the combination of different biologics and/or small molecules are yet missing.

This review aims to provide a comprehensive and clinical-based overview of available treatment options in HS.

2. Classification of Disease and Evaluation of Treatment Response

Several classification systems have been described to assess the disease severity of HS. However, a standardized and internationally accepted score is yet missing, resulting in the utilization of different classification tools in clinical studies for the evaluation of treatments. In the following, we briefly describe frequently used scoring systems.

The Hurley staging system was first described in 1989 and due to its simplicity is the most widely used classification system for HS in routine clinical practice [23]. The classification of HS into three stages, mainly based on the presence of sinus tracts and scarring, enables a fast and simple clinical based evaluation. However, the Hurley staging system is not applicable for monitoring of HS, as it represents a static and non-quantitative tool and inflammation activity is not captured [24]. A revised Hurley staging system, that takes account of inflammation activity and subcategorizes Hurley stages I and II into mild, moderate and severe disease, has been described recently; however, clinical application is limited [25].

The modified Sartorius score (mSS) represents a more detailed, open-scaled scoring system, which takes account of the number of involved body regions, the number and types of lesions, and the distance between lesions [26]. Although the mSS is a dynamic system, suitable for treatment monitoring, due to its complexity its use is often time-consuming and especially in severe cases difficult to apply [27].

The hidradenitis suppurativa physician global assessment (HS-PGA) score is a frequently used tool to assess disease severity. HS is classified into six severity grades by counting the numbers of inflammatory nodules, abscesses and sinus tracts [28]. As a dynamic scoring tool HS-PGA can be used for treatment evaluation, although especially in cases of extensive disease with multiple lesions the clinical correlation is limited [29].

The severity assessment of hidradenitis suppurativa (SAHS) score was developed by Hessam et al. and is another clinical based scoring tool, that considers the number of affected body regions, fistulas and other inflammatory lesions as well as HS-related pain and the number of new or flared boils in the last four weeks [30]. The SAHS score enables a dynamic evaluation of HS severity and can also be used for treatment evaluation in clinical practice and studies [31].

The hidradenitis suppurativa clinical response (HiSCR) is defined as a $\geq 50\%$ reduction in inflammatory lesion count and no increase in abscesses or draining fistulas in HS compared to baseline [32]. It is commonly used as a primary endpoint for treatment evaluation in recent studies and has been shown to be more responsive than HS-PGA [33]. According to the psoriasis area and severity index (PASI), $HiSCR_{75}$- and $HiSCR_{90}$- rates are further developed outcome parameters, assessed in current studies [34].

The international hidradenitis suppurativa severity score system (IHS4) represents a dynamic and easy-to-use scoring tool, and assesses disease severity by counting of inflammatory HS lesions (nodules 1 point, abscesses 2 points, sinus tracts 4 points). A total score of 3 or less signifies mild, 4–10 signifies moderate, and 11 or higher signifies severe disease [35]. Recently, a modified and dichotomous IHS4-55 score has been developed as a potential parameter for the measurement of treatment outcomes [36].

Most HS scoring tools are based solely on physical findings. However, clinical examination can be limited, especially in complex cases with deep tissue involvement. The addition of ultrasound to clinical examination could expand the diagnostic spectrum and enable an objective anatomical based assessment of HS lesions [37]. Moreover, a recent study correlated distinct sonographic parameters with treatment responses in HS patients [38]. Several ultrasound-based scoring systems have been developed for classification of HS lesions; however, clinical application is limited up to now [39,40].

3. Treatment

Clinical management of HS is often complex and includes medical and surgical treatments, which are often combined, especially in moderate-to-severe disease [41]. The reduction of symptoms and inflammation activity as well as prevention of formation of chronic HS lesions and scarring represent key therapeutic goals. In current guidelines, an individualized patient-oriented approach, based on the individual subjective impact and objective disease severity, is recommended [20,41].

3.1. General Recommendations

3.1.1. Smoking

The link between tobacco smoking and HS has been suggested in several studies. In a retrospective study, 92.2% of HS patients were smokers and clinical remission was more often reported among non-smoking patients [42]. Moreover, Sartorius et al. found lower disease severities, evaluated by the mSS, in non-smokers compared to active smokers [27]. At a molecular level, components of cigarette smoke have been demonstrated to further promote inflammation in HS via inhibition of the already compromised Notch signaling, induction of proinflammatory cytokine expression and causing infundibular epithelia hyperplasia and hypercornification [43,44]. Although clear evidence of tobacco as a trigger of HS has not been found yet, patients should be encouraged to quit smoking [20].

3.1.2. Weight Reduction

Overweight and obesity are considered as frequent comorbidities of HS. In two case–control studies an increment of the likelihood of HS with every BMI unit increase was reported [45]. In another retrospective study, the point prevalence of HS was much higher in an obese study population compared to the general population [46]. This may be explained by changes of the skin microbiome and increased friction of skin folds in obese patients [47,48]. However, evidence for improvement of HS after body weight reduction is limited. A retrospective study reported a significant reduction of inflammatory activity in HS patients undergoing bariatric surgery [46,49]. Moreover, obese HS patients reported lower remission rates than non-obese HS patients [42].

Obese patients should be motivated to reduce their body weight by initiating physical activity and dietary changes [50]. In cases of severe obesity, bariatric surgery may be an option [51].

3.1.3. Psychological Support

Due to its chronic recurrent course with painful lesions and purulent discharge, HS has a pronounced impact on the patient's life and professional support may be required. Esmann et al. described an increased risk of social isolation due to shame and fear of stigmatization [52]. Quality of life can be severely affected by HS and HS has been observed as one of the most distressing conditions in dermatology [53,54]. HS is associated with an increased risk for distinct psychiatric disorders including depression, anxiety disorders and substance-related abuse [55]. Moreover, a meta-analysis found a more than two-fold increased risk for suicide in HS patients [55]. For this reason, physicians treating HS patients should perform a screening for psychiatric comorbidities and initiate psychiatric referral if necessary.

3.2. Medical Therapy

3.2.1. Topical and Intralesional Therapy

In cases of mild-to-moderate disease with limited extent, topical therapy can be considered. Topical clindamycin 1%, applied twice daily on involved areas, is the first-line treatment option for mild-to-moderate disease, especially in absence of deep inflammation or sinus tracts [20,56]. In a small prospective study, topical clindamycin effectively reduced inflammatory lesions compared to placebo [57]. In case of refractory disease after three months of treatment, other treatment options should be considered [20].

Resorchinol is a topical agent with keratinolytic, antipruritic and anti-inflammatory properties and can be applied twice daily on active inflammatory lesions [20]. In a retrospective study with 134 patients, topical resorchinol showed a significant improvement of HiSCR and pain compared to topical clindamycin use [58]. A case series assessing the efficacy of topical resorchinol for mild HS reported significant reduction of inflammatory activity and pain in all treated patients [59].

A current phase II study assesses the efficacy of the topical JAK1/JAK2-inhibitor ruxolitinib (NCT 04414514) [60].

Intralesional injections with glucocorticosteroids as triamcinolonacetonid can be considered for the treatment of solitary acute inflammatory nodules, when rapid reduction of inflammation is desired [61,62]. Clinical response with reduction of inflammation is regularly seen after 48–72 h [20].

3.2.2. Systemic Therapies

Zinc Gluconate

Zinc salts (zinc gluconate) show anti-inflammatory effects in HS, probably through inhibition of chemotaxis of neutrophil granulocytes, modulation of cytokine expression and anti-androgen properties [63]. In HS, a high-dose therapy with 90 mg zinc gluconate per day in gradual dose escalation can be considered as a maintenance therapy for limited disease [20]. In several small studies, zinc gluconate showed promising results in mild-to-moderate HS [64–66]. As zinc competes with copper in gastrointestinal resorption, long-term use of high doses of zinc may cause hypocupremia and anemia; thus, routine monitoring of copper levels and hemoglobin is recommended [67]. Gastrointestinal discomfort is a frequent reported side effect.

Systemic Antibiotic Therapy

Patients with refractory disease under topical therapies or with severe inflammation activity are potential candidates for systemic antibiotic therapy (Table 1). A current study assessed the duration of antibiotic treatments in HS patients and showed that in the majority of oral antibiotic courses the duration of treatment was less than 12 weeks [68].

Recent guideline recommendations recognize tetracyclines as the first-line treatment for more widely spread HS in Hurley stage I/II [20]. Established tetracycline antibiotics include tetracycline, doxycycline and minocycline [69]. A prospective study comparing the efficacy of the different tetracycline antibiotics tetracycline, doxycycline and lymecycline showed a reduction of HSS in all treatment groups with greatest response in the tetracycline group. Moreover, a reduction of pain, formation of new inflammatory lesions and an improvement of quality of life was observed in all treatment groups [70].

An antibiotic combination therapy with clindamycin and rifampicin is recommended as first-line therapy for patients with Hurley stage II and moderate-to-severe disease and as second-line therapy for patients who do not respond on oral tetracycline treatment [20,56]. In an open-label prospective study with 56 patients, the combination of clindamycin and rifampicin showed an overall clinical response with reduction of HSS in 79.6%. HSS_{50} was 37% and complete remission (HSS_{100}) was observed in 13%. Side effects were observed in 55.6% of patients with diarrhea, abdominal pain and nausea being the most commonly reported [71]. This data is strengthened by several retrospective trials, which came to similar results; however, the majority of patients with initial complete remission relapsed after discontinuation of treatment [72–74]. However, due to the role of rifampicin as a potent inductor of the hepatic CYP system, metabolization of clindamycin is intensified within the combination therapy [75,76]. In one study clindamycin blood levels were decreased by around 90% within two weeks after treatment initiation, raising the question of whether the observed response rates under combination antibiotic therapy may be traced to rifampicin alone [77,78]. More research with prospective randomized trials is needed to address this topic.

For more extensive disease with severe inflammation and widespread distribution of inflammatory lesions some intensified antibiotic treatment regimens have been described; however, up to now evidence is based on case report and retrospective analyses, and these therapies have not been evaluated in prospective trials.

Join-Lambert et al. described a broad-spectrum antibiotic combination therapy consisting of rifampicin, moxifloxacin and metronidazole leading to high rates of complete remissions, defined as clearance of all inflammatory lesions, especially in Hurley stage I/II patients [79].

Ertapenem, another broad-spectrum antibiotic, showed rapid improvement in treatment-refractory cases of HS as a rescue therapy [80]. In a retrospective pilot study with 30 patients, a 6 week course of ertapenem led to a significant and sustained improvement of disease severity, assessed with the Sartorius score [81]. Through its rapid clinical improvement, ertapenem may be initiated in severe HS as neoadjuvant therapy for bridging to surgery or other maintenance therapies [80,82,83].

Table 1. Overview of systemic antibiotic regimens in clinical studies.

References	Study Design (Level of Evidence, Oxford Criteria [84])	Treatment Regimen	Efficacy Data/Results
Tetracyclines			
Jemec et al., 1996 [85]	randomized double-blind trial (n = 46) (*evidence level: 1b*)	top. clindamycin (0.1%) b.i.d. vs. tetracycline 500 mg b.i.d.	- no significant differences between treatment groups
Vural et al., 2019 [86]	retrospective analysis of different HS treatments (n = 139) (*evidence level: 4*)	doxycycline 100 mg b.i.d. for 3 months	- HiSCR achieved in 60% - doxycycline as preferred treatment regimen in Hurley stage I/II
Jørgensen et al., 2021 [70]	prospective follow-up study (n = 108) (*evidence level: 2b*)	tetracycline 500 mg b.i.d. (n = 32) vs. doxycycline 100 mg b.i.d. (n = 31) vs. lymecycline 300 mg b.i.d. (n = 45) median treatment duration: 3.2 months	- significant clinical improvements (reductions of HSS) in approx. 30%; - no significant differences between treatment groups (greatest HSS reduction observed in tetracycline group)
Armyra et al., 2017 [87]	prospective study/case series (n = 20) (*evidence level: 4*)	minocycline 100 mg q.d. + colchicine 0.5 mg b.i.d. for 3 months followed by colchicine 0.5 mg b.i.d. for 6 months	- significant clinical improvements (HS-PGA and DLQI)
Clindamycin–Rifampicin Combination Therapy			
Yao et al., 2021 [71]	prospective open-label study (n = 56) (*evidence level: 4*)	clindamycin 300 mg b.i.d. + rifampicin 300 mg b.i.d. for 10 weeks	- at 6 month follow-up: overall response rate 79.6%; HSS_{50} 37%; HSS_{100} 13% - Side effects 55.6% (esp. gastrointestinal)
van der Zee et al., 2009 [73]	retrospective study (n = 34) (*evidence level: 4*)	clindamycin 600 mg b.i.d. + rifampicin 600 mg b.i.d. varying treatment duration (<10 weeks/>10 weeks)	- overall response rate 82.4%; partial remission 35.3%; total remission 47.1% - side effects 38.2% (esp. gastrointestinal)
Gener et al., 2009 [72]	retrospective study (n = 116) (*evidence level: 4*)	clindamycin 300 mg b.i.d. + rifampicin 600 mg q.d. for 10 weeks	- significant reduction of Sartorius score; complete remission in 11% - significant down-staging (Hurley) and reduction of pain
Mendonça et al., 2006 [74]	retrospective study (n = 14) (*evidence level: 4*)	clindamycin 300 mg b.i.d. + rifampicin 300 mg b.i.d for 10 weeks	- overall response rate 82%; complete remission 66.7%

Table 1. Cont.

References	Study Design (Level of Evidence, Oxford Criteria [84])	Treatment Regimen	Efficacy Data/Results
Intensified Antibiotic Treatments			
Join-Lambert et al., 2016 [81]	retrospective study (n = 30) (evidence level: 4)	ertapenem 1 g iv. q.d. for 6 weeks followed by antibiotic consolidation treatment (rifampicin, moxifloxacin, metronidazole)	after 6 weeks (ertapenem): - significant reduction of median Sartorius score - clinical remission in 67%/26% in Hurley stage I/II after 6 months (consolidation): - further significant clinical improvement - clinical remission 100%/96%/27% in Hurley stage I/II/III
Join-Lambert et al., 2011 [79]	retrospective study (n = 28) (evidence level: 4)	rifampicin 10 mg/Kg q.d. + moxifloxacin 400 mg q.d. + metronidazole 500 mg t.i.d. for 6 weeks *, followed by consolidation with rifampicin + moxifloxacin for ≥6 weeks	- complete remission 57% (esp. in Hurley I/II) - most common side effects: gastrointestinal symptoms 64%; vaginal candidiasis 35% (of female pat.)

* In 14 patients initiation therapy with ceftriaxone 1 g iv. q.d. + metronidazole 500 mg t.i.d. for 2 weeks due to severe inflammation.

Hormonal Treatment Approaches

Clinical observations in female HS patients with premenstrual flares and cyclic alterations of inflammation activity led to the suggestion that hormonal alterations may influence the course of HS [88]. Moreover, HS is associated with endocrine disorders such as polycystic ovary syndrome (PCOS) and metabolic syndrome [89,90]. However, the role of hormonal influences on the pathogenesis of HS is still unclear [91]. Most data regarding antiandrogenic treatment approaches for HS are based on retrospective analyses, and case reports and prospective trials are rare (Table 2).

Successful disease control with an antiandrogenic therapy containing ethinylestradiol and cyproteronacetate (CPA) has been described in a case series [92]. In a double-blind controlled cross-over trial comparing two contraceptive regimens containing ethinylestradiol and norgestrel or cyproterone acetate, both treatments produced substantial improvement of disease activity; however, there was no significant difference [93]. In a retrospective study, Kraft et al. compared an antiandrogen treatment approach with antibiotic therapies in 66 female HS patients and found significantly superior response rates, 55% vs. 26%, suggesting that antiandrogen therapy should be considered for all women presenting with HS. Moreover, the authors concluded that female HS patients should be investigated for underlying PCOS and insulin resistance [94].

Spironolactone is a potassium-sparing diuretic with antiandrogen properties due to the inhibition of mineralocorticoid receptors [95]. In several retrospective analyses of female HS patients, spironolactone treatment led to a significant reduction of pain and inflammatory lesions, and improved quality of life [96–98].

The antidiabetic agent metformin reduces insulin resistance by improving peripheral insulin sensitivity and may have some antiandrogen properties [83]. In several retrospective trials and case reports, metformin showed promising clinical response rates and thus may contribute to disease control in HS as an adjunctive treatment option [99–101].

Retinoids

Retinoids influence cell differentiation and may have a beneficial impact in HS by reducing keratinocyte proliferation and subsequently preventing the plugging of the pilosebaceous unit (Table 3) [20]. Moreover, retinoids show anti-inflammatory properties by modifying monocyte chemotaxis [102]. The most common adverse events are retinoid dermatitis and, among women, hair loss. Retinoids have a teratogenic effect and effective contraception must be ensured in patients prior to treatment initiation [20].

Table 2. Clinical studies evaluating hormonal treatment approaches in HS patients.

References	Study Design (Level of Evidence, Oxford Criteria [84])	Treatment Regimen	Efficacy Data/Results
Antiandrogen Treatments			
Kraft et al., 2007 [94]	retrospective chart review patients (n = 64, all female) (*evidence level: 3b*)	various antihormonal treatments (n = 29) - ethinylestradiol 50 µg q.d. + CPA 25 mg q.d. - CPA 25 mg q.d. - Spironolactone 100 mg q.d. - CPA 25 mg q.d. + spironolactone 100 mg q.d.	- antiandrogen therapy superior to oral antibiotics (clinical response 55% vs. 26%) - prevalence of PCOS 38.1%
Sawers et al., 1986 [92]	case series (n = 4, all female) (*evidence level: 4*)	CPA 100 mg q.d. + ethinylestradiol 30–50 mg q.d.	- successful disease control in all patients - reduction of CPA dose led to HS deterioration in 75%
Mortimer et al., 1986 [93]	randomized double-blind crossover trial (n = 24, all female) (*evidence level: 2b*)	- ethinylestradiol 50 µg q.d. + CPA 50 mg q.d. - ethinylestradiol 50 µg q.d. + norgestrel 500 mg q.d.	- substantial improvement of HS in both treatment regimens; no significant difference - antiandrogen therapy may be beneficial in HS treatment
Spironolactone			
Lee et al., 2015 [97]	case series (n = 20, all female) (*evidence level: 4*)	spironolactone 100–150 mg/d ± minocycline ± CPA	- clinical improvement (reduction of HS-PGA) in 85% after 3 months; complete remission in 55% - spironolactone was well tolerated and patients were satisfied with treatment
Golbari et al., 2019 [96]	retrospective single-center chart review (n = 67, all female) (*evidence level: 4*)	spironolactone 25–200 mg/d (average dose 75 mg/d)	- significant reduction of HS-PGA, pain and inflammatory lesions - no significant difference in HS improvement between spironolactone ≤75 mg/d and ≥100 mg/d
Quinlan et al., 2020 [98]	retrospective study (n = 26, all female) (*evidence level: 4*)	spironolactone 50–100 mg/d ± metformin	- reduction of DLQI >5 in 35% - no further clinical data
Metformin			
Verdolini et al., 2013 [101]	prospective study (n = 25) (*evidence level: 4*)	metformin 1000–1700 mg/d over 24 weeks	- significant clinical improvement (reduction of Sartorius score and number of work days lost) in 72% - significant improvement of DLQI in 64%
Jennings et al., 2020 [99]	retrospective chart review (n = 53) (*evidence level: 4*)	metformin; mean dose 1.5 g/d; mean treatment duration 11.3 months	- subjective clinical response in 68%; complete remission of inflammatory skin lesions in 19% - insulin resistance present in 75%, but not predictive for treatment response
Moussa et al., 2020 [100]	retrospective study (n = 16, pediatric HS patients) (*evidence level: 4*)	metformin as adjunctive treatment (dose not specified)	- clinical improvement in 5/16 (31.3%); no improvement in 5/16 (31.3%); 6/16 patients (37.5%) lost to follow-up

Acitretin has been evaluated for the treatment of moderate-to-severe HS in a small prospective trial with 17 patients and showed an overall response rate of 47%; however, another 47% of patients dropped out due to lack of efficacy or adverse events [103]. In a retrospective study with 12 patients, acitretin showed promising results with all treated patients achieving clinical remission and reduction of pain [104]. Another recent retrospective cohort study reported significant clinical responses under acitretin treatment and identified the follicular HS phenotype, a history of follicular plugging diseases and a family history of HS as potential predictive markers for treatment response [105].

Isotretinoin has only shown limited efficacy for treatment of HS and several retrospective studies reported treatment response rates between 16.1% and 35.9% [106–108]. Clinical exacerbations and occurrence of new flares of HS have been reported after initiation of isotretinoin in various cases, which could be explained by the further reduction of the size and action of sebaceous glands due to isotretinoin therapy [109,110].

Table 3. Clinical studies evaluating retinoids for HS treatment.

References	Study Design (Level of Evidence, Oxford Criteria [84])	Treatment Regimen	Efficacy Data/Results
Acitretin			
Boer et al., 2011 [104]	retrospective study (n = 12) (*evidence level: 4*)	acitretin monotherapy; mean dose 0.59 mg/Kg/d; duration 9–12 months (mean 10.8 months)	- all patients achieved clinical remission and reduction of pain - 75% showed prolonged clinical responses
Matusiak et al., 2014 [103]	prospective study (n = 17) (*evidence level: 4*)	acitretin; mean dose 0.56 ± 0.08 mg/Kg/d; treatment duration 9 months	- HSSI ($\geq$50% reduction from baseline) reached in 47% - relapse in most patients after discontinuation of acitretin
Tan et al., 2016 [111]	retrospective study (n = 14) (*evidence level: 4*)	acitretin as monotherapy (43%) or adjunctive to other systemic treatments (57%) (dose not specified)	- no patient under acitretin monotherapy achieved clinical response compared to 87.5% in combination group - acitretin ineffective as monotherapy for HS
Sánchez-Díaz et al., 2022 [105]	retrospective cohort study (n = 62) (*evidence level: 4*)	acitretin (dose not specified)	- significant reduction of IHS4 score - follicular HS phenotype and history of follicular plugging as positive predictive markers
Isotretinoin			
Boer et al., 1999 [106]	retrospective study (n = 68) (*evidence level: 4*)	low-dose isotretinoin; mean dose 0.56 mg/Kg/d; for 4–6 months	- limited efficacy with clinical response in 23.5% and 16.2% maintained responses during follow-up - isotretinoin more effective in mild HS
Soria et al., 2009 [108]	survey-based retrospective study (n = 87) (*evidence level: 4*)	isotretinoin (dose and treatment duration not specified)	- 16.1% of patients reported clinical improvement; 83.9% reported no improvement or worsening of HS symptoms
Patel et al., 2019 [107]	survey-based retrospective study (n = 39) (*evidence level: 4*)	isotretinoin (dose and treatment duration not specified)	- clinical improvement reported by 35.9%; no response reported by 64.1% - presence of pilonidal cyst associated with clinical response

Adalimumab and Other TNFα Inhibitors

Adalimumab, a fully human, IgG1 monoclonal antibody specific for TNFα, is currently the only biologic therapy approved for the treatment of moderate-to-severe HS in adults and adolescent patients $\geq$12 years (Table 4) [20,22,112]. In two phase III multicenter, double-blind, placebo-controlled studies (PIONEER I and PIONEER II) adalimumab showed a significant effectivity compared to placebo with HiSCR rates of 41.8% and 58.9% (vs. 26.0% and 27.6% in placebo groups), respectively [113]. In open-label extension studies patients under adalimumab therapy were followed up for a minimum of 60 weeks and showed maintained treatment responses with HiSCR rates of 62.5% at week 36 and 52.3% at week 168, respectively [114]. Moreover, an improvement of quality of life, measured with the DLQI score, was observed under adalimumab [114,115].

In a retrospective study by Marzano et al. an inverse correlation between therapeutic delay and clinical response on adalimumab was found, suggesting the concept of a "window of opportunity" and supporting an early initiation of adalimumab [116]. Moreover, the efficacy and safety of adalimumab in patients undergoing wide-excision surgery was investigated in a prospective multicenter phase IV trial. Patients with perioperative use of adalimumab showed significant higher HiSCR rates compared to placebo (48% vs. 34%, $p = 0.049$) and adalimumab treatment was not associated with an increased risk of peri- and postoperative complications, supporting combined treatment approaches in extensive disease [117].

Adalimumab can be administered in subcutaneous injections in two treatment regimens with 40 mg every week or 80 mg every other week after an initial loading dose [20]. The therapy is usually well tolerated with injection side reactions being the most common side effects and large meta-analyses have shown non-significant safety issues compared to placebo [118]. In very rare cases malignancies (esp. lymphomas) have been reported under therapy [119,120].

In recent years, adalimumab biosimilars have become a frequently used alternative to the adalimumab originator agent and currently six adalimumab biosimilars are approved by the FDA and EMA [121]. Several studies have demonstrated the bioequivalence and similar safety profiles of the adalimumab biosimilars compared to the originator agent [122,123]. However, a loss of treatment efficacy has been observed after switching from adalimumab originator to biosimilars in clinical studies [124–126]. Kirsten et al. evaluated the clinical responses of 94 patients after switching from adalimumab originator to biosimilar ABP 501, and reported a loss of response or new onset of adverse events in 33.3% [127]. Another retrospective cohort study observed a more rapid loss of efficacy in patients taking adalimumab biosimilars compared to the originator agent and additionally found a greater risk for loss of efficacy in switchers compared to non-switchers, suggesting that, in the management of HS, treatment should begin and continue with the same drug [128]. Prospective studies are needed to further clarify this issue [129].

Infliximab is a chimeric mouse/human IgG1 monoclonal antibody with high affinity to soluble and transmembrane bound TNFα. A recent metanalysis calculated a pooled response rate for infliximab of 83% in patients with moderate-to-severe HS and described a low toxicity with a rate of 2.9% for severe adverse events [130]. In a phase II placebo-controlled crossover study, 57% of patients under infliximab treatment reached a reduction of the HS Severity index (HSSI) of >50% compared to 5% in the placebo group. Additionally, improvements in pain intensity and quality of life were observed with concomitant reduction in clinical markers of inflammation [131]. In another prospective trial, sustained treatment responses were observed in HS patients after a single course of infliximab [132]. Overall, infliximab is a promising treatment option for HS; however, larger prospective randomized trials are needed to investigate its efficacy compared to other biologic therapies [130].

Etanercept, a fusion protein consisting of the extracellular ligand-binding domain of the 75 kDa TNFα receptor and the Fc portion of human IgG1, inhibits TNFα signaling through competitive binding of its ligand [133]. In a small prospective placebo-controlled phase II trial, etanercept showed no significant efficacy compared to placebo [134].

Other TNFα inhibitors like golimumab and certolizumab pegol showed inconstant response rates, and evidence is limited on several case reports and small retrospective studies [135–140].

Table 4. Clinical studies evaluating adalimumab (ADA) for HS treatment.

References	Study Design (Level of Evidence, Oxford Criteria [84])	Treatment Regimen	Efficacy Data/Results
Kimball et al., 2012 [28]	phase II randomized placebo-controlled study (n = 154) (*evidence level: 1b*)	- ADA 40 mg every week from week 4, after initial doses of 160 mg at week 0 and 80 mg at week 2 - ADA 40 mg every other week (EOW) from week 1, after initial dose of 80 mg at week 0 - placebo	- clinical responses (HS-PGA reduction ≥2 from baseline) in 17.6% and 9.6% in ADA groups (weekly/EOW) vs. 3.9% in placebo at week 16 - switching from ADA weekly to ADA EOW dosing resulted in decrease in response
Kimball et al., 2016 [113]	phase III randomized placebo-controlled study (PIONEER I) (n = 307) (*evidence level: 1b*)	- ADA 40 mg every week from week 4, after initial doses of 160 mg at week 0 and 80 mg at week 2 - placebo	- HiSCR achieved in 41.8% vs. 26.0% (ADA vs. placebo) at week 12
Kimball et al., 2016 [113]	phase III randomized placebo-controlled study (PIONEER II) (n = 326) (*evidence level: 1b*)	- ADA 40 mg every week from week 4, after initial doses of 160 mg at week 0 and 80 mg at week 2 ± tetracycline antibiotics - placebo ± tetracycline antibiotics	- HiSCR achieved in 58.9% vs. 27.6% (ADA vs. placebo) at week 12 - significant reduction of inflammatory lesions, pain and modified Sartorius score
Zouboulis et al., 2019 [114]	phase III open-label extension study of PIONEER I/II (n = 88) (*evidence level: 2b*)	ADA 40 mg every week	- HiSCR achieved in 52.3% at week 168 - ADA can be considered for long-term control of HS
Marzano et al., 2021 [116]	retrospective cohort study (n = 389) (*evidence level: 2b*)	ADA 40 mg every week from week 4, after initial doses of 160 mg at week 0 and 80 mg at week 2	- HiSCR achieved in 43.7% at week 16 and in 53.9% at week 52 - significant reduction of DLQI and pain - inverse correlation between therapeutic delay and response to ADA
Bechara et al., 2021 [117]	phase IV randomized placebo-controlled study (n = 206) (*evidence level: 1b*)	HS patients undergoing wide-excision surgery - ADA 40 mg every week - placebo	- HiSCR achieved in 48% vs. 34% (ADA vs. placebo) at week 12 - continuation of ADA treatment was not associated with increased risk for peri-/postoperative complications

3.3. What's Coming Next? Promising Molecular Targets for Future HS Treatment

The increasing interest in inflammation research in recent years contributed to a deeper understanding of the pathogenesis of HS and led to the identification of potential molecular targets for new treatment options [141]. Due to capacity reasons this review focusses on the most advanced clinical approaches, namely targeting the interleukin-17, interleukin-1 axis and the JAK/STAT signaling (Table 5).

3.3.1. Interleukin-17

In recent years, interleukin 17 (IL-17) has emerged as a major player in various autoimmune and inflammatory skin disorders, and its proinflammatory isoforms IL-17A, IL-17C and IL-17F are presumed as key cytokines in HS [142,143]. IL-17A and IL-17F are mainly produced by T-helper 17 cells (T$_{H17}$) and play a major role in control of many fungal and bacterial infections, while IL-17C is released by epithelial cells like keratinocytes, and promotes further inflammation by mediation of the production of other inflammatory molecules and further enhancing the inflammation cascade through stimulation of IL-17A and IL-17F production in T$_{H17}$-cells as a feed forward loop [144,145].

The first evidence for the role of IL-17 in HS was reported by Schlapbach et al., who found a 30-fold increased expression of IL-17A in HS lesions compared to healthy skin [146]. Another study confirmed these findings and identified a dysregulated cytokine milieu in perilesional skin, suggesting that subclinical inflammation may be present in HS skin prior to the formation of active lesions [147]. Moreover, Navrazhina et al. found significantly increased expressions of the proinflammatory IL-17 isoforms A, C and F in lesional, perilesional and even unaffected skin of HS patients compared to healthy individuals [148]. Given these accumulating findings pointing toward a key role of IL-17 signaling in the pathogenesis of HS, targeting the IL-17 pathway seems like a promising treatment approach. However, as HS can be associated with inflammatory bowel disease, it should be kept in mind that paradoxical exacerbations of pre-existing IBD have been reported under anti-IL17 treatment [90,149].

Secukinumab is a recombinant human monoclonal IgG1κ antibody that selectively targets IL-17A and blocks its interaction with the IL-17 receptor [150]. In an open-label pilot study with nine patients, 78% reached HiSCR after 24 weeks of treatment with secukinumab 300 mg every 4 weeks [151]. Another open-label trial with 20 enrolled patients tested two dose levels of secukinumab (300 mg every 2 or 4 weeks after an initial loading dose) and observed pooled HiSCR rates of 70%. Interestingly, clinical responses were also observed in patients with failure to prior anti-TNFα treatment [152].

Recently, the first results of two randomized, placebo-controlled, multicenter phase III trials (SUNSHINE, SUNRISE) evaluating the efficacy of secukinumab in two dose regimens (every 2 weeks or every 4 weeks) have been presented. After 16 weeks, the primary endpoint was reached in both studies for the every 2 weeks (Q2W) regimen and in one for the every 4 weeks (Q4W) regimen, demonstrating the superiority of secukinumab over placebo in patients with moderate-to-severe HS (HiSCR rates: 45% vs. 33.7% (study 1) and 42.3% vs. 31.2% (study 2) for secukinumab 300 mg every 2 weeks, and 41.8% vs. 33.7% (study 1) and 46.1% vs. 31.2% (study 2) for secukinumab every 4 weeks). In both treatment groups secukinumab significantly reduced inflammatory lesions and pain, and improved patients' quality of life [153].

Bimekizumab is another humanized IgG1κ monoclonal antibody, targeting IL-17A and IL-17F. In a recent double-blind, placebo-controlled, phase II clinical trial (ClinicalTrials.gov NCT03248531) 90 patients were randomized to receive bimekizumab (640 mg at week 0, 320 mg every 2 weeks), adalimumab (160 mg at week 0, 80 mg at week 2 and 40 mg every week for weeks 4–10) or placebo. HiSCR was reached in 57.3% of the bimekizumab group compared to 26.1% in the placebo arm. Moreover, 46% of the patients under bimekizumab achieved $HiSCR_{75}$ and 32% achieved $HiSCR_{90}$, compared to 10% and 0% in the placebo group, respectively [34]. These promising results led to the initiation of three placebo-controlled phase III studies, which are currently ongoing (NCT04901195, NCT04242498, NCT04242446).

Nanobodies represent a novel innovative class of antibody-derived targeted therapies. Consisting of one or more domains based on the small antigen binding variable regions of heavy chain antibodies, they are much smaller compared to conventional monoclonal antibodies, facilitating their tissue penetration [154]. Moreover, several nanobodies can be linked to obtain multi-specific molecules [154,155].

Sonelokimab is a trivalent nanobody containing three domains with specificity for IL-17A, IL-17F and human serum albumin, and has already showed clinical efficacy in the treatment of plaque psoriasis in a recent phase II study [156]. An ongoing randomized placebo-controlled trial evaluates the efficacy of sonelokimab in patients with moderate-to-severe hidradenitis suppurativa (ClinicalTrials.gov NCT05322473) [157].

Izokibep, another small, molecular, antibody-mimetic IL-17A inhibitor has recently shown significant clinical responses in patients with psoriatic arthritis and is currently in a placebo-controlled phase II trial in HS (ClinicalTrials.gov NCT05355805) [158].

3.3.2. Interleukin-1

The proinflammatory interleukin-1 pathway is involved in promoting inflammation in HS and IL-1β has been shown to be significantly overexpressed in lesional skin of HS patients [159]. As the primary circulating isoform, IL-1β is expressed by macrophages, monocytes and dendritic cells due to activation of pattern recognition receptors in an inflammasome-dependent process [160]. IL-1β induces the expression of molecules promoting remodeling of the extracellular matrix and immune cell infiltration, making it a potential target for future HS treatments [159].

Anakinra is a recombinant IL-1 receptor antagonist, preventing its interaction with the ligands IL-1α and IL-1β [161]. In a phase II placebo-controlled trial, HiSCR rates of 78% have been described after 12 week treatment compared to 30% in the placebo group; however, the majority of patients relapsed after treatment discontinuation [162]. Another prospective open-label study with five patients reported clinical improvements of inflammation activity and quality of life after an 8 week course of anakinra [163]. Several case reports described inconstant clinical responses with partial improvements and failure of anakinra treatment [140,164–167].

Bermekimab (also known as MABp1) is a recombinant monoclonal antibody that neutralizes IL-1α. In a prospective randomized controlled phase II trial, patients with moderate-to-severe HS, that were not eligible for or failed a prior anti-TNFα treatment, showed significant clinical responses with HiSCR rates of 60% compared to 10% in the placebo group after 12 weeks [168]. Patients who were initially randomized to the placebo group were allowed to continue in an open-label extension study and 75% showed clinical response (HiSCR) after 12 weeks of bermekimab treatment [169].

In another phase II study with 42 patients with moderate-to-severe HS who were naïve to or had failed prior anti-TNFα therapy, significant clinical responses were observed in both groups with HiSCR rates of 63% in the TNFα-failure group and 61% in the TNFα-naïve group, respectively, qualifying bermekimab as potential alternative treatment option for non-responders to anti-TNFα [170].

A randomized placebo and active-comparator-controlled phase IIa/b trial evaluating the efficacy of bermekimab compared to placebo and adalimumab is currently ongoing (ClinicalTrials.gov NCT04988308) [171].

Canakinumab is a human monoclonal antibody targeting IL-1β. There is limited evidence for its efficacy in HS and case reports described contradictory responses [172–174].

Lutikizumab, a human dual variable-domain antibody that selectively binds and inhibits IL-1α and IL-1β, has been previously tested as an anti-inflammatory treatment in osteoarthritis [175,176]. A recent phase II trial studies the efficacy of lutikizumab in HS patients with failure to prior anti-TNFα therapy (ClinicalTrials.gov NCT05139602) [177].

3.3.3. JAK/STAT Inhibitors

The Janus kinase and signal transducers and activators of transcription (JAK/STAT) pathway represents a rapid membrane-to-nucleus cell signaling module, which regulates the expression of various critical mediators of cancer and inflammation [178]. Inhibitors of the JAK/STAT pathway are a potential approach for future treatment of HS, as they enable the simultaneous modulation of expression of different cytokines that are involved in the complex inflammatory process of HS [141,179].

The efficacy of the JAK1 inhibitor INCB054707 was evaluated in two phase II studies (ClinicalTrials.gov NCT03569371, NCT03607487) in patients with moderate-to-severe HS. INCB054707 was well tolerated and clinical improvement of disease was observed; however, the effect was only significant in the high-dose group with 90 mg (HiSCR 88% vs. 57% placebo) [180].

Upadacitinib is a second-generation JAK inhibitor with selectivity for JAK1. In a retrospective cohort study 75% and 100% of patients treated with upadacitinib reached HiSCR after 4 and 12 weeks of treatment, respectively. $HiSCR_{75}$ rates were 30% and 95% after 4 weeks and 12 weeks [181]. These promising observations led to the initiation of a phase II randomized controlled trial with results unpublished (ClinicalTrials.gov NCT04430855) [182].

A phase II trial for topical treatment of early-stage HS lesions with the JAK1/JAK2 inhibitor ruxolitinib is currently ongoing (ClinicalTrials.gov NCT04414514) [60].

Table 5. Results of clinical studies evaluating new treatment approaches for HS (only completed studies with reported study results).

References	Study Design (Level of Evidence, Oxford Criteria [84])	Treatment Regimen	Efficacy Data/Results
IL-17 (Secukinumab)			
Prussick et al., 2019 [151]	open-label pilot study (n = 9) *(evidence level: 4)*	secukinumab 300 mg weekly for 5 weeks (loading dose) followed by 300 mg every 4 weeks for 24 weeks	- HiSCR achieved in 78% after 24 weeks - improvement of Sartorius score and DLQI
Casseres et al., 2020 [152]	open-label study (n = 20) *(evidence level: 4)*	secukinumab 300 mg weekly for 5 weeks (loading dose) followed by 300 mg every 2 or 4 weeks	- pooled HiSCR rate of 70% after 24 weeks - clinical responses were also observed in patients with failure to prior anti-TNFα treatment
Reguiaï et al., 2020 [183]	retrospective study (n = 20) *(evidence level: 4)*	secukinumab 300 mg weekly for 5 weeks (loading dose) followed by 300 mg every 4 weeks	- HiSCR achieved in 75% after 16 weeks - maintained clinical responses during follow-up - 2 patients developed Crohn disease after 3 and 5 months of treatment
Ribero et al., 2021 [184]	retrospective multicenter study (n = 31) *(evidence level: 4)*	secukinumab 300 mg weekly for 5 weeks (loading dose) followed by 300 mg every 4 weeks	- HiSCR achieved in 41% after 28 weeks
Kimball et al., 2022 [153]	2 phase III randomized placebo-controlled trials (n = 1084) - NCT03713619 (SUNSHINE) - NCT03713632 (SUNRISE) *(evidence level: 1b)*	- secukinumab 300 mg every 2 weeks (Q2W) - secukinumab 300 mg every 4 weeks (Q4W) - placebo	- HiSCR rates at week 16: SUNSHINE: 45.0% (Q2W); 41.8% (QW4); 33.7% (placebo) SUNRISE: 42.3% (Q2W); 46.1% (QW4); 31.2% (placebo) - superiority of secukinumab over placebo in moderate-to-severe HS - rapid clinical responses (observed from week 2) - acceptable safety profile
IL-17 (Bimekizumab)			
Glatt et al., 2021 [34]	phase II randomized placebo- and active-comparator-controlled trial (n = 90) *(evidence level: 1b)*	- bimekizumab 640 mg at week 0 followed by 320 mg every 2 weeks - adalimumab 160 mg at week 0, 80 mg at week 2, followed by 40 mg every week - placebo	- HiSCR was achieved in 57.3% in the bimekizumab group at week 12 (vs. 26.1% in placebo group) - HiSCR75 rates of 46.0% in bimekizumab group at week 12 (vs. 10% in placebo group; 35% in adalimumab group) - HiSCR90 reached in 32% of patients with bimekizumab (vs. 0% in placebo group; 15% in adalimumab group)

Table 5. Cont.

References	Study Design (Level of Evidence, Oxford Criteria [84])	Treatment Regimen	Efficacy Data/Results
IL-1 (Anakinra)			
Leslie et al., 2014 [163]	open-label study (n = 6) (*evidence level: 4*)	anakinra 100 mg daily for 8 weeks	- clinical responses with reduction of mSS and improvement of DLQI - rapid relapses after treatment discontinuation in the follow-up period
Tzanetakou et al., 2016 [162]	phase II randomized placebo-controlled trial (n = 20) (*evidence level: 2b*)	- anakinra 100 mg daily for 12 weeks - placebo	- HiSCR achieved in 78% after 12 weeks (vs. 30% in placebo group) - modulation of cytokine production in peripheral blood mononuclear cells - majority of patients relapse after treatment discontinuation
IL-1α (MABp1/Bermekimab)			
Kanni et al., 2018 [168]	phase II randomized placebo-controlled trial (n = 20); patients not eligible for anti-TNFα treatment (*evidence level: 2b*)	- MABp1 (bermekimab) 7.5 mg/Kg every 2 weeks for 12 weeks - placebo	- HiSCR achieved in 60% vs. 10% (MABp1 vs. placebo) at week 12 - maintained clinical responses in 40% after 24 weeks
Kanni et al., 2021 [169]	open-label extension study of NCT02643654 (n = 8 *¹) (*evidence level: 4*)	MABp1 (bermekimab) 7.5 mg/Kg every 2 weeks for 12 weeks	patients initially randomized to placebo achieved HiSCR in 75% after 12 weeks of MABp1 treatment
Gottlieb et al., 2020 [170]	phase II open-label study (n = 42) (*evidence level: 3b*)	bermekimab 400 mg every week for 12 weeks in - patients with failure to prior anti-TNFα therapy (group A) - patients naïve to anti-TNFα therapy (group B)	- comparable HiSCR rates after 12 weeks with 63% (group A) and 61% (group B) - bermekimab as potential treatment alternative for TNFα non-responders
JAK/STAT Inhibitors			
Alavi et al., 2022 [180]	open-label study (NCT03569371) (n = 10) (*evidence level: 4*)	INCB054707 15 mg p.o. daily for 8 weeks	- HiSCR achieved in 43% at week 8 - 70% experienced at least one AE (esp. upper respiratory tract infections)
Alavi et al., 2022 [180]	phase II randomized placebo-controlled trial (NCT03607487) (n = 35) (*evidence level: 2b*)	- INCB054707 in escalating dose regimens (30/60/90 mg daily) for 8 weeks - placebo	- dose dependent clinical responses; HiSCR rates of 56%/56%/88% (30/60/90 mg group) vs. 57% (placebo) - asymptomatic thrombocytopenia occurred in 4 patients of the 90 mg group, resolved after dose interruption
Kozera et al., 2022 [181]	retrospective cohort study (n = 20) (*evidence level: 4*)	upadacitinib for 12 weeks - 15 mg p.o. daily until week 4 - at week 4: patients failing HiSCR were switched to 30 mg daily	- HiSCR rates of 75% after 4 weeks and 100% after 12 weeks - HiSCR75 achieved in 95% after 12 weeks

*¹ Patients initially randomized to placebo group.

3.4. Surgical Treatment Options

There are various options for surgical intervention, requiring an individualized strategy that considers multiple factors such as the types of lesions, inflammation activity and patients' preferences [185,186]. In general, surgical intervention in HS is mostly reserved for advanced cases with irreversible tissue destruction, such as sinus tracts, scars and contractions [187]. Malignancies, especially cutaneous squamous cell carcinoma, represent a rare, yet severe complication in HS patients and, in suspected cases, an early surgical excision is recommended [188]. Moreover, surgery can be considered for chronic inflammatory lesions that do not respond on conservative therapies and for the treatment of acute inflammatory lesions when rapid symptom relief is desired [20]. However, it should be noted that there is no generally accepted consensus on the definition and application of distinct surgical techniques in HS and comparative studies are rare [22]. Moreover, a clear definition of the terminus "recurrence after surgery" is still missing.

3.4.1. Incision and Drainage

In acute cases with abscess formation, incision and drainage can be considered for acute pain relief, although this is only a symptom treatment with nearly 100% recurrence rates [189]. As deroofing can be performed approximately in the same amount of time, coming with higher recurrence-free rates, experts recommend deroofing over incision and drainage [41].

3.4.2. Deroofing

Deroofing describes a superficial removal of the skin covering an inflammatory nodule or a solitary sinus tract, exposing the partially epithelialized basis of the lesion with subsequently curettage of the gelatinous granulation tissue [190–192]. The advantages of this procedure are its simplicity, cost-effectiveness and that it can be performed under local anesthesia, qualifying this method for treatment of inflammatory nodules, abscesses and solitary sinus tracts [186]. In a small study with 44 patients undergoing deroofing of axillary or inguinal HS lesions, 87% were recurrence-free in the follow-up interval of five years [193].

The skin-tissue-sparing excision with electrosurgical peeling (STEEP) method represents a similar surgical approach and was first described by Blok et al. [194]. Here, successive tangential excisions are performed with an electrosurgical wire loop until the epithelialized bottom of the lesion is exposed, whilst saving as much healthy tissue as possible. Although this surgical technique is associated with a short time to wound healing and a low risk of wound contraction, no long-term outcomes are reported and evidence is limited on small case series [195].

3.4.3. Excision

Excision describes the complete removal of the affected tissue and represents a more invasive surgical approach in HS. Depending on the extent of resection experts differentiate between limited, wide and radical excisions; however, there are no generally accepted definitions and distinctions between surgical interventions are blurred [186]. Van Rappard et al. defined limited or localized excisions as the complete excision of the affected tissue, beyond the borders of activity, leaving clear margins [196]. Limited excisions represent a low-invasive surgical approach, appropriate for the treatment of recurrent inflammatory nodules or abscesses and solitary sinus tracts in Hurley stage I or II, and can be performed under local anesthesia in an outpatient setting [196]. Wide excisions are understood as the surgical removal of the affected tissue including the surrounding subcutaneous fat and perilesional skin with an additional resection margin [197,198]. In severe cases, radical excisions with the complete removal of the entire hair bearing area including the subcutaneous fat to the underlying fascia of an affected body region can be performed [20]. Nesmith et al. suggested an additional superficial lymphadenectomy for a further reduction of the risk of recurrence [199].

In cases of extensive disease with multiple or confluent sinus tracts, preoperative MRI- or ultrasound-based imaging methods or an intraoperative use of dye mapping methods, such as methyl violet or iodine starch, can contribute to an improved visualization of the surgical site [200–202].

Although there are no accepted definitions for surgical techniques and recurrence in HS, it is generally considered that more extensive resections are associated with a lower risk of recurrence [203].

3.4.4. Laser-Based Therapies

Various laser and light-based therapies have gained increasing attention as a possible treatment modality for HS [204].

The carbon dioxide (CO_2) laser acts at a wavelength of 10,600 nm and can be used for tissue ablation in different modalities, namely vaporization and excision. CO_2-laser vaporization represents a tissue-sparing treatment option, that aims on a focal destruction of chronic or inflammatory HS lesions, and was first described by Dalrymple et al. for the treatment of sinus tracts [205]. In two case series, Lapins et al. reported low local recurrence rates and satisfactory postoperative outcomes after a stepwise horizontal CO_2-laser evaporation of sinus tracts in Hurley stage II patients [206,207]. Another retrospective study showed similar outcomes, but described local recurrence rates of 29% [208]. A retrospective study evaluated the outcomes of 185 treated sites of 61 HS patients after CO2-laser excision or marsupialization with secondary intention healing, and demonstrated fast healing rates and a local recurrence rate of 1% [209].

Summarizing, CO_2-laser interventions are tissue-sparing treatment options for HS lesions with fast postoperative wound healing and low complication rates. As they can be performed under local anesthesia and wounds are generally allowed to heal by secondary intention, these treatments seem suitable for an outpatient setting [204].

Neodymium-doped yttrium aluminum garnet (Nd:YAG) lasers act as non-ablative lasers at a wavelength of 1064 nm and enable a selective photothermolysis of hair follicles [210]. Their efficacy has been demonstrated in several randomized controlled studies, leading to significant clinical improvements and prevention of new inflammatory lesions in the treated body areas of HS patients [211,212]. In a histopathologic study, an initially increased perifollicular inflammation, observed after 1 week of treatment, was followed by a fibrotic tissue transformation after 4–8 weeks of treatment [213]. Axillary and inguinal areas have been shown to be more responsive to Nd:YAG-laser treatment compared to inframammary and gluteal regions [212].

Moreover, combination treatments consisting of Nd:YAG-laser-mediated hair follicle destruction and CO_2-laser ablation of HS lesions have shown superior clinical responses [214,215].

3.4.5. Postoperative Wound Management and Wound Closure Options

There are various options for wound closure after surgical intervention, including healing by secondary intention, application of skin grafts and primary wound closure techniques [20]. Rompel et al. analyzed the outcomes of 106 HS patients undergoing radical excision and found no correlation between recurrence rates and the type of surgical reconstruction [201]. However, a current meta-analysis reported recurrence rates following wide surgical excision with 15% after primary wound closure, 8% after skin flap reconstruction and 6% after application of skin grafts, respectively [216]. Ovadja et al. described similar results with the highest recurrence rates after primary wound closure and lowest recurrence rates after skin graft coverage [217].

Negative pressure wound therapy (NPWT) has been shown to improve wound healing and wound granulation by increasing tissue oxygenation and reducing the bacterial load [218]. In HS, NPWT can be considered for postoperative wound management following wide or radical excisions. After completion of NPWT-assisted wound granulation, healing by secondary intention or defect coverage with skin grafts can be performed [219].

A small study analyzing NPWT for axillary wound management following wide excisions in HS patients reported a reduced time of hospitalization, and low recurrence and complication rates [220].

Postoperative secondary intention healing is a well established approach for wounds after surgical intervention with low recurrence rates and favorable functional outcomes [221]. However, the time to complete wound healing is generally longer than in primary wound closure options and frequent follow-up visits should be recommended to ensure optimal results [222].

Skin grafts can be considered for defect coverage following extensive excisions or in critical areas with a high risk for postoperative scar contraction. In HS split-thickness skin grafts (STSG) are the most frequently used skin grafts, as in comparison to full thickness skin grafts harvesting is easier and less invasive [223]. If required, meshing of STSG can achieve coverage of larger wound areas [224]. In a comparative study by Morgan et al. split-thickness skin grafts showed faster wound healing than healing by secondary intention. However, secondary healing with frequent wound dressing resulted in certain healing with good cosmetic results and avoided the need for immobilization and a painful donor site. Most patients in this study preferred secondary wound healing to skin grafting [222]. Another retrospective study analyzed the outcomes of HS patients after axillary reconstruction with STSG and skin flaps, and found no significant differences in postoperative outcome and recurrence rates [225].

Primary wound closure represents an option for closure of small excision wounds, especially in cases with limited disease [196]. However, primary wound closure is associated with a high risk of local recurrence [216,226].

Skin flaps can be considered as a more complex reconstructive approach for wounds after larger excisions, especially when critical anatomical structures, such as nerves or blood vessels, are exposed or when there is a risk for postoperative scarring and contraction [227]. As local flaps bear the risk of containing HS affected skin, reconstruction with skin flaps should only be performed after wide surgical excisions [228]. Currently, there is a large number of different skin flaps that have been described for HS reconstruction and frequently used flaps are lateral thoracic island fasciocutaneous flaps [229], Limberg transposition flaps [230], fasciocutaneous perforator-based flaps [231], myocutaneous flaps [232,233] and thoracodorsal artery perforator flaps [234,235].

4. Conclusions

Treatment of hidradenitis suppurativa is often challenging and should be performed with an individualized, patient-oriented approach considering medical and surgical treatment modalities. Several promising novel treatment approaches, including antibodies, nanobodies, small molecules and hormonal treatments, are currently being investigated in clinical studies and could enrich the therapeutic spectrum for HS.

Author Contributions: Conceptualization, L.O. and F.G.B.; methodology, L.O. and F.G.B.; validation L.O., N.A.R., C.S. (Caroline Seifert), C.S. (Christina Scheel) and F.G.B., formal analysis L.O. and F.G.B.; resources, L.O. and F.G.B.; writing—original draft preparation, L.O.; writing—review and editing, L.O., F.G.B., N.A.R., C.S. (Caroline Seifert) and C.S. (Christina Scheel); visualization, L.O.; supervision, F.G.B.; project administration, L.O. and F.G.B.; funding acquisition, L.O. All authors have read and agreed to the published version of the manuscript.

Funding: This research received no external funding, except for the Open Access Publication Funds of the Ruhr-Universität Bochum.

Institutional Review Board Statement: Not applicable.

Data Availability Statement: Not applicable.

Acknowledgments: We acknowledge support by the Open Access Publication Funds of the Ruhr-Universität Bochum.

Conflicts of Interest: F.G.B. has received honoraria for participation in advisory boards, in clinical trials and/or as a speaker from AbbVie Inc., AbbVie Deutschland GmbH & Co. KG, Boehringer Ingelheim Pharma GmbH & Co. KG, Novartis Pharma GmbH, UCB Pharma, Incyte Corporation and JanssenCilag GmbH, MoonLake. The other authors declare no conflict of interest. The funders had no role in the design of the study; in the collection, analyses, or interpretation of data; in the writing of the manuscript; or in the decision to publish the results.

References

1. Garg, A.; Kirby, J.S.; Lavian, J.; Lin, G.; Strunk, A. Sex- and Age-Adjusted Population Analysis of Prevalence Estimates for Hidradenitis Suppurativa in the United States. *JAMA Dermatol.* **2017**, *153*, 760–764. [CrossRef] [PubMed]
2. Theut Riis, P.; Pedersen, O.B.; Sigsgaard, V.; Erikstrup, C.; Paarup, H.M.; Nielsen, K.R.; Burgdorf, K.S.; Hjalgrim, H.; Rostgaard, K.; Banasik, K.; et al. Prevalence of Patients with Self-Reported Hidradenitis Suppurativa in a Cohort of Danish Blood Donors: A Cross-Sectional Study. *Br. J. Dermatol.* **2019**, *180*, 774–781. [CrossRef] [PubMed]
3. Jfri, A.; Nassim, D.; O'Brien, E.; Gulliver, W.; Nikolakis, G.; Zouboulis, C.C. Prevalence of Hidradenitis Suppurativa: A Systematic Review and Meta-Regression Analysis. *JAMA Dermatol.* **2021**, *157*, 924–931. [CrossRef]
4. Jemec, G.B.; Heidenheim, M.; Nielsen, N.H. The Prevalence of Hidradenitis Suppurativa and Its Potential Precursor Lesions. *J. Am. Acad. Dermatol.* **1996**, *35*, 191–194. [CrossRef]
5. Mac Mahon, J.; Kirthi, S.; Byrne, N.; O'Grady, C.; Tobin, A. An Update on Health-Related Quality of Life and Patient-Reported Outcomes in Hidradenitis Suppurativa. *Patient Relat. Outcome Meas.* **2020**, *11*, 21–26. [CrossRef] [PubMed]
6. Sampogna, F.; Abeni, D.; Gieler, U.; Tomas-Aragones, L.; Lien, L.; Titeca, G.; Jemec, G.B.E.; Misery, L.; Szabó, C.; Linder, M.D.; et al. Impairment of Sexual Life in 3485 Dermatological Outpatients From a Multicentre Study in 13 European Countries. *Acta Derm. Venereol.* **2017**, *97*, 478–482. [CrossRef]
7. Savage, K.T.; Singh, V.; Patel, Z.S.; Yannuzzi, C.A.; McKenzie-Brown, A.M.; Lowes, M.A.; Orenstein, L.A.V. Pain Management in Hidradenitis Suppurativa and a Proposed Treatment Algorithm. *J. Am. Acad. Dermatol.* **2021**, *85*, 187–199. [CrossRef] [PubMed]
8. Smith, H.S.; Chao, J.D.; Teitelbaum, J. Painful Hidradenitis Suppurativa. *Clin. J. Pain* **2010**, *26*, 435–444. [CrossRef] [PubMed]
9. Theut Riis, P.; Thorlacius, L.; Knudsen List, E.; Jemec, G.B.E. A Pilot Study of Unemployment in Patients with Hidradenitis Suppurativa in Denmark. *Br. J. Dermatol.* **2017**, *176*, 1083–1085. [CrossRef] [PubMed]
10. Saunte, D.M.; Boer, J.; Stratigos, A.; Szepietowski, J.C.; Hamzavi, I.; Kim, K.H.; Zarchi, K.; Antoniou, C.; Matusiak, L.; Lim, H.W.; et al. Diagnostic Delay in Hidradenitis Suppurativa Is a Global Problem. *Br. J. Dermatol.* **2015**, *173*, 1546–1549. [CrossRef] [PubMed]
11. Kokolakis, G.; Wolk, K.; Schneider-Burrus, S.; Kalus, S.; Barbus, S.; Gomis-Kleindienst, S.; Sabat, R. Delayed Diagnosis of Hidradenitis Suppurativa and Its Effect on Patients and Healthcare System. *Dermatology* **2020**, *236*, 421–430. [CrossRef]
12. Shlyankevich, J.; Chen, A.J.; Kim, G.E.; Kimball, A.B. Hidradenitis Suppurativa Is a Systemic Disease with Substantial Comorbidity Burden: A Chart-Verified Case-Control Analysis. *J. Am. Acad. Dermatol.* **2014**, *71*, 1144–1150. [CrossRef] [PubMed]
13. Deckers, I.E.; Benhadou, F.; Koldijk, M.J.; Del Marmol, V.; Horváth, B.; Boer, J.; van der Zee, H.H.; Prens, E.P. Inflammatory Bowel Disease Is Associated with Hidradenitis Suppurativa: Results from a Multicenter Cross-Sectional Study. *J. Am. Acad. Dermatol.* **2017**, *76*, 49–53. [CrossRef]
14. Egeberg, A.; Gislason, G.H.; Hansen, P.R. Risk of Major Adverse Cardiovascular Events and All-Cause Mortality in Patients With Hidradenitis Suppurativa. *JAMA Dermatol.* **2016**, *152*, 429–434. [CrossRef]
15. Patel, K.R.; Lee, H.H.; Rastogi, S.; Vakharia, P.P.; Hua, T.; Chhiba, K.; Singam, V.; Silverberg, J.I. Association between Hidradenitis Suppurativa, Depression, Anxiety, and Suicidality: A Systematic Review and Meta-Analysis. *J. Am. Acad. Dermatol.* **2020**, *83*, 737–744. [CrossRef] [PubMed]
16. Richette, P.; Molto, A.; Viguier, M.; Dawidowicz, K.; Hayem, G.; Nassif, A.; Wendling, D.; Aubin, F.; Lioté, F.; Bachelez, H. Hidradenitis Suppurativa Associated with Spondyloarthritis—Results from a Multicenter National Prospective Study. *J. Rheumatol.* **2014**, *41*, 490–494. [CrossRef] [PubMed]
17. Sabat, R.; Chanwangpong, A.; Schneider-Burrus, S.; Metternich, D.; Kokolakis, G.; Kurek, A.; Philipp, S.; Uribe, D.; Wolk, K.; Sterry, W. Increased Prevalence of Metabolic Syndrome in Patients with Acne Inversa. *PLoS ONE* **2012**, *7*, e31810. [CrossRef] [PubMed]
18. Garg, A.; Malviya, N.; Strunk, A.; Wright, S.; Alavi, A.; Alhusayen, R.; Alikhan, A.; Daveluy, S.D.; Delorme, I.; Goldfarb, N.; et al. Comorbidity Screening in Hidradenitis Suppurativa: Evidence-Based Recommendations from the US and Canadian Hidradenitis Suppurativa Foundations. *J. Am. Acad. Dermatol.* **2022**, *86*, 1092–1101. [CrossRef] [PubMed]
19. Timila Touhouche, A.; Chaput, B.; Marie Rouquet, R.; Montastier, E.; Caron, P.; Gall, Y.; Aquilina, C.; Boulinguez, S.; Claude Marguery, M.; Giordano-Labadie, F.; et al. Integrated Multidisciplinary Approach to Hidradenitis Suppurativa in Clinical Practice. *Int. J. Womens Dermatol.* **2020**, *6*, 164–168. [CrossRef]
20. Zouboulis, C.C.; Desai, N.; Emtestam, L.; Hunger, R.E.; Ioannides, D.; Juhász, I.; Lapins, J.; Matusiak, L.; Prens, E.P.; Revuz, J.; et al. European S1 Guideline for the Treatment of Hidradenitis Suppurativa/Acne Inversa. *J. Eur. Acad. Dermatol. Venereol.* **2015**, *29*, 619–644. [CrossRef]
21. Seyed Jafari, S.M.; Hunger, R.E.; Schlapbach, C. Hidradenitis Suppurativa: Current Understanding of Pathogenic Mechanisms and Suggestion for Treatment Algorithm. *Front. Med.* **2020**, *7*, 68. [CrossRef] [PubMed]

22. Sabat, R.; Jemec, G.B.E.; Matusiak, Ł.; Kimball, A.B.; Prens, E.; Wolk, K. Hidradenitis Suppurativa. *Nat. Rev. Dis. Primer* **2020**, *6*, 18. [CrossRef]
23. Harry, J. Hurley Axillary Hyperhidrosis, Apocrine Bromhidrosis, Hidradenitis Suppurativa and Familial Benign Pemphigus: Surgical Approach. In *Roenigk & Roenigk's Dermatologic Surgery: Principles and Practice*, 2nd ed.; Marcel Dekker Inc.: New York, NY, USA, 1996; pp. 623–646. ISBN 978-0-8247-9503-0.
24. Napolitano, M.; Megna, M.; Timoshchuk, E.A.; Patruno, C.; Balato, N.; Fabbrocini, G.; Monfrecola, G. Hidradenitis Suppurativa: From Pathogenesis to Diagnosis and Treatment. *Clin. Cosmet. Investig. Dermatol.* **2017**, *10*, 105–115. [CrossRef] [PubMed]
25. Rondags, A.; van Straalen, K.R.; van Hasselt, J.R.; Janse, I.C.; Ardon, C.B.; Vossen, A.R.; Prens, E.P.; van der Zee, H.H.; Horváth, B. Correlation of the Refined Hurley Classification for Hidradenitis Suppurativa with Patient-Reported Quality of Life and Objective Disease Severity Assessment. *Br. J. Dermatol.* **2019**, *180*, 1214–1220. [CrossRef]
26. Sartorius, K.; Lapins, J.; Emtestam, L.; Jemec, G.B.E. Suggestions for Uniform Outcome Variables When Reporting Treatment Effects in Hidradenitis Suppurativa. *Br. J. Dermatol.* **2003**, *149*, 211–213. [CrossRef] [PubMed]
27. Sartorius, K.; Emtestam, L.; Jemec, G.B.E.; Lapins, J. Objective Scoring of Hidradenitis Suppurativa Reflecting the Role of Tobacco Smoking and Obesity. *Br. J. Dermatol.* **2009**, *161*, 831–839. [CrossRef]
28. Kimball, A.B.; Kerdel, F.; Adams, D.; Mrowietz, U.; Gelfand, J.M.; Gniadecki, R.; Prens, E.P.; Schlessinger, J.; Zouboulis, C.C.; van der Zee, H.H.; et al. Adalimumab for the Treatment of Moderate to Severe Hidradenitis Suppurativa: A Parallel Randomized Trial. *Ann. Intern. Med.* **2012**, *157*, 846–855. [CrossRef]
29. Monfrecola, G.; Megna, M. Classification and Severity Scales. In *Hidradenitis Suppurativa*; John Wiley & Sons, Ltd.: Hoboken, NJ, USA, 2017; pp. 39–45. ISBN 978-1-119-42429-1.
30. Hessam, S.; Scholl, L.; Sand, M.; Schmitz, L.; Reitenbach, S.; Bechara, F.G. A Novel Severity Assessment Scoring System for Hidradenitis Suppurativa. *JAMA Dermatol.* **2018**, *154*, 330–335. [CrossRef] [PubMed]
31. Kokolakis, G.; Sabat, R. Distinguishing Mild, Moderate, and Severe Hidradenitis Suppurativa. *JAMA Dermatol.* **2018**, *154*, 971–972. [CrossRef] [PubMed]
32. Kimball, A.B.; Jemec, G.B.E.; Yang, M.; Kageleiry, A.; Signorovitch, J.E.; Okun, M.M.; Gu, Y.; Wang, K.; Mulani, P.; Sundaram, M. Assessing the Validity, Responsiveness and Meaningfulness of the Hidradenitis Suppurativa Clinical Response (HiSCR) as the Clinical Endpoint for Hidradenitis Suppurativa Treatment. *Br. J. Dermatol.* **2014**, *171*, 1434–1442. [CrossRef]
33. Kimball, A.B.; Sobell, J.M.; Zouboulis, C.C.; Gu, Y.; Williams, D.A.; Sundaram, M.; Teixeira, H.D.; Jemec, G.B.E. HiSCR (Hidradenitis Suppurativa Clinical Response): A Novel Clinical Endpoint to Evaluate Therapeutic Outcomes in Patients with Hidradenitis Suppurativa from the Placebo-Controlled Portion of a Phase 2 Adalimumab Study. *J. Eur. Acad. Dermatol. Venereol. JEADV* **2016**, *30*, 989–994. [CrossRef]
34. Glatt, S.; Jemec, G.B.E.; Forman, S.; Sayed, C.; Schmieder, G.; Weisman, J.; Rolleri, R.; Seegobin, S.; Baeten, D.; Ionescu, L.; et al. Efficacy and Safety of Bimekizumab in Moderate to Severe Hidradenitis Suppurativa: A Phase 2, Double-Blind, Placebo-Controlled Randomized Clinical Trial. *JAMA Dermatol.* **2021**, *157*, 1279–1288. [CrossRef] [PubMed]
35. Zouboulis, C.C.; Tzellos, T.; Kyrgidis, A.; Jemec, G.B.E.; Bechara, F.G.; Giamarellos-Bourboulis, E.J.; Ingram, J.R.; Kanni, T.; Karagiannidis, I.; Martorell, A.; et al. Development and Validation of the International Hidradenitis Suppurativa Severity Score System (IHS4), a Novel Dynamic Scoring System to Assess HS Severity. *Br. J. Dermatol.* **2017**, *177*, 1401–1409. [CrossRef]
36. Tzellos, T.; van Straalen, K.R.; Kyrgidis, A.; Alavi, A.; Goldfarb, N.; Gulliver, W.; Jemec, G.B.E.; Lowes, M.A.; Marzano, A.V.; Prens, E.P.; et al. Development and Validation of IHS4-55, an IHS4 Dichotomous Outcome to Assess Treatment Effect for Hidradenitis Suppurativa. *J. Eur. Acad. Dermatol. Venereol.* **2022**, 1–7. [CrossRef]
37. Kelekis, N.L.; Efstathopoulos, E.; Balanika, A.; Spyridopoulos, T.N.; Pelekanou, A.; Kanni, T.; Savva, A.; Brountzos, E.; Giamarellos-Bourboulis, E.J. Ultrasound Aids in Diagnosis and Severity Assessment of Hidradenitis Suppurativa. *Br. J. Dermatol.* **2010**, *162*, 1400–1402. [CrossRef]
38. Nazzaro, G.; Calzari, P.; Passoni, E.; Vaienti, S.; Moltrasio, C.; Barbareschi, M.; Muratori, S.; Veraldi, S.; Marzano, A.V. Vascularization and Fibrosis Are Important Ultrasonographic Tools for Assessing Response to Adalimumab in Hidradenitis Suppurativa: Prospective Study of 32 Patients. *Dermatol. Ther.* **2021**, *34*, e14706. [CrossRef] [PubMed]
39. Wortsman, X.; Moreno, C.; Soto, R.; Arellano, J.; Pezo, C.; Wortsman, J. Ultrasound In-Depth Characterization and Staging of Hidradenitis Suppurativa. *Dermatol. Surg.* **2013**, *39*, 1835–1842. [CrossRef] [PubMed]
40. Nazzaro, G.; Passoni, E.; Muratori, S.; Moltrasio, C.; Guanziroli, E.; Barbareschi, M.; Veraldi, S.; Marzano, A.V. Comparison of Clinical and Sonographic Scores in Hidradenitis Suppurativa and Proposal of a Novel Ultrasound Scoring System. *Ital. J. Dermatol. Venereol.* **2021**, *156*, 235–239. [CrossRef]
41. Alikhan, A.; Sayed, C.; Alavi, A.; Alhusayen, R.; Brassard, A.; Burkhart, C.; Crowell, K.; Eisen, D.B.; Gottlieb, A.B.; Hamzavi, I.; et al. North American Clinical Management Guidelines for Hidradenitis Suppurativa: A Publication from the United States and Canadian Hidradenitis Suppurativa Foundations: Part II: Topical, Intralesional, and Systemic Medical Management. *J. Am. Acad. Dermatol.* **2019**, *81*, 91–101. [CrossRef]
42. Kromann, C.B.; Deckers, I.E.; Esmann, S.; Boer, J.; Prens, E.P.; Jemec, G.B.E. Risk Factors, Clinical Course and Long-Term Prognosis in Hidradenitis Suppurativa: A Cross-Sectional Study. *Br. J. Dermatol.* **2014**, *171*, 819–824. [CrossRef]
43. Bukvić Mokos, Z.; Miše, J.; Balić, A.; Marinović, B. Understanding the Relationship Between Smoking and Hidradenitis Suppurativa. *Acta Dermatovenerol. Croat. ADC* **2020**, *28*, 9–13. [PubMed]

44. Melnik, B.C.; John, S.M.; Chen, W.; Plewig, G. T Helper 17 Cell/Regulatory T-Cell Imbalance in Hidradenitis Suppurativa/Acne Inversa: The Link to Hair Follicle Dissection, Obesity, Smoking and Autoimmune Comorbidities. *Br. J. Dermatol.* **2018**, *179*, 260–272. [CrossRef] [PubMed]
45. Revuz, J.E.; Canoui-Poitrine, F.; Wolkenstein, P.; Viallette, C.; Gabison, G.; Pouget, F.; Poli, F.; Faye, O.; Roujeau, J.C.; Bonnelye, G.; et al. Prevalence and Factors Associated with Hidradenitis Suppurativa: Results from Two Case-Control Studies. *J. Am. Acad. Dermatol.* **2008**, *59*, 596–601. [CrossRef] [PubMed]
46. Kromann, C.B.; Ibler, K.S.; Kristiansen, V.B.; Jemec, G.B.E. The Influence of Body Weight on the Prevalence and Severity of Hidradenitis Suppurativa. *Acta Derm. Venereol.* **2014**, *94*, 553–557. [CrossRef]
47. Brandwein, M.; Katz, I.; Katz, A.; Kohen, R. Beyond the Gut: Skin Microbiome Compositional Changes Are Associated with BMI. *Hum. Microbiome J.* **2019**, *13*, 100063. [CrossRef]
48. Darlenski, R.; Mihaylova, V.; Handjieva-Darlenska, T. The Link Between Obesity and the Skin. *Front. Nutr.* **2022**, *9*, 855573. [CrossRef]
49. Gallagher, C.; Kirthi, S.; Burke, T.; O'Shea, D.; Tobin, A.-M. Remission of Hidradenitis Suppurativa after Bariatric Surgery. *JAAD Case Rep.* **2017**, *3*, 436–437. [CrossRef]
50. Khan, A.; Chang, M.W. The Role of Nutrition in Acne Vulgaris and Hidradenitis Suppurativa. *Clin. Dermatol.* **2022**, *40*, 114–121. [CrossRef] [PubMed]
51. Canard, C.; Cives, A.D.; Gaubil-Kaladjian, I.; Bertin, E.; Viguier, M. Impact of Bariatric Surgery on Hidradenitis Suppurativa. *Acta Derm. Venereol.* **2021**, *101*, adv00471. [CrossRef] [PubMed]
52. Esmann, S.; Jemec, G.B.E. Psychosocial Impact of Hidradenitis Suppurativa: A Qualitative Study. *Acta Derm. Venereol.* **2011**, *91*, 328–332. [CrossRef]
53. Matusiak, Ł.; Bieniek, A.; Szepietowski, J.C. Hidradenitis Suppurativa Markedly Decreases Quality of Life and Professional Activity. *J. Am. Acad. Dermatol.* **2010**, *62*, 706–708.e1. [CrossRef]
54. Wolkenstein, P.; Loundou, A.; Barrau, K.; Auquier, P.; Revuz, J. Quality of Life Impairment in Hidradenitis Suppurativa: A Study of 61 Cases. *J. Am. Acad. Dermatol.* **2007**, *56*, 621–623. [CrossRef] [PubMed]
55. Phan, K.; Huo, Y.R.; Smith, S.D. Hidradenitis Suppurativa and Psychiatric Comorbidities, Suicides and Substance Abuse: Systematic Review and Meta-Analysis. *Ann. Transl. Med.* **2020**, *8*, 821. [CrossRef] [PubMed]
56. Gulliver, W.; Zouboulis, C.C.; Prens, E.; Jemec, G.B.E.; Tzellos, T. Evidence-Based Approach to the Treatment of Hidradenitis Suppurativa/Acne Inversa, Based on the European Guidelines for Hidradenitis Suppurativa. *Rev. Endocr. Metab. Disord.* **2016**, *17*, 343–351. [CrossRef] [PubMed]
57. Clemmensen, O.J. Topical Treatment of Hidradenitis Suppurativa with Clindamycin. *Int. J. Dermatol.* **1983**, *22*, 325–328. [CrossRef]
58. Molinelli, E.; Brisigotti, V.; Simonetti, O.; Sapigni, C.; D'Agostino, G.M.; Rizzetto, G.; Giacchetti, A.; Offidani, A. Efficacy and Safety of Topical Resorcinol 15% versus Topical Clindamycin 1% in the Management of Mild-to-Moderate Hidradenitis Suppurativa: A Retrospective Study. *Dermatol. Ther.* **2022**, *35*, e15439. [CrossRef]
59. Boer, J.; Jemec, G.B.E. Resorcinol Peels as a Possible Self-Treatment of Painful Nodules in Hidradenitis Suppurativa. *Clin. Exp. Dermatol.* **2010**, *35*, 36–40. [CrossRef]
60. Kirby, J.S.; Milton, S. Exploratory Trial of Ruxolitinib 1.5% Cream for the Treatment of Early Stage Hidradenitis Suppurativa. 2022. Available online: https://clinicaltrials.gov/ct2/show/NCT04414514 (accessed on 6 October 2022).
61. Riis, P.T.; Boer, J.; Prens, E.P.; Saunte, D.M.L.; Deckers, I.E.; Emtestam, L.; Sartorius, K.; Jemec, G.B.E. Intralesional Triamcinolone for Flares of Hidradenitis Suppurativa (HS): A Case Series. *J. Am. Acad. Dermatol.* **2016**, *75*, 1151–1155. [CrossRef]
62. Martora, F.; Martora, L.; Fabbrocini, G.; Marasca, C. A Case of Pemphigus Vulgaris and Hidradenitis Suppurativa: May Systemic Steroids Be Considered in the Standard Management of Hidradenitis Suppurativa? *Skin Appendage Disord.* **2022**, *8*, 265–268. [CrossRef]
63. Brocard, A.; Dréno, B. Innate Immunity: A Crucial Target for Zinc in the Treatment of Inflammatory Dermatosis. *J. Eur. Acad. Dermatol. Venereol. JEADV* **2011**, *25*, 1146–1152. [CrossRef]
64. Brocard, A.; Knol, A.-C.; Khammari, A.; Dréno, B. Hidradenitis Suppurativa and Zinc: A New Therapeutic Approach. A Pilot Study. *Dermatol. Basel Switz.* **2007**, *214*, 325–327. [CrossRef] [PubMed]
65. Hessam, S.; Sand, M.; Meier, N.M.; Gambichler, T.; Scholl, L.; Bechara, F.G. Combination of Oral Zinc Gluconate and Topical Triclosan: An Anti-Inflammatory Treatment Modality for Initial Hidradenitis Suppurativa. *J. Dermatol. Sci.* **2016**, *84*, 197–202. [CrossRef] [PubMed]
66. Molinelli, E.; Brisigotti, V.; Campanati, A.; Sapigni, C.; Giacchetti, A.; Cota, C.; Offidani, A. Efficacy of Oral Zinc and Nicotinamide as Maintenance Therapy for Mild/Moderate Hidradenitis Suppurativa: A Controlled Retrospective Clinical Study. *J. Am. Acad. Dermatol.* **2020**, *83*, 665–667. [CrossRef] [PubMed]
67. Wahab, A.; Mushtaq, K.; Borak, S.G.; Bellam, N. Zinc-Induced Copper Deficiency, Sideroblastic Anemia, and Neutropenia: A Perplexing Facet of Zinc Excess. *Clin. Case Rep.* **2020**, *8*, 1666–1671. [CrossRef] [PubMed]
68. Kitts, S.; Govea, R.; Maczuga, S.; Kirby, J. Long-Term Antibiotic Use for the Treatment of Hidradenitis Suppurativa Consistent with Guideline Recommendations. *Clin. Exp. Dermatol.* **2021**, *46*, 582–583. [CrossRef]
69. Marasca, C.; Tranchini, P.; Marino, V.; Annunziata, M.C.; Napolitano, M.; Fattore, D.; Fabbrocini, G. The Pharmacology of Antibiotic Therapy in Hidradenitis Suppurativa. *Expert Rev. Clin. Pharmacol.* **2020**, *13*, 521–530. [CrossRef]

70. Jørgensen, A.-H.R.; Yao, Y.; Thomsen, S.F.; Ring, H.C. Treatment of Hidradenitis Suppurativa with Tetracycline, Doxycycline, or Lymecycline: A Prospective Study. *Int. J. Dermatol.* **2021**, *60*, 785–791. [CrossRef]
71. Yao, Y.; Jørgensen, A.-H.R.; Ring, H.C.; Thomsen, S.F. Effectiveness of Clindamycin and Rifampicin Combination Therapy in Hidradenitis Suppurativa: A 6-Month Prospective Study. *Br. J. Dermatol.* **2021**, *184*, 552–553. [CrossRef]
72. Gener, G.; Canoui-Poitrine, F.; Revuz, J.E.; Faye, O.; Poli, F.; Gabison, G.; Pouget, F.; Viallette, C.; Wolkenstein, P.; Bastuji-Garin, S. Combination Therapy with Clindamycin and Rifampicin for Hidradenitis Suppurativa: A Series of 116 Consecutive Patients. *Dermatol. Basel Switz.* **2009**, *219*, 148–154. [CrossRef] [PubMed]
73. van der Zee, H.H.; Boer, J.; Prens, E.P.; Jemec, G.B.E. The Effect of Combined Treatment with Oral Clindamycin and Oral Rifampicin in Patients with Hidradenitis Suppurativa. *Dermatol. Basel Switz.* **2009**, *219*, 143–147. [CrossRef]
74. Mendonça, C.O.; Griffiths, C.E.M. Clindamycin and Rifampicin Combination Therapy for Hidradenitis Suppurativa. *Br. J. Dermatol.* **2006**, *154*, 977–978. [CrossRef] [PubMed]
75. Niemi, M.; Backman, J.T.; Fromm, M.F.; Neuvonen, P.J.; Kivistö, K.T. Pharmacokinetic Interactions with Rifampicin: Clinical Relevance. *Clin. Pharmacokinet.* **2003**, *42*, 819–850. [CrossRef] [PubMed]
76. Wynalda, M.A.; Hutzler, J.M.; Koets, M.D.; Podoll, T.; Wienkers, L.C. In Vitro Metabolism of Clindamycin in Human Liver and Intestinal Microsomes. *Drug Metab. Dispos. Biol. Fate Chem.* **2003**, *31*, 878–887. [CrossRef] [PubMed]
77. Albrecht, J.; Barbaric, J.; Nast, A. Rifampicin Alone May Be Enough: Is It Time to Abandon the Classic Oral Clindamycin–Rifampicin Combination for Hidradenitis Suppurativa? *Br. J. Dermatol.* **2019**, *180*, 949–950. [CrossRef] [PubMed]
78. Join-Lambert, O.; Ribadeau-Dumas, F.; Jullien, V.; Kitzis, M.-D.; Jais, J.-P.; Coignard-Biehler, H.; Guet-Revillet, H.; Consigny, P.-H.; Delage, M.; Nassif, X.; et al. Dramatic Reduction of Clindamycin Plasma Concentration in Hidradenitis Suppurativa Patients Treated with the Rifampin-Clindamycin Combination. *Eur. J. Dermatol. EJD* **2014**, *24*, 94–95. [CrossRef]
79. Join-Lambert, O.; Coignard, H.; Jais, J.-P.; Guet-Revillet, H.; Poirée, S.; Fraitag, S.; Jullien, V.; Ribadeau-Dumas, F.; Thèze, J.; Le Guern, A.-S.; et al. Efficacy of Rifampin-Moxifloxacin-Metronidazole Combination Therapy in Hidradenitis Suppurativa. *Dermatol. Basel Switz.* **2011**, *222*, 49–58. [CrossRef]
80. Chahine, A.A.; Nahhas, A.F.; Braunberger, T.L.; Rambhatla, P.V.; Hamzavi, I.H. Ertapenem Rescue Therapy in Hidradenitis Suppurativa. *JAAD Case Rep.* **2018**, *4*, 482–483. [CrossRef]
81. Join-Lambert, O.; Coignard-Biehler, H.; Jais, J.-P.; Delage, M.; Guet-Revillet, H.; Poirée, S.; Duchatelet, S.; Jullien, V.; Hovnanian, A.; Lortholary, O.; et al. Efficacy of Ertapenem in Severe Hidradenitis Suppurativa: A Pilot Study in a Cohort of 30 Consecutive Patients. *J. Antimicrob. Chemother.* **2016**, *71*, 513–520. [CrossRef]
82. Braunberger, T.L.; Nartker, N.T.; Nicholson, C.L.; Nahhas, A.F.; Parks-Miller, A.; Hanna, Z.; Jayaprakash, R.; Ramesh, M.S.; Rambhatla, P.V.; Hamzavi, I.H. Ertapenem—A Potent Treatment for Clinical and Quality of Life Improvement in Patients with Hidradenitis Suppurativa. *Int. J. Dermatol.* **2018**, *57*, 1088–1093. [CrossRef]
83. Ghanian, S.; Yamanaka-Takaichi, M.; Naik, H.B.; Alavi, A. Medical Management of Hidradenitis Suppurativa with Non-Biologic Therapy: What's New? *Am. J. Clin. Dermatol.* **2022**, *23*, 167–176. [CrossRef]
84. Oxford Centre for Evidence-Based Medicine: Levels of Evidence (March 2009)—Centre for Evidence-Based Medicine (CEBM), University of Oxford. Available online: https://www.cebm.ox.ac.uk/resources/levels-of-evidence/oxford-centre-for-evidence-based-medicine-levels-of-evidence-march-2009 (accessed on 27 November 2022).
85. Jemec, G.B.; Wendelboe, P. Topical Clindamycin versus Systemic Tetracycline in the Treatment of Hidradenitis Suppurativa. *J. Am. Acad. Dermatol.* **1998**, *39*, 971–974. [CrossRef] [PubMed]
86. Vural, S.; Gündoğdu, M.; Akay, B.N.; Boyvat, A.; Erdem, C.; Koçyiğit, P.; Bostancı, S.; Sanli, H.; Kundakci, N. Hidradenitis Suppurativa: Clinical Characteristics and Determinants of Treatment Efficacy. *Dermatol. Ther.* **2019**, *32*, e13003. [CrossRef] [PubMed]
87. Armyra, K.; Kouris, A.; Markantoni, V.; Katsambas, A.; Kontochristopoulos, G. Hidradenitis Suppurativa Treated with Tetracycline in Combination with Colchicine: A Prospective Series of 20 Patients. *Int. J. Dermatol.* **2017**, *56*, 346–350. [CrossRef] [PubMed]
88. Collier, E.K.; Price, K.N.; Grogan, T.R.; Naik, H.B.; Shi, V.Y.; Hsiao, J.L. Characterizing Perimenstrual Flares of Hidradenitis Suppurativa. *Int. J. Womens Dermatol.* **2020**, *6*, 372–376. [CrossRef] [PubMed]
89. Garg, A.; Neuren, E.; Strunk, A. Hidradenitis Suppurativa Is Associated with Polycystic Ovary Syndrome: A Population-Based Analysis in the United States. *J. Investig. Dermatol.* **2018**, *138*, 1288–1292. [CrossRef] [PubMed]
90. Shalom, G.; Freud, T.; Harman-Boehm, I.; Polishchuk, I.; Cohen, A.D. Hidradenitis Suppurativa and Metabolic Syndrome: A Comparative Cross-Sectional Study of 3207 Patients. *Br. J. Dermatol.* **2015**, *173*, 464–470. [CrossRef] [PubMed]
91. Clark, A.K.; Quinonez, R.L.; Saric, S.; Sivamani, R.K. Hormonal Therapies for Hidradenitis Suppurativa: Review. *Dermatol. Online J.* **2017**, *23*, 13030. [CrossRef]
92. Sawers, R.S.; Randall, V.A.; Ebling, F.J. Control of Hidradenitis Suppurativa in Women Using Combined Antiandrogen (Cyproterone Acetate) and Oestrogen Therapy. *Br. J. Dermatol.* **1986**, *115*, 269–274. [CrossRef]
93. Mortimer, P.S.; Dawber, R.P.; Gales, M.A.; Moore, R.A. A Double-Blind Controlled Cross-over Trial of Cyproterone Acetate in Females with Hidradenitis Suppurativa. *Br. J. Dermatol.* **1986**, *115*, 263–268. [CrossRef]
94. Kraft, J.N.; Searles, G.E. Hidradenitis Suppurativa in 64 Female Patients: Retrospective Study Comparing Oral Antibiotics and Antiandrogen Therapy. *J. Cutan. Med. Surg.* **2007**, *11*, 125–131. [CrossRef] [PubMed]
95. Corvol, P.; Michaud, A.; Menard, J.; Freifeld, M.; Mahoudeau, J. Antiandrogenic Effect of Spirolactones: Mechanism of Action. *Endocrinology* **1975**, *97*, 52–58. [CrossRef] [PubMed]

96. Golbari, N.M.; Porter, M.L.; Kimball, A.B. Antiandrogen Therapy with Spironolactone for the Treatment of Hidradenitis Suppurativa. *J. Am. Acad. Dermatol.* **2019**, *80*, 114–119. [CrossRef] [PubMed]
97. Lee, A.; Fischer, G. A Case Series of 20 Women with Hidradenitis Suppurativa Treated with Spironolactone. *Australas. J. Dermatol.* **2015**, *56*, 192–196. [CrossRef] [PubMed]
98. Quinlan, C.; Kirby, B.; Hughes, R. Spironolactone Therapy for Hidradenitis Suppurativa. *Clin. Exp. Dermatol.* **2020**, *45*, 464–465. [CrossRef]
99. Jennings, L.; Hambly, R.; Hughes, R.; Moriarty, B.; Kirby, B. Metformin Use in Hidradenitis Suppurativa. *J. Dermatol. Treat.* **2020**, *31*, 261–263. [CrossRef]
100. Moussa, C.; Wadowski, L.; Price, H.; Mirea, L.; O'Haver, J. Metformin as Adjunctive Therapy for Pediatric Patients With Hidradenitis Suppurativa. *J. Drugs Dermatol. JDD* **2020**, *19*, 1231–1234. [CrossRef]
101. Verdolini, R.; Clayton, N.; Smith, A.; Alwash, N.; Mannello, B. Metformin for the Treatment of Hidradenitis Suppurativa: A Little Help along the Way. *J. Eur. Acad. Dermatol. Venereol. JEADV* **2013**, *27*, 1101–1108. [CrossRef]
102. Layton, A. The Use of Isotretinoin in Acne. *Derm.-Endocrinol.* **2009**, *1*, 162–169. [CrossRef] [PubMed]
103. Matusiak, L.; Bieniek, A.; Szepietowski, J.C. Acitretin Treatment for Hidradenitis Suppurativa: A Prospective Series of 17 Patients. *Br. J. Dermatol.* **2014**, *171*, 170–174. [CrossRef]
104. Boer, J.; Nazary, M. Long-Term Results of Acitretin Therapy for Hidradenitis Suppurativa. Is Acne Inversa Also a Misnomer? *Br. J. Dermatol.* **2011**, *164*, 170–175. [CrossRef] [PubMed]
105. Sánchez-Díaz, M.; Díaz-Calvillo, P.; Rodríguez-Pozo, J.Á.; Arias-Santiago, S.; Molina-Leyva, A. Effectiveness and Safety of Acitretin for the Treatment of Hidradenitis Suppurativa, Predictors of Clinical Response: A Cohort Study. *Dermatology* **2022**, 1–8. [CrossRef]
106. Boer, J.; van Gemert, M.J. Long-Term Results of Isotretinoin in the Treatment of 68 Patients with Hidradenitis Suppurativa. *J. Am. Acad. Dermatol.* **1999**, *40*, 73–76. [CrossRef] [PubMed]
107. Patel, N.; McKenzie, S.A.; Harview, C.L.; Truong, A.K.; Shi, V.Y.; Chen, L.; Grogan, T.R.; Bennett, R.G.; Hsiao, J.L. Isotretinoin in the Treatment of Hidradenitis Suppurativa: A Retrospective Study. *J. Dermatol. Treat.* **2021**, *32*, 473–475. [CrossRef] [PubMed]
108. Soria, A.; Canoui-Poitrine, F.; Wolkenstein, P.; Poli, F.; Gabison, G.; Pouget, F.; Viallette, C.; Revuz, J. Absence of Efficacy of Oral Isotretinoin in Hidradenitis Suppurativa: A Retrospective Study Based on Patients' Outcome Assessment. *Dermatology* **2009**, *218*, 134–135. [CrossRef] [PubMed]
109. Gallagher, C.G.; Kirthi, S.K.; Cotter, C.C.; Revuz, J.R.; Tobin, A.M.T. Could Isotretinoin Flare Hidradenitis Suppurativa? A Case Series. *Clin. Exp. Dermatol.* **2019**, *44*, 777–780. [CrossRef] [PubMed]
110. Kamp, S.; Fiehn, A.M.; Stenderup, K.; Rosada, C.; Pakkenberg, B.; Kemp, K.; Dam, T.N.; Jemec, G.B. Hidradenitis Suppurativa: A Disease of the Absent Sebaceous Gland? Sebaceous Gland Number and Volume Are Significantly Reduced in Uninvolved Hair Follicles from Patients with Hidradenitis Suppurativa. *Br. J. Dermatol.* **2011**, *164*, 1017–1022. [CrossRef] [PubMed]
111. Tan, M.G.; Shear, N.H.; Walsh, S.; Alhusayen, R. Acitretin. *J. Cutan. Med. Surg.* **2017**, *21*, 48–53. [CrossRef]
112. Markota Čagalj, A.; Marinović, B.; Bukvić Mokos, Z. New and Emerging Targeted Therapies for Hidradenitis Suppurativa. *Int. J. Mol. Sci.* **2022**, *23*, 3753. [CrossRef]
113. Kimball, A.B.; Okun, M.M.; Williams, D.A.; Gottlieb, A.B.; Papp, K.A.; Zouboulis, C.C.; Armstrong, A.W.; Kerdel, F.; Gold, M.H.; Forman, S.B.; et al. Two Phase 3 Trials of Adalimumab for Hidradenitis Suppurativa. *N. Engl. J. Med.* **2016**, *375*, 422–434. [CrossRef]
114. Zouboulis, C.C.; Okun, M.M.; Prens, E.P.; Gniadecki, R.; Foley, P.A.; Lynde, C.; Weisman, J.; Gu, Y.; Williams, D.A.; Jemec, G.B.E. Long-Term Adalimumab Efficacy in Patients with Moderate-to-Severe Hidradenitis Suppurativa/Acne Inversa: 3-Year Results of a Phase 3 Open-Label Extension Study. *J. Am. Acad. Dermatol.* **2019**, *80*, 60–69.e2. [CrossRef] [PubMed]
115. Muralidharan, V.; Pathmarajah, P.; Peterknecht, E.; Qazi, E.; Barlow, R.; Muralidharan, V.; Abdullah, A.; McDonald, B.; Bewley, A. Real Life Data on the Biopsychosocial Effects of Adalimumab in the Management of Hidradenitis Suppurativa: A Multicenter Cross Sectional Analysis and Consideration of a Multisystem Monitoring Approach to Follow Up. *Dermatol. Ther.* **2021**, *34*, e14643. [CrossRef]
116. Marzano, A.V.; Genovese, G.; Casazza, G.; Moltrasio, C.; Dapavo, P.; Micali, G.; Sirna, R.; Gisondi, P.; Patrizi, A.; Dini, V.; et al. Evidence for a 'Window of Opportunity' in Hidradenitis Suppurativa Treated with Adalimumab: A Retrospective, Real-Life Multicentre Cohort Study*. *Br. J. Dermatol.* **2021**, *184*, 133–140. [CrossRef]
117. Bechara, F.G.; Podda, M.; Prens, E.P.; Horváth, B.; Giamarellos-Bourboulis, E.J.; Alavi, A.; Szepietowski, J.C.; Kirby, J.; Geng, Z.; Jean, C.; et al. Efficacy and Safety of Adalimumab in Conjunction With Surgery in Moderate to Severe Hidradenitis Suppurativa: The SHARPS Randomized Clinical Trial. *JAMA Surg.* **2021**, *156*, 1001–1009. [CrossRef] [PubMed]
118. Lu, J.-W.; Huang, Y.-W.; Chen, T.-L. Efficacy and Safety of Adalimumab in Hidradenitis Suppurativa. *Medicine* **2021**, *100*, e26190. [CrossRef]
119. Alballa, N.; Alyousef, A.; Alamari, A.; Alhumidi, A.A.; Zayed, M.A.; Zeitouni, L.; Alsaif, F.M. Hodgkin's Lymphoma in a Patient on Adalimumab Treatment for Psoriasis. *AME Case Rep.* **2018**, *2*, 49. [CrossRef]
120. Wong, A.K.; Kerkoutian, S.; Said, J.; Rashidi, H.; Pullarkat, S.T. Risk of Lymphoma in Patients Receiving Antitumor Necrosis Factor Therapy: A Meta-Analysis of Published Randomized Controlled Studies. *Clin. Rheumatol.* **2012**, *31*, 631–636. [CrossRef] [PubMed]

121. Coghlan, J.; He, H.; Schwendeman, A.S. Overview of Humira® Biosimilars: Current European Landscape and Future Implications. *J. Pharm. Sci.* **2021**, *110*, 1572–1582. [CrossRef] [PubMed]
122. Gimeno-Gracia, M.; Gargallo-Puyuelo, C.J.; Gomollón, F. Bioequivalence Studies with Anti-TNF Biosimilars. *Expert Opin. Biol. Ther.* **2019**, *19*, 1031–1043. [CrossRef]
123. Wynne, C.; Altendorfer, M.; Sonderegger, I.; Gheyle, L.; Ellis-Pegler, R.; Buschke, S.; Lang, B.; Assudani, D.; Athalye, S.; Czeloth, N. Bioequivalence, Safety and Immunogenicity of BI 695501, an Adalimumab Biosimilar Candidate, Compared with the Reference Biologic in a Randomized, Double-Blind, Active Comparator Phase I Clinical Study (VOLTAIRE®-PK) in Healthy Subjects. *Expert Opin. Investig. Drugs* **2016**, *25*, 1361–1370. [CrossRef] [PubMed]
124. Montero-Vilchez, T.; Cuenca-Barrales, C.; Rodriguez-Tejero, J.; Martinez-Lopez, A.; Arias-Santiago, S.; Molina-Leyva, A. Switching from Adalimumab Originator to Biosimilar: Clinical Experience in Patients with Hidradenitis Suppurativa. *J. Clin. Med.* **2022**, *11*, 1007. [CrossRef] [PubMed]
125. Ricceri, F.; Rosi, E.; Di Cesare, A.; Pescitelli, L.; Fastame, M.T.; Prignano, F. Clinical Experience with Adalimumab Biosimilar Imraldi in Hidradenitis Suppurativa. *Dermatol. Ther.* **2020**, *33*, e14387. [CrossRef] [PubMed]
126. Roccuzzo, G.; Rozzo, G.; Burzi, L.; Repetto, F.; Dapavo, P.; Ribero, S.; Quaglino, P. Switching from Adalimumab Originator to Biosimilars in Hidradenitis Suppurativa: What's beyond Cost-Effectiveness? *Dermatol. Ther.* **2022**, *35*, e15803. [CrossRef] [PubMed]
127. Kirsten, N.; Ohm, F.; Gehrdau, K.; Girbig, G.; Stephan, B.; Ben-Anaya, N.; Pinter, A.; Bechara, F.G.; Presser, D.; Zouboulis, C.C.; et al. Switching from Adalimumab Originator to Biosimilar in Patients with Hidradenitis Suppurativa Results in Losses of Response-Data from the German HS Registry HSBest. *Life Basel Switz.* **2022**, *12*, 1518. [CrossRef] [PubMed]
128. Burlando, M.; Fabbrocini, G.; Marasca, C.; Dapavo, P.; Chiricozzi, A.; Malvaso, D.; Dini, V.; Campanati, A.; Offidani, A.; Dattola, A.; et al. Adalimumab Originator vs. Biosimilar in Hidradenitis Suppurativa: A Multicentric Retrospective Study. *Biomedicines* **2022**, *10*, 2522. [CrossRef] [PubMed]
129. Martora, F.; Marasca, C.; Fabbrocini, G.; Ruggiero, A. Strategies Adopted in a Southern Italian Referral Centre to Reduce Adalimumab Discontinuation: Comment on 'Can We Increase the Drug Survival Time of Biologic Therapies in Hidradenitis Suppurativa'? *Clin. Exp. Dermatol.* **2022**, *47*, 1864–1865. [CrossRef]
130. Shih, T.; Lee, K.; Grogan, T.; De, D.R.; Shi, V.Y.; Hsiao, J.L. Infliximab in Hidradenitis Suppurativa: A Systematic Review and Meta-Analysis. *Dermatol. Ther.* **2022**, *35*, e15691. [CrossRef] [PubMed]
131. Grant, A.; Gonzalez, T.; Montgomery, M.O.; Cardenas, V.; Kerdel, F.A. Infliximab Therapy for Patients with Moderate to Severe Hidradenitis Suppurativa: A Randomized, Double-Blind, Placebo-Controlled Crossover Trial. *J. Am. Acad. Dermatol.* **2010**, *62*, 205–217. [CrossRef]
132. Mekkes, J.R.; Bos, J.D. Long-Term Efficacy of a Single Course of Infliximab in Hidradenitis Suppurativa. *Br. J. Dermatol.* **2008**, *158*, 370–374. [CrossRef]
133. Jarvis, B.; Faulds, D. Etanercept. *Drugs* **1999**, *57*, 945–966. [CrossRef]
134. Adams, D.R.; Yankura, J.A.; Fogelberg, A.C.; Anderson, B.E. Treatment of Hidradenitis Suppurativa With Etanercept Injection. *Arch. Dermatol.* **2010**, *146*, 501–504. [CrossRef]
135. Esme, P.; Akoglu, G.; Caliskan, E. Rapid Response to Certolizumab Pegol in Hidradenitis Suppurativa: A Case Report. *Skin Appendage Disord.* **2021**, *7*, 58–61. [CrossRef]
136. Holm, J.G.; Jørgensen, A.-H.R.; Yao, Y.; Thomsen, S.F. Certolizumab Pegol for Hidradenitis Suppurativa: Case Report and Literature Review. *Dermatol. Ther.* **2020**, *33*, e14494. [CrossRef] [PubMed]
137. Melendez-Gonzalez, M.D.M.; Hamad, J.; Sayed, C. Golimumab for the Treatment of Hidradenitis Suppurativa in Patients with Previous TNF-α Treatment Failure. *J. Investig. Dermatol.* **2021**, *141*, 2975–2979. [CrossRef] [PubMed]
138. Sand, F.L.; Thomsen, S.F. Off-Label Use of TNF-Alpha Inhibitors in a Dermatological University Department: Retrospective Evaluation of 118 Patients. *Dermatol. Ther.* **2015**, *28*, 158–165. [CrossRef] [PubMed]
139. Tursi, A. Concomitant Hidradenitis Suppurativa and Pyostomatitis Vegetans in Silent Ulcerative Colitis Successfully Treated with Golimumab. *Dig. Liver Dis. Off. J. Ital. Soc. Gastroenterol. Ital. Assoc. Study Liver* **2016**, *48*, 1511–1512. [CrossRef] [PubMed]
140. van der Zee, H.H.; Prens, E.P. Failure of Anti-Interleukin-1 Therapy in Severe Hidradenitis Suppurativa: A Case Report. *Dermatol. Basel Switz.* **2013**, *226*, 97–100. [CrossRef]
141. Zouboulis, C.C.; Frew, J.W.; Giamarellos-Bourboulis, E.J.; Jemec, G.B.E.; Marmol, V.; Marzano, A.V.; Nikolakis, G.; Sayed, C.J.; Tzellos, T.; Wolk, K.; et al. Target Molecules for Future Hidradenitis Suppurativa Treatment. *Exp. Dermatol.* **2021**, *30*, 8–17. [CrossRef]
142. Fletcher, J.M.; Moran, B.; Petrasca, A.; Smith, C.M. IL-17 in Inflammatory Skin Diseases Psoriasis and Hidradenitis Suppurativa. *Clin. Exp. Immunol.* **2020**, *201*, 121–134. [CrossRef]
143. Yao, Y.; Thomsen, S.F. The Role of Interleukin-17 in the Pathogenesis of Hidradenitis Suppurativa. *Dermatol. Online J.* **2017**, *23*, 1. [CrossRef]
144. Johnston, A.; Fritz, Y.; Dawes, S.M.; Diaconu, D.; Al-Attar, P.M.; Guzman, A.M.; Chen, C.S.; Fu, W.; Gudjonsson, J.E.; McCormick, T.S.; et al. Keratinocyte Overexpression of IL-17C Promotes Psoriasiform Skin Inflammation. *J. Immunol. Baltim. Md 1950* **2013**, *190*, 2252–2262. [CrossRef]
145. Mills, K.H.G. IL-17 and IL-17-Producing Cells in Protection versus Pathology. *Nat. Rev. Immunol.* **2022**, 1–17. [CrossRef]

146. Schlapbach, C.; Hänni, T.; Yawalkar, N.; Hunger, R.E. Expression of the IL-23/Th17 Pathway in Lesions of Hidradenitis Suppurativa. *J. Am. Acad. Dermatol.* **2011**, *65*, 790–798. [CrossRef] [PubMed]
147. Kelly, G.; Hughes, R.; McGarry, T.; van den Born, M.; Adamzik, K.; Fitzgerald, R.; Lawlor, C.; Tobin, A.M.; Sweeney, C.M.; Kirby, B. Dysregulated Cytokine Expression in Lesional and Nonlesional Skin in Hidradenitis Suppurativa. *Br. J. Dermatol.* **2015**, *173*, 1431–1439. [CrossRef]
148. Navrazhina, K.; Frew, J.; Krueger, J. Research Letter: IL-17C Is Elevated in Lesional Tissue of Hidradenitis Suppurativa. *Br. J. Dermatol.* **2020**, *182*, 1045–1047. [CrossRef] [PubMed]
149. Fauny, M.; Moulin, D.; D'Amico, F.; Netter, P.; Petitpain, N.; Arnone, D.; Jouzeau, J.-Y.; Loeuille, D.; Peyrin-Biroulet, L. Paradoxical Gastrointestinal Effects of Interleukin-17 Blockers. *Ann. Rheum. Dis.* **2020**, *79*, 1132–1138. [CrossRef] [PubMed]
150. Frieder, J.; Kivelevitch, D.; Menter, A. Secukinumab: A Review of the Anti-IL-17A Biologic for the Treatment of Psoriasis. *Ther. Adv. Chronic Dis.* **2018**, *9*, 5–21. [CrossRef]
151. Prussick, L.; Rothstein, B.; Joshipura, D.; Saraiya, A.; Turkowski, Y.; Abdat, R.; Alomran, A.; Zancanaro, P.; Kachuk, C.; Dumont, N.; et al. Open-Label, Investigator-Initiated, Single-Site Exploratory Trial Evaluating Secukinumab, an Anti-Interleukin-17A Monoclonal Antibody, for Patients with Moderate-to-Severe Hidradenitis Suppurativa. *Br. J. Dermatol.* **2019**, *181*, 609–611. [CrossRef]
152. Casseres, R.G.; Prussick, L.; Zancanaro, P.; Rothstein, B.; Joshipura, D.; Saraiya, A.; Turkowski, Y.; Au, S.C.; Alomran, A.; Abdat, R.; et al. Secukinumab in the Treatment of Moderate to Severe Hidradenitis Suppurativa: Results of an Open-Label Trial. *J. Am. Acad. Dermatol.* **2020**, *82*, 1524–1526. [CrossRef]
153. Kimball, A.B. Secukinumab in Moderate-to-Severe Hidradenitis Suppurativa: Primary Endpoint Analysis from the SUNSHINE and SUNRISE Phase III Trials. In Proceedings of the 31st European Academy of Dermatology and Venereology (EADV) Congress, Milan, Italy, 7–10 September 2022; Available online: https://www.emjreviews.com/dermatology/abstract/secukinumab-in-moderate-to-severe-hidradenitis-suppurativa-primary-endpoint-analysis-from-the-sunshine-and-sunrise-phase-iii-trials-j030122/ (accessed on 25 October 2022).
154. Science—MoonLake. Available online: https://moonlaketx.com/science/ (accessed on 25 October 2022).
155. Svecova, D.; Lubell, M.W.; Casset-Semanaz, F.; Mackenzie, H.; Grenningloh, R.; Krueger, J.G. A Randomized, Double-Blind, Placebo-Controlled Phase 1 Study of Multiple Ascending Doses of Subcutaneous M1095, an Anti–Interleukin 17A/F Nanobody, in Moderate-to-Severe Psoriasis. *J. Am. Acad. Dermatol.* **2019**, *81*, 196–203. [CrossRef]
156. Papp, K.A.; Weinberg, M.A.; Morris, A.; Reich, K. IL17A/F Nanobody Sonelokimab in Patients with Plaque Psoriasis: A Multicentre, Randomised, Placebo-Controlled, Phase 2b Study. *Lancet* **2021**, *397*, 1564–1575. [CrossRef]
157. MoonLake Immunotherapeutics, A.G. Phase 2, Randomized, Parallel-Group, Double-Blind, Placebo-Controlled Study of Sonelokimab in Patients With Active Moderate to Severe Hidradenitis Suppurativa. 2022. Available online: https://ichgcp.net/clinical-trials-registry/NCT05322473 (accessed on 25 October 2022).
158. Behrens, F.; Taylor, P.C.; Wetzel, D.; Brun, N.C.; Brandt-Juergens, J.; Drescher, E.; Dokoupilova, E.; Rowińska-Osuch, A.; Martin, N.A.-K.; Vlam, K. de Op0258 Izokibep (Aby-035) in Patients with Active Psoriatic Arthritis—16-Week Results from a Phase 2 Study. *Ann. Rheum. Dis.* **2022**, *81*, 170–171. [CrossRef]
159. Witte-Händel, E.; Wolk, K.; Tsaousi, A.; Irmer, M.L.; Mößner, R.; Shomroni, O.; Lingner, T.; Witte, K.; Kunkel, D.; Salinas, G.; et al. The IL-1 Pathway Is Hyperactive in Hidradenitis Suppurativa and Contributes to Skin Infiltration and Destruction. *J. Investig. Dermatol.* **2019**, *139*, 1294–1305. [CrossRef] [PubMed]
160. Iznardo, H.; Puig, L. IL-1 Family Cytokines in Inflammatory Dermatoses: Pathogenetic Role and Potential Therapeutic Implications. *Int. J. Mol. Sci.* **2022**, *23*, 9479. [CrossRef] [PubMed]
161. Mertens, M.; Singh, J.A. Anakinra for Rheumatoid Arthritis. *Cochrane Database Syst. Rev.* **2009**, *36*, 1118–1125. [CrossRef]
162. Tzanetakou, V.; Kanni, T.; Giatrakou, S.; Katoulis, A.; Papadavid, E.; Netea, M.G.; Dinarello, C.A.; van der Meer, J.W.M.; Rigopoulos, D.; Giamarellos-Bourboulis, E.J. Safety and Efficacy of Anakinra in Severe Hidradenitis Suppurativa: A Randomized Clinical Trial. *JAMA Dermatol.* **2016**, *152*, 52–59. [CrossRef] [PubMed]
163. Leslie, K.S.; Tripathi, S.V.; Nguyen, T.V.; Pauli, M.; Rosenblum, M.D. An Open-Label Study of Anakinra for the Treatment of Moderate to Severe Hidradenitis Suppurativa. *J. Am. Acad. Dermatol.* **2014**, *70*, 243–251. [CrossRef] [PubMed]
164. André, R.; Marescassier, H.; Gabay, C.; Pittet, B.; Laffitte, E. Long-Term Therapy with Anakinra in Hidradenitis Suppurativa in Three Patients. *Int. J. Dermatol.* **2019**, *58*, e208–e209. [CrossRef]
165. Menis, D.; Maroñas-Jiménez, L.; Delgado-Marquez, A.M.; Postigo-Llorente, C.; Vanaclocha-Sebastián, F. Two Cases of Severe Hidradenitis Suppurativa with Failure of Anakinra Therapy. *Br. J. Dermatol.* **2015**, *172*, 810–811. [CrossRef] [PubMed]
166. Russo, V.; Alikhan, A. Failure of Anakinra in a Case of Severe Hidradenitis Suppurativa. *J. Drugs Dermatol. JDD* **2016**, *15*, 772–774.
167. Zarchi, K.; Dufour, D.N.; Jemec, G.B.E. Successful Treatment of Severe Hidradenitis Suppurativa With Anakinra. *JAMA Dermatol.* **2013**, *149*, 1192–1194. [CrossRef] [PubMed]
168. Kanni, T.; Argyropoulou, M.; Spyridopoulos, T.; Pistiki, A.; Stecher, M.; Dinarello, C.A.; Simard, J.; Giamarellos-Bourboulis, E.J. MABp1 Targeting IL-1α for Moderate to Severe Hidradenitis Suppurativa Not Eligible for Adalimumab: A Randomized Study. *J. Investig. Dermatol.* **2018**, *138*, 795–801. [CrossRef] [PubMed]
169. Kanni, T.; Argyropoulou, M.; Dinarello, C.A.; Simard, J.; Giamarellos-Bourboulis, E.J. MABp1 Targeting Interleukin-1α in Hidradenitis Suppurativa Ineligible for Adalimumab Treatment: Results of the Open-Label Extension Period. *Clin. Exp. Dermatol.* **2021**, *46*, 162–163. [CrossRef] [PubMed]

170. Gottlieb, A.; Natsis, N.E.; Kerdel, F.; Forman, S.; Gonzalez, E.; Jimenez, G.; Hernandez, L.; Kaffenberger, J.; Guido, G.; Lucas, K.; et al. A Phase II Open-Label Study of Bermekimab in Patients with Hidradenitis Suppurativa Shows Resolution of Inflammatory Lesions and Pain. *J. Investig. Dermatol.* **2020**, *140*, 1538–1545.e2. [CrossRef] [PubMed]
171. Janssen Research & Development, LLC. A Phase 2a/2b, Multicenter, Randomized, Placebo and Active Comparator-Controlled, Double-Blind, Dose-Ranging Study to Evaluate the Safety and Efficacy of Bermekimab (JNJ-77474462) for the Treatment of Subjects With Moderate to Severe Hidradenitis Suppurativa. 2022. Available online: https://ichgcp.net/clinical-trials-registry/NCT04988308 (accessed on 27 September 2022).
172. Houriet, C.; Seyed Jafari, S.M.; Thomi, R.; Schlapbach, C.; Borradori, L.; Yawalkar, N.; Hunger, R.E. Canakinumab for Severe Hidradenitis Suppurativa: Preliminary Experience in 2 Cases. *JAMA Dermatol.* **2017**, *153*, 1195–1197. [CrossRef] [PubMed]
173. Sun, N.Z.; Ro, T.; Jolly, P.; Sayed, C.J. Non-Response to Interleukin-1 Antagonist Canakinumab in Two Patients with Refractory Pyoderma Gangrenosum and Hidradenitis Suppurativa. *J. Clin. Aesthet. Dermatol.* **2017**, *10*, 36–38.
174. Tekin, B.; Salman, A.; Ergun, T. Hidradenitis Suppurativa Unresponsive to Canakinumab Treatment: A Case Report. *Indian J. Dermatol. Venereol. Leprol.* **2017**, *83*, 615. [CrossRef] [PubMed]
175. Fleischmann, R.M.; Bliddal, H.; Blanco, F.J.; Schnitzer, T.J.; Peterfy, C.; Chen, S.; Wang, L.; Feng, S.; Conaghan, P.G.; Berenbaum, F.; et al. A Phase II Trial of Lutikizumab, an Anti–Interleukin-1α/β Dual Variable Domain Immunoglobulin, in Knee Osteoarthritis Patients With Synovitis. *Arthritis Rheumatol.* **2019**, *71*, 1056–1069. [CrossRef]
176. Lacy, S.E.; Wu, C.; Ambrosi, D.J.; Hsieh, C.-M.; Bose, S.; Miller, R.; Conlon, D.M.; Tarcsa, E.; Chari, R.; Ghayur, T.; et al. Generation and Characterization of ABT-981, a Dual Variable Domain Immunoglobulin (DVD-Ig(TM)) Molecule That Specifically and Potently Neutralizes Both IL-1α and IL-1β. *mAbs* **2015**, *7*, 605–619. [CrossRef]
177. AbbVie. A Phase 2 Multicenter, Randomized, Double-Blind Placebo-Controlled Study to Evaluate the Safety and Efficacy of Lutikizumab (ABT-981) in Adult Subjects With Moderate to Severe Hidradenitis Suppurativa Who Have Failed Anti-TNF Therapy. 2022. Available online: https://ichgcp.net/clinical-trials-registry/NCT05139602 (accessed on 18 October 2022).
178. Hu, X.; Li, J.; Fu, M.; Zhao, X.; Wang, W. The JAK/STAT Signaling Pathway: From Bench to Clinic. *Signal Transduct. Target. Ther.* **2021**, *6*, 402. [CrossRef]
179. Damsky, W.; King, B.A. JAK Inhibitors in Dermatology: The Promise of a New Drug Class. *J. Am. Acad. Dermatol.* **2017**, *76*, 736–744. [CrossRef]
180. Alavi, A.; Hamzavi, I.; Brown, K.; Santos, L.L.; Zhu, Z.; Liu, H.; Howell, M.D.; Kirby, J.S. Janus Kinase 1 Inhibitor INCB054707 for Patients with Moderate-to-Severe Hidradenitis Suppurativa: Results from Two Phase II Studies. *Br. J. Dermatol.* **2022**, *186*, 803–813. [CrossRef] [PubMed]
181. Kozera, E.; Flora, A.; Frew, J.W. Real-World Safety and Clinical Response of Janus Kinase Inhibitor Upadacitinib in the Treatment of Hidradenitis Suppurativa: A Retrospective Cohort Study. *J. Am. Acad. Dermatol.* **2022**, *87*, 1440–1442. [CrossRef] [PubMed]
182. AbbVie. A Phase 2, Multicenter, Randomized, Placebo-Controlled, Double-Blind Study to Evaluate Upadacitinib in Adult Subjects With Moderate to Severe Hidradenitis Suppurativa. 2022. Available online: https://ichgcp.net/clinical-trials-registry/NCT04430855 (accessed on 22 March 2022).
183. Reguiaï, Z.; Fougerousse, A.C.; Maccari, F.; Bécherel, P.A. Effectiveness of Secukinumab in Hidradenitis Suppurativa: An Open Study (20 Cases). *J. Eur. Acad. Dermatol. Venereol.* **2020**, *34*, e750–e751. [CrossRef]
184. Ribero, S.; Ramondetta, A.; Fabbrocini, G.; Bettoli, V.; Potenza, C.; Chiricozzi, A.; Licciardello, M.; Marzano, A.V.; Bianchi, L.; Rozzo, G.; et al. Effectiveness of Secukinumab in the Treatment of Moderate-Severe Hidradenitis Suppurativa: Results from an Italian Multicentric Retrospective Study in a Real-Life Setting. *J. Eur. Acad. Dermatol. Venereol. JEADV* **2021**, *35*, e441–e442. [CrossRef] [PubMed]
185. Scholl, L.; Hessam, S.; Reitenbach, S.; Bechara, F.G. Operative Behandlungsoptionen bei Hidradenitis suppurativa/Acne inversa. *Hautarzt* **2018**, *69*, 149–161. [CrossRef]
186. Shukla, R.; Karagaiah, P.; Patil, A.; Farnbach, K.; Ortega-Loayza, A.G.; Tzellos, T.; Szepietowski, J.C.; Giulini, M.; Schepler, H.; Grabbe, S.; et al. Surgical Treatment in Hidradenitis Suppurativa. *J. Clin. Med.* **2022**, *11*, 2311. [CrossRef] [PubMed]
187. Cramer, P.; Schneider-Burrus, S.; Kovács, M.; Scholl, L.; Podda, M.; Bechara, F.G. Hidradenitis suppurativa/acne inversa-surgical options, reconstruction and combinations with drug therapies-an update. *Hautarzt Z. Dermatol. Venerol. Verwandte Geb.* **2021**, *72*, 692–699. [CrossRef] [PubMed]
188. Maclean, G.M.; Coleman, D.J. Three Fatal Cases of Squamous Cell Carcinoma Arising in Chronic Perineal Hidradenitis Suppurativa. *Ann. R. Coll. Surg. Engl.* **2007**, *89*, 709–712. [CrossRef]
189. Kohorst, J.J.; Baum, C.L.; Otley, C.C.; Roenigk, R.K.; Schenck, L.A.; Pemberton, J.H.; Dozois, E.J.; Tran, N.V.; Senchenkov, A.; Davis, M.D.P. Surgical Management of Hidradenitis Suppurativa: Outcomes of 590 Consecutive Patients. *Dermatol. Surg. Off. Publ. Am. Soc. Dermatol. Surg. Al* **2016**, *42*, 1030–1040. [CrossRef] [PubMed]
190. Dahmen, R.A.; Gkalpakiotis, S.; Mardesicova, L.; Arenberger, P.; Arenbergerova, M. Deroofing Followed by Thorough Sinus Tract Excision: A Modified Surgical Approach for Hidradenitis Suppurativa. *J. Dtsch. Dermatol. Ges. J. Ger. Soc. Dermatol. JDDG* **2019**, *17*, 698–702. [CrossRef]
191. Lin, C.-H.; Chang, K.-P.; Huang, S.-H. Deroofing: An Effective Method for Treating Chronic Diffuse Hidradenitis Suppurativa. *Dermatol. Surg. Off. Publ. Am. Soc. Dermatol. Surg. Al* **2016**, *42*, 273–275. [CrossRef] [PubMed]
192. van Hattem, S.; Spoo, J.R.; Horváth, B.; Jonkman, M.F.; Leeman, F.W.J. Surgical Treatment of Sinuses by Deroofing in Hidradenitis Suppurativa. *Dermatol. Surg. Off. Publ. Am. Soc. Dermatol. Surg. Al* **2012**, *38*, 494–497. [CrossRef]

193. van der Zee, H.H.; Prens, E.P.; Boer, J. Deroofing: A Tissue-Saving Surgical Technique for the Treatment of Mild to Moderate Hidradenitis Suppurativa Lesions. *J. Am. Acad. Dermatol.* **2010**, *63*, 475–480. [CrossRef] [PubMed]
194. Blok, J.L.; Spoo, J.R.; Leeman, F.W.J.; Jonkman, M.F.; Horváth, B. Skin-Tissue-Sparing Excision with Electrosurgical Peeling (STEEP): A Surgical Treatment Option for Severe Hidradenitis Suppurativa Hurley Stage II/III. *J. Eur. Acad. Dermatol. Venereol. JEADV* **2015**, *29*, 379–382. [CrossRef] [PubMed]
195. Janse, I.C.; Hellinga, J.; Blok, J.L.; van den Heuvel, E.R.; Spoo, J.R.; Jonkman, M.F.; Terra, J.B.; Horváth, B. Skin-Tissue-Sparing Excision with Electrosurgical Peeling: A Case Series in Hidradenitis Suppurativa. *Acta Derm. Venereol.* **2016**, *96*, 390–391. [CrossRef]
196. van Rappard, D.C.; Mooij, J.E.; Mekkes, J.R. Mild to Moderate Hidradenitis Suppurativa Treated with Local Excision and Primary Closure. *J. Eur. Acad. Dermatol. Venereol.* **2012**, *26*, 898–902. [CrossRef]
197. Alharbi, Z.; Kauczok, J.; Pallua, N. A Review of Wide Surgical Excision of Hidradenitis Suppurativa. *BMC Dermatol.* **2012**, *12*, 9. [CrossRef]
198. Deckers, I.E.; Dahi, Y.; van der Zee, H.H.; Prens, E.P. Hidradenitis Suppurativa Treated with Wide Excision and Second Intention Healing: A Meaningful Local Cure Rate after 253 Procedures. *J. Eur. Acad. Dermatol. Venereol.* **2018**, *32*, 459–462. [CrossRef] [PubMed]
199. Nesmith, R.B.; Merkel, K.L.; Mast, B.A. Radical Surgical Resection Combined With Lymphadenectomy-Directed Antimicrobial Therapy Yielding Cure of Severe Axillary Hidradenitis. *Ann. Plast. Surg.* **2013**, *70*, 538–541. [CrossRef]
200. Elkin, K.; Daveluy, S.; Avanaki, K. Review of Imaging Technologies Used in Hidradenitis Suppurativa. *Skin Res. Technol.* **2020**, *26*, 3–10. [CrossRef]
201. Rompel, R.; Petres, J. Long-Term Results of Wide Surgical Excision in 106 Patients with Hidradenitis Suppurativa. *Dermatol. Surg. Off. Publ. Am. Soc. Dermatol. Surg. Al* **2000**, *26*, 638–643. [CrossRef] [PubMed]
202. Scuderi, N.; Monfrecola, A.; Dessy, L.A.; Fabbrocini, G.; Megna, M.; Monfrecola, G. Medical and Surgical Treatment of Hidradenitis Suppurativa: A Review. *Skin Appendage Disord.* **2017**, *3*, 95–110. [CrossRef]
203. Ritz, J.-P.; Runkel, N.; Haier, J.; Buhr, H.J. Extent of Surgery and Recurrence Rate of Hidradenitis Suppurativa. *Int. J. Colorectal Dis.* **1998**, *13*, 164–168. [CrossRef] [PubMed]
204. Hamzavi, I.H.; Griffith, J.L.; Riyaz, F.; Hessam, S.; Bechara, F.G. Laser and Light-Based Treatment Options for Hidradenitis Suppurativa. *J. Am. Acad. Dermatol.* **2015**, *73*, S78–S81. [CrossRef]
205. Dalrymple, J.C.; Monaghan, J.M. Treatment of Hidradenitis Suppurativa with the Carbon Dioxide Laser. *Br. J. Surg.* **1987**, *74*, 420. [CrossRef] [PubMed]
206. Lapins, J.; Marcusson, J.A.; Emtestam, L. Surgical Treatment of Chronic Hidradenitis Suppurativa: CO2 Laser Stripping-Secondary Intention Technique. *Br. J. Dermatol.* **1994**, *131*, 551–556. [CrossRef]
207. Lapins, J.; Sartorius, K.; Emtestam, L. Scanner-Assisted Carbon Dioxide Laser Surgery: A Retrospective Follow-up Study of Patients with Hidradenitis Suppurativa. *J. Am. Acad. Dermatol.* **2002**, *47*, 280–285. [CrossRef] [PubMed]
208. Mikkelsen, P.R.; Dufour, D.N.; Zarchi, K.; Jemec, G.B.E. Recurrence Rate and Patient Satisfaction of CO2 Laser Evaporation of Lesions in Patients with Hidradenitis Suppurativa: A Retrospective Study. *Dermatol. Surg. Off. Publ. Am. Soc. Dermatol. Surg. Al* **2015**, *41*, 255–260. [CrossRef] [PubMed]
209. Hazen, P.G.; Hazen, B.P. Hidradenitis Suppurativa: Successful Treatment Using Carbon Dioxide Laser Excision and Marsupialization. *Dermatol. Surg. Off. Publ. Am. Soc. Dermatol. Surg. Al* **2010**, *36*, 208–213. [CrossRef]
210. Jfri, A.; Saxena, A.; Rouette, J.; Netchiporouk, E.; Barolet, A.; O'Brien, E.; Barolet, D.; Litvinov, I.V. The Efficacy and Effectiveness of Non-Ablative Light-Based Devices in Hidradenitis Suppurativa: A Systematic Review and Meta-Analysis. *Front. Med.* **2020**, *7*, 591580. [CrossRef] [PubMed]
211. Mahmoud, B.H.; Tierney, E.; Hexsel, C.L.; Pui, J.; Ozog, D.M.; Hamzavi, I.H. Prospective Controlled Clinical and Histopathologic Study of Hidradenitis Suppurativa Treated with the Long-Pulsed Neodymium:Yttrium-Aluminium-Garnet Laser. *J. Am. Acad. Dermatol.* **2010**, *62*, 637–645. [CrossRef]
212. Tierney, E.; Mahmoud, B.H.; Hexsel, C.; Ozog, D.; Hamzavi, I. Randomized Control Trial for the Treatment of Hidradenitis Suppurativa with a Neodymium-Doped Yttrium Aluminium Garnet Laser. *Dermatol. Surg. Off. Publ. Am. Soc. Dermatol. Surg. Al* **2009**, *35*, 1188–1198. [CrossRef] [PubMed]
213. Xu, L.Y.; Wright, D.R.; Mahmoud, B.H.; Ozog, D.M.; Mehregan, D.A.; Hamzavi, I.H. Histopathologic Study of Hidradenitis Suppurativa Following Long-Pulsed 1064-Nm Nd:YAG Laser Treatment. *Arch. Dermatol.* **2011**, *147*, 21–28. [CrossRef] [PubMed]
214. Abdel Azim, A.A.; Salem, R.T.; Abdelghani, R. Combined Fractional Carbon Dioxide Laser and Long-Pulsed Neodymium: Yttrium-Aluminium-Garnet (1064 Nm) Laser in Treatment of Hidradenitis Suppurativa; a Prospective Randomized Intra-Individual Controlled Study. *Int. J. Dermatol.* **2018**, *57*, 1135–1144. [CrossRef]
215. Jain, V.; Jain, A. Use of Lasers for the Management of Refractory Cases of Hidradenitis Suppurativa and Pilonidal Sinus. *J. Cutan. Aesthetic Surg.* **2012**, *5*, 190–192. [CrossRef] [PubMed]
216. Mehdizadeh, A.; Hazen, P.G.; Bechara, F.G.; Zwingerman, N.; Moazenzadeh, M.; Bashash, M.; Sibbald, R.G.; Alavi, A. Recurrence of Hidradenitis Suppurativa after Surgical Management: A Systematic Review and Meta-Analysis. *J. Am. Acad. Dermatol.* **2015**, *73*, S70–S77. [CrossRef]

217. Ovadja, Z.N.; Zugaj, M.; Jacobs, W.; van der Horst, C.M.A.M.; Lapid, O. Recurrence Rates Following Reconstruction Strategies After Wide Excision of Hidradenitis Suppurativa: A Systematic Review and Meta-Analysis. *Dermatol. Surg. Off. Publ. Am. Soc. Dermatol. Surg. Al* **2021**, *47*, e106–e110. [CrossRef]
218. Morykwas, M.J.; Argenta, L.C.; Shelton-Brown, E.I.; McGuirt, W. Vacuum-Assisted Closure: A New Method for Wound Control and Treatment: Animal Studies and Basic Foundation. *Ann. Plast. Surg.* **1997**, *38*, 553–562. [CrossRef]
219. Chen, E.; Friedman, H.I. Management of Regional Hidradenitis Suppurativa with Vacuum-Assisted Closure and Split Thickness Skin Grafts. *Ann. Plast. Surg.* **2011**, *67*, 397–401. [CrossRef]
220. Ezanno, A.; Fougerousse, A.; Guillem, P. The Role of Negative-pressure Wound Therapy in the Management of Axillary Hidradenitis Suppurativa. *Int. Wound J.* **2021**, *19*, 802–810. [CrossRef]
221. Humphries, L.S.; Kueberuwa, E.; Beederman, M.; Gottlieb, L.J. Wide Excision and Healing by Secondary Intent for the Surgical Treatment of Hidradenitis Suppurativa: A Single-Center Experience. *J. Plast. Reconstr. Aesthetic Surg. JPRAS* **2016**, *69*, 554–566. [CrossRef] [PubMed]
222. Morgan, W.P.; Harding, K.G.; Hughes, L.E. A Comparison of Skin Grafting and Healing by Granulation, Following Axillary Excision for Hidradenitis Suppurativa. *Ann. R. Coll. Surg. Engl.* **1983**, *65*, 235–236. [PubMed]
223. Janse, I.; Bieniek, A.; Horváth, B.; Matusiak, Ł. Surgical Procedures in Hidradenitis Suppurativa. *Dermatol. Clin.* **2016**, *34*, 97–109. [CrossRef] [PubMed]
224. Pope, E.R. Mesh Skin Grafting. *Vet. Clin. North Am. Small Anim. Pract.* **1990**, *20*, 177–187. [CrossRef] [PubMed]
225. Afsharfard, A.; Khodaparast, M.B.; Zarrintan, S.; Yavari, N. Comparison of Split Thickness Skin Grafts and Flaps in Bilateral Chronic Axillary Hidradenitis Suppurativa. *World J. Plast. Surg.* **2020**, *9*, 55–61. [CrossRef] [PubMed]
226. Mandal, A.; Watson, J. Experience with Different Treatment Modules in Hidradenitis Suppuritiva: A Study of 106 Cases. *The Surgeon* **2005**, *3*, 23–26. [CrossRef]
227. Civelek, B.; Aksoy, K.; Bilgen, E.; İnal, I.; Sahin, U.; Çelebioğlu, S. Reconstructive Options in Severe Cases of Hidradenitis Suppurativa. *Open Med.* **2010**, *5*, 674–678. [CrossRef]
228. Menderes, A.; Sunay, O.; Vayvada, H.; Yilmaz, M. Surgical Management of Hidradenitis Suppurativa. *Int. J. Med. Sci.* **2010**, *7*, 240–247. [CrossRef]
229. Schwabegger, A.H.; Herczeg, E.; Piza, H. The Lateral Thoracic Fasciocutaneous Island Flap for Treatment of Recurrent Hidradenitis Axillaris Suppurativa and Other Axillary Skin Defects. *Br. J. Plast. Surg.* **2000**, *53*, 676–678. [CrossRef]
230. Varkarakis, G.; Daniels, J.; Coker, K.; Oswald, T.; Akdemir, O.; Lineaweaver, W.C. Treatment of Axillary Hidradenitis with Transposition Flaps: A 6-Year Experience. *Ann. Plast. Surg.* **2010**, *64*, 592–594. [CrossRef]
231. Geh, J.L.C.; Niranjan, N.S. Perforator-Based Fasciocutaneous Island Flaps for the Reconstruction of Axillary Defects Following Excision of Hidradenitis Suppurativa. *Br. J. Plast. Surg.* **2002**, *55*, 124–128. [CrossRef] [PubMed]
232. Gorkisch, K.; Boese-Landgraf, J.; Vaubel, E. Hidradenitis suppurativa—Treatment with myocutaneous island flap or the traditional method. *Handchir. Mikrochir. Plast. Chir. Organ Deutschsprachigen Arbeitsgemeinschaft Handchir. Organ Deutschsprachigen Arbeitsgemeinschaft Mikrochir. Peripher. Nerven Gefasse Organ V* **1984**, *16*, 135–138.
233. Solanki, N.S.; Roshan, A.; Malata, C.M. Pedicled Gracilis Myocutaneous Flap for Treatment of Recalcitrant Hidradenitis Suppurativa of the Groin and Perineum. *J. Wound Care* **2009**, *18*, 111–112. [CrossRef] [PubMed]
234. Busnardo, F.F.; Coltro, P.S.; Olivan, M.V.; Busnardo, A.P.V.; Ferreira, M.C. The Thoracodorsal Artery Perforator Flap in the Treatment of Axillary Hidradenitis Suppurativa: Effect on Preservation of Arm Abduction. *Plast. Reconstr. Surg.* **2011**, *128*, 949–953. [CrossRef]
235. Vaillant, C.; Berkane, Y.; Lupon, E.; Atlan, M.; Rousseau, P.; Lellouch, A.G.; Duisit, J.; Bertheuil, N. Outcomes and Reliability of Perforator Flaps in the Reconstruction of Hidradenitis Suppurativa Defects: A Systemic Review and Meta-Analysis. *J. Clin. Med.* **2022**, *11*, 5813. [CrossRef]

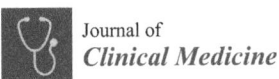

Review

Acne Vulgaris—Novel Treatment Options and Factors Affecting Therapy Adherence: A Narrative Review

Aleksandra Tobiasz, Danuta Nowicka * and Jacek C. Szepietowski

Department of Dermatology, Venereology and Allergology, Wrocław Medical University, Chałubińskiego 1, 50-368 Wrocław, Poland
* Correspondence: danuta.nowicka@umed.wroc.pl; Tel.: +48-609-03-42-48

Abstract: Acne vulgaris is an extremely common skin condition, affecting a large population of adolescents, but at the same time, remaining a quite common issue in the group of adult patients. Its complex pathogenesis includes increased sebum secretion, impaired follicular keratinization, colonization of sebaceous glands with *Cutibacterium acne* bacteria, and the development of inflammation in pilosebaceous units. Although there are many methods of treatment available targeting the mechanisms mentioned above, a large percentage of patients remain undertreated or non-compliant with treatment. Ineffective treatment results in the formation of acne scars, which has a major impact on the well-being and quality of life of the patients. The aim of this publication was a review of available evidence on widely used and novel methods of topical and systemic treatment of acne, additionally including current literature-based analysis of factors affecting patients' compliance. The strengths and limitations of novel substances for treating acne were discussed. We conclude that an effective acne treatment remains a challenge. A better understanding of current treatment options and factors affecting patients' compliance could be a helpful tool in choosing a proper treatment option.

Keywords: acne vulgaris; dermatology; treatment; compliance; persistence

1. Introduction

Acne vulgaris, very common in adolescence, is a condition of complex pathogenesis with a wide variety of treatment options with different mechanisms of action [1–3]. Because of its long duration and exposure to affected areas, acne is associated with a major deterioration in a patient's quality of life and well-being [4–6]. According to the European evidence-based (S3) guideline for the treatment of acne [7], certain topical and systemic treatment options remain a standard. Nevertheless, there is still a need for novel treatment options. According to the guidelines, the intensity of treatment depends on the severity of the acne and should start with topical agents only—the combination of adapalene and benzyl peroxide or clindamycin with benzyl peroxide. In severe cases, it is recommended to begin treatment with systemic isotretinoin. Long-term therapy is essential for achieving certain therapeutic goals. Therefore, patient cooperation and adherence to doctor recommendations are of great importance. Since the largest group of patients struggling with acne are adolescents, achieving good cooperation can be a challenge [8].

2. Topical Treatment

Topical treatment of acne is widely used and effective, especially in cases of mild and moderate acne [7]. Various agents are commonly used, such as topical retinoids, antibiotics, benzoyl peroxide, azelaic acid, and salicylic acid [9]. Even though some of them are used in monotherapy, the advantage of various combinations of the above-mentioned substances in therapy has shown superior effects in many studies and is included in European guidelines [7,10,11]. What is more, many research studies indicate that agents such as topical antibiotics should not be used in monotherapy because of growing bacterial resistance and the limited action of such treatment [12,13].

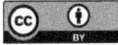

In recent years, novel promising drugs have been introduced in topical form. Furthermore, medications used in dermatology to treat inflammatory disorders have attracted the attention of researchers due to their possible usefulness in the treatment of acne.

2.1. Retinoids

Topical retinoids have been used in the treatment of acne for more than 50 years, with all-trans retinoic acid (tretinoin, ATRA) being their first natural representative [14]. Activation of retinoic receptors by retinoids (RARα, RARβ and RARγ) results in gene transcription, which affects the growth and differentiation of skin cells. As a result, a comedolytic effect is reached, which is desired in the treatment of acne [15]. Over the years, new synthetic retinoids such as tazarotene and adapalene have been introduced in the treatment of acne [15–17]. In the last decade, the FDA has approved a new fourth-generation retinoid, trifarotene [18], which is a selective retinoic receptor gamma agonist characterized by better tolerability. It was initially approved for treating lamellar ichthyosis and later for treating acne vulgaris [19]. Many studies have proven its effectiveness and a favorable safety profile. In the study by Aubert et al. [20], its high pharmacological potency was confirmed in the pluristratified RHE model. In addition, in vivo, it eliminated almost all comedones using ten times lower dosages than used in the case of tazarotene and ATRA (classical retinoid-responsive rhino mouse model). The study by Tan et al. [21] was designed as a vehicle-controlled, double-blind, randomized, phase III study of 50 µg/g trifarotene cream once-daily vs. vehicle. This study lasted 12 weeks and included 1208 subjects with moderate facial and truncal acne. Trifarotene proved to be effective and safe with manageable tolerability. Another multicenter study by Blume-Peytavi et al. [22] and post-hoc analysis of two large-scale phase III pivotal trials by Eichenfield et al. [23] also confirmed the effectiveness, safety and tolerability of trifarotene. Not only are new synthetic retinol derivatives of great interest, but so are novel delivery systems. In recent years, various delivery systems of topical retinoids have been introduced, including polymeric nanoparticles, solid lipid nanoparticles, nanostructured lipid carriers, flexible liposomes, nanoemulsions, and microemulsions [24–27].

Microsponges are microscopic spheres with a diameter of 5–300 µm, which contain up to 250,000 pores. Therefore, they have specific properties; they slowly release the substance that is encapsulated in them, avoiding the accumulation of excessive amounts of the drug. The microsponge particles are too large to be absorbed through the skin, which increases their safety [28], resulting in a reduction of side effects characteristic of topical medication, such as skin irritation. Microsponge technology was patented in 1987 [29]. Regarding acne therapy, some products using this technology and containing retinoids have been introduced [30]. Numerous studies have shown that microsponge formulations allow the release of active substances in a controlled manner [31]. Two double-blind, randomized, split-face studies compared 0.1% tazarotene gel once daily versus 0.1% tretinoin microsponge gel once daily for the treatment of facial acne vulgaris. Tazarotene showed higher efficacy and similar tolerability, which made this medication a cost-effective alternative to 0.1% tretinoin microsponge gel [32,33]. Other studies focused on the properties of benzyl peroxide microsponge formulations [34,35]. Microsponges are definitely a very interesting and novel technology which could be used more frequently in the future.

2.2. Clascoterone

Clascoterone is a novel topical agent approved by the FDA in 2020 for the treatment of acne in patients 12 years of age and older [36]. It is a monoester of cortexolone (cortexolone 17alpha-propionate) with topical antiandrogenic activity. First, studies on rats indicated its apparent absence of systemic effects [37]. The study by Mazzetti et al. [38] investigated clascoterone cream in various concentrations (0.1%, 0.5%, and 1%) and confirmed its favorable safety and tolerability profile. In this study, the 1% cream proved to be the most effective, and it was selected for further clinical studies and development. Another study of the 1% cream in a group of patients with acne vulgaris showed the safety and tolerability of such a treatment [39]. Finally, a study by Hebert et al. [40] on the effects of treatment with 1% clascoterone cream in a group of 1440 patients with facial acne proved its efficacy and safety with low rates of adverse.

2.3. Dapsone

Another drug widely used in dermatology that has promising effects in the treatment of acne is dapsone. It is known to have a broad spectrum of action, including inhibition of neutrophil and eosinophil myeloperoxidase, inhibition of neutrophil adhesion to vascular endothelium integrins, inhibition of chemotaxis and generation of 5-lipogenase products in neutrophils and macrophages [15]. A 5% gel was approved by the FDA for the treatment of acne in 2005, and later, in 2016, its higher concentration of 7.5% also received such approval [41]. A 5% gel should be used twice a day [42], whereas a 7.5% gel is effective, safe, and well tolerated with once-a-day use [43]. Interestingly, a posthoc analysis of two clinical trials conducted by Tanghetti et al. [44] on the effect of 7.5% dapsone gel used for 12 weeks by patients with facial acne reported superior efficacy of such treatment in a female group and similar tolerability in male and female groups. Furthermore, a study by Taylor et al. [44] revealed the effectiveness of 7.5% dapsone gel in patients of all skin phototypes and good tolerability and safety of use. Finally, a study by Grove et al. [45] aimed to compare tolerability and irritation during topical use of benzyl peroxide 5%-clindamycin phosphate 1.2% versus benzyl peroxide 2.5%-clindamycin phosphate versus dapsone 5% and benzyl peroxide 2.5%-adapalene 0.1% in a group of healthy subjects indicated good tolerability of all the preparations mentioned above with higher frequency of adverse perceptions in the group of patients which used benzylperoxide 2.5%-adapalene 0.1%. Taking all studies into consideration, dapsone is a highly effective and well-tolerated form of topical treatment for acne vulgaris.

2.4. Calcipotriol

Calcipotriol, an analog of calcitriol, is widely used in the topical treatment of psoriasis in combination with betamethasone. Its mechanism of action involves binding to the vitamin D receptor of the nuclei of keratinocytes and suppression of keratinocyte proliferation [46]. A study by Abdel-Wahab et al. [47] performed between December 2021 and February 2022 investigated its use among 40 patients with mild and moderate acne vulgaris. In this study, patients were treated with 0.005% calcipotriol cream on the right side of the face and with 0.1% adapalene gel on the left side of the face once a day for two months. After two months of treatment, a significant reduction in comedones, inflammatory lesions, and total acne lesions was observed on each side of the face, with no statistically significant difference between the sides of the face. The analysis of skin biopsy showed greater anti-inflammatory potential of calcipotriol in comparison with adapalene. Additionally, calcipotriol was better tolerated by the patients than adapalene. The results of this study, although conducted in a small group of patients, are promising, proposing calcipotriol as a noteworthy form of topical treatment of acne.

2.5. Photodynamic Therapy

Photodynamic therapy uses the energy of visible light and a photosensitive drug such as aminolaevulinic acid, which is converted to protoporphyrin [48,49]. This process results in the production of 1O2, which has a highly reactive cytocidal action. It has been mostly used in the treatment of actinic keratosis, basal cell skin cancer, cutaneous T-cell lymphoma, etc. [50–53].

Many recent studies showed its effectiveness in the treatment of severe acne vulgaris. According to Yang et al. [54], photodynamic therapy with 5% ALA-PDT and red light is effective in the treatment of acne conglobate with a high response rate and reduced scar formation. A study by Liu et al. [55] investigating a combination of 5-aminolevulinic acid photodynamic therapy and isotretinoin in a group of 67 patients showed its effectiveness in the treatment of moderate to severe acne.

Pain seems to be the most bothering side effect [56], while other side effects include edema, erythema, and hyperpigmentation [57]. A study by Wojewoda et al. [58] indicated that the use of methyl aminolevulinate (MAL-PDT), shorter incubation time, and smaller doses could increase the tolerability of treatment. Interestingly, Zhang et al. [59] noted that the use of 5% and 10% ALA-PDT on different sides of the face of patients with severe facial acne vulgaris resulted in a slightly higher pain level with 10% gel on the pain score, but there were no differences in experienced pain between used concentrations during the second, third and fourth session of photodynamic therapy.

There is a high need for a protocol with fixed concentrations of photosensitizing agents, light dose, number of sessions, and incubation time, which would combine the highest possible effectiveness with the least bothersome side effects.

3. Systemic Treatment

Although isotretinoin remains a golden standard for the systemic treatment of severe acne, because of its adverse effects [15] and teratogenic action [53], there is still a need for a systemic drug with a better safety profile and fewer side effects. According to European guidelines [7], another option for systemic treatment of severe acne is antibiotics in combination with topical adapalene or azelaic acid. The antibiotics of choice remain doxycycline and lymecycline but are limited to a treatment period of three months.

3.1. Sarecycline

The development of bacterial resistance during the treatment with systemic antibiotics has become a great concern. In recent years, a higher resistance of *Cutibacterium acnes* to antibiotics was described in various studies [60–62]. That is why novel antibiotics with safer action profiles are being developed. An example of such an antibiotic is sarecycline, a tetracycline-derived oral antibiotic, which was approved by the FDA in 2018 for the treatment of moderate to severe acne vulgaris [63]. It shows higher selectivity for *C. acnes* compared to older-generation tetracyclines because there is a lower risk of developing bacterial resistance during treatment [64]. According to clinical studies, sarecycline has shown good effectiveness in the treatment of severe facial and truncal acne, with a relatively low rate of side effects and good tolerability [65–67].

3.2. Montelukast

An interesting acne therapeutic option described in various studies is montelukast. Montelukast is a selective CysLT1 receptor antagonist with an anti-inflammatory effect of action [68]. In Poland, this drug is registered for the treatment of asthma [69]. A 2015 study by Behrangi et al. [70] in a group of 52 patients with moderate acne comparing the treatment with oral doxycycline 100mg/day plus topical 1% clindamycin and with montelukast 5mg plus 1% topical clindamycin reported a significant reduction in the acne severity index in both groups, without significant differences between the groups. Another study by Rokni et al. [71] in a group of 65 women with moderate acne vulgaris evaluating treatment with the combination of oral montelukast and finasteride with topical clindamycin showed good efficacy of both treatment methods with the advantage of finasteride. Whereas the study by Fazelzadeh-Haghighi et al. [72] in a group of 108 patients with moderate acne vulgaris comparing a treatment with doxycycline 100mg/day with montelukast 10mg/day and doxycycline 100 mg/day with placebo showed a superior effect of the montelukast/doxycycline combination versus doxycycline alone. Both groups also received a topical 5% benzyl peroxide gel to use once every night. Surely montelukast is an interesting agent, but its effectiveness as an adjuvant in the therapy of acne requires further studies.

3.3. Hormonal Therapy

Hormonal therapy for acne, particularly in women, is an important option because women after 25 years of age suffer from frequent relapses of acne following standard treatment. There are several hormones that can contribute to the development of acne, including androgens. Although in those women, symptoms of acne appear even if androgens remain within the normal range. This group of patients shows good results after hormonal treatment [73].

4. Adherence

An issue without which successful therapy is impossible is the compliance of the patients. Furthermore, Cramer et al. [74] indicate that for treatment to be successful, not only is compliance (adherence) key, but persistence is also of great importance. In this study, after three years of review and discussion by the ISPOR Work Group, the following definitions were proposed according to which medication compliance " ... refers to the act of conforming to the recommendations made by the provider with respect to timing, dosage, and frequency of medication taking." And medication persistence " ... refers to the act of conforming to a recommendation of continuing treatment for the prescribed length of time."

Considering the long duration of acne treatment, the visibility of the lesions, and the struggle with various side effects, these two concepts are especially important. A large observational study on the adherence to acne therapy by Dreno et al. [75] on more than 3000 patients from all over the world using multivariate analysis indicated eight factors that had predictive power in relationship to adherence (two historical factors, three clinical factors, and three related to the current treatment). It permitted the establishment of a patient profile more likely to be poorly adherent to acne treatment. Historical factors were the severity of the disease and previous consultation with a general practitioner about acne. Clinical factors included patients' age, satisfaction with treatment, and knowledge about acne treatment. Patients with poor adherence were more often school-aged, single, with symptom onset before puberty, and with lower levels of knowledge about acne. Characteristics of the current treatment regarded the additional anti-acne cosmetics prescription, the degree of clinical improvement evaluated by the physician, and the occurrence of side effects. The study resulted in the Elaboration d'un outil d'evaluation de l'observance des traitements medicamenteux (ESOB) questionnaire, which can help doctors to identify patients with poor adherence. Another study by Hayran et al. [76] included a group of 500 patients and reported poor treatment adherence to treatment in 64.4% of the patients. Identified factors related to better adherence to treatment were the use of oral isotretinoin and satisfaction with treatment.

Comparing adherence between topical and systemic acne vulgaris treatment results vary between available studies. A study by Hayran et al. [76] mentions better adherence of patients using oral isotretinoin (83.7% of patients). Interestingly the study by Salamzadeh et al. [77], which investigated adherence in a group of 200 patients with mild, moderate, and severe acne vulgaris in Iran, indicated no significant difference between adherence to topical versus systemic treatment. On the other hand, studies by Dreno et al. [75] as well as Miyachi et al. [78] indicated higher adherence to topical treatment. Even though mentioned studies described general adherence to the treatment of patients with acne vulgaris as poor, a study by Alsubeeh et al. [79] included a group of 2330 patients with psoriasis, chronic dermatitis, acne vulgaris, hair growth disorders, and vitiligo, indicated better adherence of patients with acne vulgaris than the ones with psoriasis or chronic dermatitis. The duration of the treatment might be a possible explanation. In the study of Yentzer et al. [80], in the group of teenagers using 5% gel with benzoyl peroxide, a large decline in adherence during six weeks of treatment was described. Even such a short duration of treatment affected patients' adherence.

Patients' persistence, on the other hand, has fewer studies than adherence. Nevertheless, some interesting observations have been described. A study by Grada et al. [81]

investigated persistence in a group of 230,552 patients with acne, and it indicated a relatively high Medication Possession Ratio (percentage of patients for whom medication is available) but poor treatment persistence.

Considering all the above-mentioned information, proper education of the patient is of great importance. Regarding choosing a proper medium study by Hung et al. [82] showed that a larger group of patients preferred educational videos over pamphlets. That is why educational videos are a useful tool in the education of patients about the treatment.

5. Conclusions

Acne is a multi-factorial skin disease that requires long-term treatment. Over the years, many topical and systemic treatment options have been introduced; however, many patients do not see satisfactory treatment results and experience difficulties adhering to treatment recommendations. Therefore, selecting the appropriate treatment is of great importance for achieving satisfactory treatment outcomes that match patient needs and ensure patient cooperation.

Author Contributions: Conceptualization and methodology A.T. and D.N.; formal analysis, A.T. and D.N.; writing—original draft preparation A.T. and D.N.; writing—review and editing, A.T., D.N., and J.C.S.; visualization A.T.; supervision, A.T., and D.N. All authors have read and agreed to the published version of the manuscript.

Funding: This research received no external funding.

Institutional Review Board Statement: Not applicable.

Informed Consent Statement: Not applicable.

Data Availability Statement: Not applicable.

Conflicts of Interest: The authors declare no conflict of interest.

References

1. Hay, R.J.; Johns, N.E.; Williams, H.C.; Bolliger, I.W.; Dellavalle, R.P.; Margolis, D.J.; Marks, R.; Naldi, L.; Weinstock, M.A.; Wulf, S.K.; et al. The global burden of skin disease in 2010: An analysis of the prevalence and impact of skin conditions. *J. Investig. Dermatol.* **2014**, *134*, 1527–1534. [CrossRef] [PubMed]
2. Williams, H.C.; Dellavalle, R.P.; Garner, S. Acne vulgaris. *Lancet* **2012**, *379*, 361–372. [CrossRef] [PubMed]
3. Tuchayi, S.M.; Makrantonaki, E.; Ganceviciene, R.; Dessinioti, C.; Feldman, S.R.; Zouboulis, C.C. Acne vulgaris. *Nat. Rev. Dis. Primers* **2015**, *1*, 15033. [CrossRef]
4. Szepietowska, M.; Dąbrowska, A.; Nowak, B.; Skinderowicz, K.; Wilczyński, B.; Krajewski, P.K.; Jankowska-Konsur, A. Facial acne causes stigmatization among adolescents: A cross-sectional study. *J. Cosmet. Dermatol.* **2022**, in press. [CrossRef] [PubMed]
5. Lim, T.H.; Badaruddin, N.S.F.; Foo, S.Y.; Bujang, M.A.; Muniandy, P. Prevalence and psychosocial impact of acne vulgaris among high school and university students in Sarawak, Malaysia. *Med. J. Malaysia* **2022**, *77*, 446–453.
6. Andersen, R.K.; Bouazzi, D.; Erikstrup, C.; Nielsen, K.R.; Burgdorf, K.S.; Bruun, M.T.; Hjalgrim, H.; Mikkelsen, S.; Ullum, H.; Pedersen, O.B.; et al. The Social and Psychological Impact of Acne Treatment: A Cross-Sectional Study of Blood Donors. *J. Cutan. Med. Surg.* **2022**, *26*, 485–493. [CrossRef] [PubMed]
7. Nast, A.; Dréno, B.; Bettoli, V.; Bukvic Mokos, Z.; Degitz, K.; Dressler, C.; Finlay, A.Y.; Haedersdal, M.; Lambert, J.; Layton, A.; et al. European evidence-based (S3) guideline for the treatment of acne—Update 2016—Short version. *J. Eur. Acad. Dermatol. Venereol.* **2016**, *30*, 1261–1268. [CrossRef] [PubMed]
8. Hester, C.; Park, C.; Chung, J.; Balkrishnan, R.; Feldman, S.; Chang, J. Medication Adherence in Children and Adolescents with Acne Vulgaris in Medicaid: A Retrospective Study Analysis. *Pediatr. Dermatol.* **2016**, *33*, 49–55. [CrossRef]
9. Afarideh, M.; Rodriguez Baisi, K.E.; Davis, D.M.R.; Hand, J.L.; Tollefson, M.M. Trends in utilization of non-first-line topical acne medications among children, adolescents, and adults in the United States, 2012–2016. *Pediatr. Dermatol.* **2021**, *38*, 1066–1073. [CrossRef]
10. Berenbaum, M.C. What is synergy? *Pharmacol. Rev.* **1989**, *41*, 93–141.
11. Thiboutot, D.M.; Weiss, J.; Bucko, A.; Eichenfield, L.; Jones, T.; Clark, S.; Liu, Y.; Graeber, M.; Kang, S. Adapalene-benzoyl peroxide, a fixed-dose combination for the treatment of acne vulgaris: Results of a multicenter, randomized double-blind, controlled study. *J. Am. Acad. Dermatol.* **2007**, *57*, 791–799. [CrossRef]
12. Austin, B.A.; Fleischer, A.B., Jr. The extinction of topical erythromycin therapy for acne vulgaris and concern for the future of topical clindamycin. *J. Dermatolog. Treat.* **2017**, *28*, 145–148. [CrossRef] [PubMed]

13. Xu, J.H.; Lu, Q.J.; Huang, J.H.; Hao, F.; Sun, Q.N.; Fang, H.; Gu, J.; Dong, X.Q.; Zheng, J.; Luo, D.; et al. A multicentre, randomized, single-blind comparison of topical clindamycin 1%/benzoyl peroxide 5% once-daily gel versus clindamycin 1% twice-daily gel in the treatment of mild to moderate acne vulgaris in Chinese patients. *J. Eur. Acad. Dermatol. Venereol.* **2016**, *30*, 1176–1182. [CrossRef] [PubMed]
14. Kligman, A.M.; Fulton, J.E., Jr.; Plewig, G. Topical vitamin A acid in acne vulgaris. *Arch. Dermatol.* **1969**, *99*, 469–476. [CrossRef]
15. Wolverton, S.E.; Wu, J.J. *Comprehensive Dermatologic Drug Therapy*, 4th ed.; Elsevier: Amsterdam, The Netherlands, 2020; p. 1.
16. Ioannides, D.; Rigopoulos, D.; Katsambas, A. Topical adapalene gel 0.1% vs. isotretinoin gel 0.05% in the treatment of acne vulgaris: A randomized open-label clinical trial. *Br. J. Dermatol.* **2002**, *147*, 523–527. [CrossRef]
17. Thiboutot, D.; Arsonnaud, S.; Soto, P. Efficacy and tolerability of adapalene 0.3% gel compared to tazarotene 0.1% gel in the treatment of acne vulgaris. *J. Drugs Dermatol.* **2008**, *7*, s3–s10.
18. AKLIEF® (Trifarotene) Cream, for Topical Use. Available online: https://www.accessdata.fda.gov/drugsatfda_docs/label/2019/211527s000lbl.pdf (accessed on 30 October 2022).
19. De Ruiter, J.; Holston, P.L. Trifarotene (Aklief, Galderma). *New Drug Rev.* **2020**, *45*, 26–33.
20. Aubert, J.; Piwnica, D.; Bertino, B.; Blanchet-Réthoré, S.; Carlavan, I.; Déret, S.; Dreno, B.; Gamboa, B.; Jomard, A.; Luzy, A.P.; et al. Nonclinical and human pharmacology of the potent and selective topical retinoic acid receptor-γ agonist trifarotene. *Br. J. Dermatol.* **2018**, *179*, 442–456. [CrossRef] [PubMed]
21. Tan, J.; Thiboutot, D.; Popp, G.; Gooderham, M.; Lynde, C.; Del Rosso, J.; Weiss, J.; Blume-Peytavi, U.; Weglovska, J.; Johnson, S.; et al. Randomized phase 3 evaluation of trifarotene 50 μg/g cream treatment of moderate facial and truncal acne. *J. Am. Acad. Dermatol.* **2019**, *80*, 1691–1699. [CrossRef]
22. Blume-Peytavi, U.; Fowler, J.; Kemény, L.; Draelos, Z.; Cook-Bolden, F.; Dirschka, T.; Eichenfield, L.; Graeber, M.; Ahmad, F.; Alió Saenz, A.; et al. Long-term safety and efficacy of trifarotene 50 μg/g cream, a first-in-class RAR-γ selective topical retinoid, in patients with moderate facial and truncal acne. *J. Eur. Acad. Dermatol. Venereol.* **2020**, *34*, 166–173. [CrossRef]
23. Eichenfield, L.; Kwong, P.; Lee, S.; Krowchuk, D.; Arekapudi, K.; Hebert, A. Advances in Topical Management of Adolescent Facial and Truncal Acne: A Phase 3 Pooled Analysis of Safety and Efficacy of Trifarotene 0.005% Cream. *J. Drugs Dermatol.* **2022**, *21*, 582–586. [CrossRef] [PubMed]
24. Samadi, A.; Sartipi, Z.; Ahmad Nasrollahi, S.; Sheikholeslami, B.; Nassiri Kashani, M.; Rouini, M.R.; Dinarvand, R.; Firooz, A. Efficacy assessments of tretinoin-loaded nano lipid carriers in acne vulgaris: A double blind, split-face randomized clinical study. *Arch Dermatol. Res.* **2022**, *314*, 553–561. [CrossRef] [PubMed]
25. Sabouri, M.; Samadi, A.; Ahmad Nasrollahi, S.; Farboud, E.S.; Mirrahimi, B.; Hassanzadeh, H.; Nassiri Kashani, M.; Dinarvand, R.; Firooz, A. Tretinoin Loaded Nanoemulsion for Acne Vulgaris: Fabrication, Physicochemical and Clinical Efficacy Assessments. *Skin Pharmacol. Physiol.* **2018**, *31*, 316–323. [CrossRef] [PubMed]
26. Prasad, S.; Mukhopadhyay, A.; Kubavat, A.; Kelkar, A.; Modi, A.; Swarnkar, B.; Bajaj, B.; Vedamurthy, M.; Sheikh, S.; Mittal, R. Efficacy and safety of a nano-emulsion gel formulation of adapalene 0.1% and clindamycin 1% combination in acne vulgaris: A randomized, open label, active-controlled, multicentric, phase IV clinical trial. *Indian J. Dermatol. Venereol. Leprol.* **2012**, *78*, 459–467. [CrossRef]
27. Najafi-Taher, R.; Jafarzadeh Kohneloo, A.; Eslami Farsani, V.; Mehdizade Rayeni, N.; Moghimi, H.R.; Ehsani, A.; Amani, A. A topical gel of tea tree oil nanoemulsion containing adapalene versus adapalene marketed gel in patients with acne vulgaris: A randomized clinical trial. *Arch Dermatol. Res.* **2022**, *314*, 673–679. [CrossRef]
28. Kaity, S.; Maiti, S.; Ghosh, A.K.; Pal, D.; Ghosh, A.; Banerjee, S. Microsponges: A novel strategy for drug delivery system. *J. Adv. Pharm. Technol. Res.* **2010**, *1*, 283–290. [CrossRef]
29. Won, R. Method for Delivering an Active Ingredient by Controlled Time Release Utilizing a Novel Delivery Vehicle Which Can Be Prepared by a Process Utilizing the Active Ingredient as a Porogen. U.S. Patent 4,690,825, 1987. Available online: https://patents.google.com/patent/US4690825A/en (accessed on 30 October 2022).
30. Mahant, S.; Kumar, S.; Nanda, S.; Rao, R. Microsponges for dermatological applications: Perspectives and challenges. *Asian J. Pharm. Sci.* **2020**, *15*, 273–291. [CrossRef]
31. Khattab, A.; Nattouf, A. Microsponge based gel as a simple and valuable strategy for formulating and releasing Tazarotene in a controlled manner. *Sci. Rep.* **2022**, *12*, 11414. [CrossRef]
32. Leyden, J.J.; Tanghetti, E.A.; Miller, B.; Ung, M.; Berson, D.; Lee, J. Once-daily tazarotene 0.1 % gel versus once-daily tretinoin 0.1 % microsponge gel for the treatment of facial acne vulgaris: A double-blind randomized trial. *Cutis* **2002**, *69*, 12–19.
33. Leyden, J.; Grove, G.L. Randomized facial tolerability studies comparing gel formulations of retinoids used to treat acne vulgaris. *Cutis* **2001**, *67*, 17–27.
34. Jelvehgari, M.; Siahi-Shadbad, M.R.; Azarmi, S.; Martin, G.P.; Nokhodchi, A. The microsponge delivery system of benzoyl peroxide: Preparation, characterization and release studies. *Int. J. Pharm.* **2006**, *308*, 124–132. [CrossRef] [PubMed]
35. Nokhodchi, A.; Jelvehgari, M.; Siahi, M.R.; Mozafari, M.R. Factors affecting the morphology of benzoyl peroxide microsponges. *Micron* **2007**, *38*, 834–840. [CrossRef] [PubMed]
36. WINLEVI® (Clascoterone) Cream, for Topical Use. Available online: https://www.accessdata.fda.gov/drugsatfda_docs/label/2020/213433s000lbl.pdf (accessed on 30 October 2022).

37. Celasco, G.; Moro, L.; Bozzella, R.; Ferraboschi, P.; Bartorelli, L.; Quattrocchi, C.; Nicoletti, F. Biological profile of cortexolone 17alpha-propionate (CB-03-01), a new topical and peripherally selective androgen antagonist. *Arzneimittelforschung* **2004**, *54*, 881–886. [CrossRef]
38. Mazzetti, A.; Moro, L.; Gerloni, M.; Cartwright, M. A Phase 2b, Randomized, Double-Blind Vehicle Controlled, Dose Escalation Study Evaluating Clascoterone 0.1%, 0.5%, and 1% Topical Cream in Subjects with Facial Acne. *J. Drugs Dermatol.* **2019**, *18*, 570. [PubMed]
39. Mazzetti, A.; Moro, L.; Gerloni, M.; Cartwright, M. Pharmacokinetic Profile, Safety, and Tolerability of Clascoterone (Cortexolone 17-alpha propionate, CB-03-01) Topical Cream, 1% in Subjects with Acne Vulgaris: An Open-Label Phase 2a Study. *J. Drugs Dermatol.* **2019**, *18*, 563.
40. Hebert, A.; Thiboutot, D.; Stein Gold, L.; Cartwright, M.; Gerloni, M.; Fragasso, E.; Mazzetti, A. Efficacy and Safety of Topical Clascoterone Cream, 1%, for Treatment in Patients with Facial Acne: Two Phase 3 Randomized Clinical Trials. *JAMA Dermatol.* **2020**, *156*, 621–630. [CrossRef]
41. Brown, P.C. ACZONE® (Dapsone) Gel, 7.5%–Clinical Review. Available online: https://www.fda.gov/media/104709/download (accessed on 30 October 2022).
42. Draelos, Z.D.; Carter, E.; Maloney, J.M.; Elewski, B.; Poulin, Y.; Lynde, C.; Garrett, S. Two randomized studies demonstrate the efficacy and safety of dapsone gel, 5% for the treatment of acne vulgaris. *J. Am. Acad. Dermatol.* **2007**, *56*, 439.e1–439.e10. [CrossRef]
43. Eichenfield, L.F.; Lain, T.; Frankel, E.H.; Jones, T.M.; Chang-Lin, J.E.; Berk, D.R.; Ruan, S.; Kaoukhov, A. Efficacy and Safety of Once-Daily Dapsone Gel, 7.5% for Treatment of Adolescents and Adults with Acne Vulgaris: Second of Two Identically Designed, Large, Multicenter, Randomized, Vehicle-Controlled Trials. *J. Drugs Dermatol.* **2016**, *15*, 962–969.
44. Taylor, S.C.; Cook-Bolden, F.E.; McMichael, A.; Downie, J.B.; Rodriguez, D.A.; Alexis, A.F.; Callender, V.D.; Alvandi, N. Efficacy, Safety, and Tolerability of Topical Dapsone Gel, 7.5% for Treatment of Acne Vulgaris by Fitzpatrick Skin Phototype. *J. Drugs Dermatol.* **2018**, *17*, 160–167.
45. Grove, G.; Zerweck, C.; Gwazdauskas, J. Tolerability and irritation potential of four topical acne regimens in healthy subjects. *J. Drugs Dermatol.* **2013**, *12*, 644–649.
46. Wang, R.C.; Levine, B. Calcipotriol induces autophagy in HeLa cells and keratinocytes. *J. Invest Dermatol.* **2011**, *131*, 990–993. [CrossRef] [PubMed]
47. Abdel-Wahab, H.M.; Ali, A.K.; Ragaie, M.H. Calcipotriol: A novel tool in treatment of acne vulgaris. *Dermatol. Ther.* **2022**, *35*, e15690. [CrossRef] [PubMed]
48. Chen, J.; Keltner, L.; Christophersen, J.; Zheng, F.; Krouse, M.; Singhal, A.; Wang, S.S. New technology for deep light distribution in tissue for phototherapy. *Cancer J.* **2002**, *8*, 154–163. [CrossRef] [PubMed]
49. Hongcharu, W.; Taylor, C.R.; Chang, Y.; Aghassi, D.; Suthamjariya, K.; Anderson, R.R. Topical ALA-photodynamic therapy for the treatment of acne vulgaris. *J. Invest Dermatol.* **2000**, *115*, 183–192. [CrossRef]
50. Sáenz-Guirado, S.; Cuenca-Barrales, C.; Vega-Castillo, J.; Linares-Gonzalez, L.; Ródenas-Herranz, T.; Molina-Leyva, A.; Ruiz-Villaverde, R. Combined versus conventional photodynamic therapy with 5-aminolaevulinic acid nanoemulsion (BF-200 ALA) for actinic keratosis: A randomized, single-blind, prospective study. *Photodermatol. Photoimmunol. Photomed.* **2022**, *38*, 334–342. [CrossRef]
51. Steeb, T.; Wessely, A.; Petzold, A.; Brinker, T.J.; Schmitz, L.; Leiter, U.; Garbe, C.; Schöffski, O.; Berking, C.; Heppt, M.V. Evaluation of Long-term Clearance Rates of Interventions for Actinic Keratosis: A Systematic Review and Network Meta-analysis. *JAMA Dermatol.* **2021**, *157*, 1066–1077. [CrossRef]
52. Buzzá, H.H.; Moriyama, L.T.; Vollet-Filho, J.D.; Inada, N.M.; da Silva, A.P.; Stringasci, M.D.; Requena, M.B.; de Andrade, C.T.; Blanco, K.C.; Ramirez, D.P.; et al. Overall Results for a National Program of Photodynamic Therapy for Basal Cell Carcinoma: A Multicenter Clinical Study to Bring New Techniques to Social Health Care. *Cancer Control* **2019**, *26*, 1073274819856885. [CrossRef]
53. Kim, E.J.; Mangold, A.R.; DeSimone, J.A.; Wong, H.K.; Seminario-Vidal, L.; Guitart, J.; Appel, J.; Geskin, L.; Lain, E.; Korman, N.J. Efficacy and Safety of Topical Hypericin Photodynamic Therapy for Early-Stage Cutaneous T-Cell Lymphoma (Mycosis Fungoides): The FLASH Phase 3 Randomized Clinical Trial. *JAMA Dermatol.* **2022**, *158*, 1031–1039. [CrossRef]
54. Yang, G.L.; Zhao, M.; Wang, J.M.; He, C.F.; Luo, Y.; Liu, H.Y.; Gao, J.; Long, C.Q.; Bai, J.R. Short-term clinical effects of photodynamic therapy with topical 5-aminolevulinic acid for facial acne conglobata: An open, prospective, parallel-arm trial. *Photodermatol. Photoimmunol. Photomed.* **2013**, *29*, 233–238. [CrossRef]
55. Liu, L.; Liu, P.; Wei, G.; Meng, L.; Zhang, C.; Zhang, C. Combination of 5-Aminolevulinic acid photodynamic therapy and isotretinoin to treat moderate-to-severe acne. *Photodiagnosis. Photodyn. Ther.* **2021**, *34*, 102215. [CrossRef]
56. Warren, C.B.; Karai, L.J.; Vidimos, A.; Maytin, E.V. Pain associated with aminolevulinic acid-photodynamic therapy of skin disease. *J. Am. Acad. Dermatol.* **2009**, *61*, 1033–1043. [CrossRef] [PubMed]
57. Boen, M.; Brownell, J.; Patel, P.; Tsoukas, M.M. The Role of Photodynamic Therapy in Acne: An Evidence-Based Review. *Am. J. Clin. Dermatol.* **2017**, *18*, 311–321. [CrossRef] [PubMed]
58. Wojewoda, K.; Gillstedt, M.; Tovi, J.; Salah, L.; Wennberg Larkö, A.M.; Sjöholm, A.; Sandberg, C. Optimizing treatment of acne with photodynamic therapy (PDT) to achieve long-term remission and reduce side effects. A prospective randomized controlled trial. *J. Photochem. Photobiol. B* **2021**, *223*, 112299. [CrossRef] [PubMed]

59. Zhang, J.; Zhang, X.; He, Y.; Wu, X.; Huang, J.; Huang, H.; Lu, C. Photodynamic therapy for severe facial acne vulgaris with 5% 5-aminolevulinic acid vs 10% 5-aminolevulinic acid: A split-face randomized controlled study. *J. Cosmet. Dermatol.* **2020**, *19*, 368–374. [CrossRef]
60. Alvarez-Sánchez, M.; Rodríguez-Ayala, E.; Ponce-Olivera, R.M.; Tirado-Sánchez, A.; Arellano-Mendoza, M.I. Bacterial resistance in acne? A meta-analysis of the controversy. *Cir. Cir.* **2016**, *84*, 190–195. [CrossRef]
61. Tan, H.H.; Goh, C.L.; Yeo, M.G.; Tan, M.L. Antibiotic sensitivity of Propionibacterium acnes isolates from patients with acne vulgaris in a tertiary dermatological referral centre in Singapore. *Ann. Acad. Med. Singap.* **2001**, *30*, 22–25.
62. Dessinioti, C.; Katsambas, A. Propionibacterium acnes and antimicrobial resistance in acne. *Clin. Dermatol.* **2017**, *35*, 163–167. [CrossRef]
63. SEYSARA™ (Sarecycline) Tablets for Oral Use. Available online: https://www.accessdata.fda.gov/drugsatfda_docs/label/2018/209521s000lbl.pdf (accessed on 30 October 2022).
64. Zhanel, G.; Critchley, I.; Lin, L.Y.; Alvandi, N. Microbiological Profile of Sarecycline, a Novel Targeted Spectrum Tetracycline for the Treatment of Acne Vulgaris. *Antimicrob. Agents Chemother.* **2019**, *63*, e01297-18. [CrossRef]
65. Moore, A.; Green, L.J.; Bruce, S.; Sadick, N.; Tschen, E.; Werschler, P.; Cook-Bolden, F.E.; Dhawan, S.S.; Forsha, D.; Gold, M.H.; et al. Once-Daily Oral Sarecycline 1.5 mg/kg/day Is Effective for Moderate to Severe Acne Vulgaris: Results from Two Identically Designed, Phase 3, Randomized, Double-Blind Clinical Trials. *J. Drugs Dermatol.* **2018**, *17*, 987–996. [CrossRef]
66. Del Rosso, J.Q.; Stein Gold, L.; Baldwin, H.; Harper, J.C.; Zeichner, J.; Obagi, S.; Graber, E.; Jimenez, X.; Vicente, F.H.; Grada, A. Management of Truncal Acne with Oral Sarecycline: Pooled Results from Two Phase-3 Clinical Trials. *J. Drugs Dermatol.* **2021**, *20*, 634–640. [CrossRef]
67. Pariser, D.M.; Green, L.J.; Lain, E.L.; Schmitz, C.; Chinigo, A.S.; McNamee, B.; Berk, D.R. Safety and Tolerability of Sarecycline for the Treatment of Acne Vulgaris: Results from a Phase III, Multicenter, Open-Label Study and a Phase I Phototoxicity Study. *J. Clin. Aesthet. Dermatol.* **2019**, *12*, E53–E62. [CrossRef] [PubMed]
68. Zhao, R.; Shi, W.Z.; Zhang, Y.M.; Fang, S.H.; Wei, E.Q. Montelukast, a cysteinyl leukotriene receptor-1 antagonist, attenuates chronic brain injury after focal cerebral ischaemia in mice and rats. *J. Pharm. Pharmacol.* **2011**, *63*, 550–557. [CrossRef] [PubMed]
69. Montelukast 10 mg Film Coated Tablets. EMC. Available online: https://www.medicines.org.uk/emc/product/1243/ (accessed on 30 October 2022).
70. Behrangi, E.; Arasteh, E.; Tavakoli, T.; Mehran, G.; Atefi, N.; Esmaeeli, S.; Azizian, Z. Comparing efficacy of Montelukast versus doxycycline in treatment of moderate acne. *J. Res. Med. Sci.* **2015**, *20*, 379–382. [PubMed]
71. Rokni, G.R.; Mohammadnezhad, F.; Saeedi, M.; Shadi, S.; Sharma, A.; Sandhu, S.; Gupta, A.; Goldust, M. Efficacy, tolerability, and safety of montelukast versus finasteride for the treatment of moderate acne in women: A prospective, randomized, single-blinded, active-controlled trial. *J. Cosmet. Dermatol.* **2021**, *20*, 3580–3585. [CrossRef]
72. Fazelzadeh Haghighi, N.; Dastgheib, L.; Saki, N.; Alipour, S.; Ranjbar, S. Montelukast as an effective adjuvant in the treatment of moderate acne vulgaris. *Dermatol. Ther.* **2022**, *35*, e15770. [CrossRef]
73. George, R.; Clarke, S.; Thiboutot, D. Hormonal therapy for acne. *Semin. Cutan. Med. Surg.* **2008**, *27*, 188–196. [CrossRef]
74. Cramer, J.A.; Roy, A.; Burrell, A.; Fairchild, C.J.; Fuldeore, M.J.; Ollendorf, D.A.; Wong, P.K. Medication compliance and persistence: Terminology and definitions. *Value Health* **2008**, *11*, 44–47. [CrossRef]
75. Dréno, B.; Thiboutot, D.; Gollnick, H.; Finlay, A.Y.; Layton, A.; Leyden, J.J.; Leutenegger, E.; Perez, M. Large-scale worldwide observational study of adherence with acne therapy. *Int. J. Dermatol.* **2010**, *49*, 448–456. [CrossRef]
76. Hayran, Y.; İncel Uysal, P.; Öktem, A.; Aksoy, G.G.; Akdoğan, N.; Yalçın, B. Factors affecting adherence and patient satisfaction with treatment: A cross-sectional study of 500 patients with acne vulgaris. *J. Dermatol. Treat.* **2021**, *32*, 64–69. [CrossRef]
77. Salamzadeh, J.; Torabi Kachousangi, S.; Hamzelou, S.; Naderi, S.; Daneshvar, E. Medication adherence and its possible associated factors in patients with acne vulgaris: A cross-sectional study of 200 patients in Iran. *Dermatol. Ther.* **2020**, *33*, e14408. [CrossRef]
78. Miyachi, Y.; Hayashi, N.; Furukawa, F.; Akamatsu, H.; Matsunaga, K.; Watanabe, S.; Kawashima, M. Acne management in Japan: Study of patient adherence. *Dermatology* **2011**, *223*, 174–181. [CrossRef] [PubMed]
79. Alsubeeh, N.A.; Alsharafi, A.A.; Ahamed, S.S.; Alajlan, A. Treatment Adherence among Patients with Five Dermatological Diseases and Four Treatment Types—A Cross-Sectional Study. *Patient Prefer. Adherence* **2019**, *13*, 2029–2038. [CrossRef]
80. Yentzer, B.A.; Alikhan, A.; Teuschler, H.; Williams, L.L.; Tusa, M.; Fleischer, A.B., Jr.; Kaur, M.; Balkrishnan, R.; Feldman, S.R. An exploratory study of adherence to topical benzoyl peroxide in patients with acne vulgaris. *J. Am. Acad. Dermatol.* **2009**, *60*, 879–880. [CrossRef]
81. Grada, A.; Perche, P.; Feldman, S. Adherence and Persistence to Acne Medications: A Population-Based Claims Database Analysis. *J. Drugs Dermatol.* **2022**, *21*, 758–764. [CrossRef] [PubMed]
82. Hung, C.T.; Chen, Y.H.; Hung, T.L.; Chiang, C.P.; Chen, C.Y.; Wang, W.M. Clinician-created educational video for shared decision-making in the outpatient management of acne. *PLoS ONE* **2022**, *17*, e0271100. [CrossRef] [PubMed]

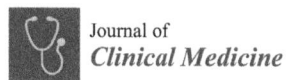

Review

Revisiting the Role of Local Cryotherapy for Acne Treatment: A Review and Update

Nark-Kyoung Rho

Leaders Aesthetic Laser & Cosmetic Surgery Center, Seoul 06014, Republic of Korea; rhonark@hanmail.net

Abstract: Acne vulgaris is a well-recognized condition among adolescents and adults that adversely affects their quality of life. Local cryotherapy has long been reported to be effective in treating acne vulgaris, inducing a more rapid involution of acne than topical medications. However, the use of cryotherapy has been limited for acne treatment due to several drawbacks, including procedural pain and pigmentary alterations. Currently, newer cryotherapy devices are gaining attention in dermatology due to their ability to monitor and precisely control the target temperature. In this narrative review, a brief history and the latest update on acne cryotherapy will be presented. Additionally, a special emphasis is placed on the role of cryotherapy, alone or in combination with intralesional steroid injections for nodulocystic acne.

Keywords: acne vulgaris; analgesia; cryosurgery; cryotherapy; hidradenitis suppurativa; intralesional injections; pain; sebaceous gland

Citation: Rho, N.-K. Revisiting the Role of Local Cryotherapy for Acne Treatment: A Review and Update. *J. Clin. Med.* **2023**, *12*, 26. https://doi.org/10.3390/jcm12010026

Academic Editor: Stamatis Gregoriou

Received: 20 November 2022
Revised: 7 December 2022
Accepted: 16 December 2022
Published: 20 December 2022

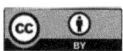

Copyright: © 2022 by the author. Licensee MDPI, Basel, Switzerland. This article is an open access article distributed under the terms and conditions of the Creative Commons Attribution (CC BY) license (https://creativecommons.org/licenses/by/4.0/).

1. Introduction

Since acne vulgaris is a multifactorial disorder, dermatologists often provide different treatment modalities to attack as many factors as possible. Along with topical or systemic medications, physical procedures have been employed for many years to complement medical therapy for acne, from simple extraction to energy-based treatments [1]. Dermatologists use cryotherapy as an inexpensive, safe, and easy way to treat skin lesions in a clinical setting. However, it is still relatively unknown today that local cryotherapy is one of the most frequently used physical modalities to treat acne and has been used for several decades. In this review, we provide a historical perspective and recent updates on the use of cryotherapy to treat acne and related conditions.

2. Brief History and Early Reports of Acne Cryotherapy

Dermatologic cryosurgery textbooks and scholarly reviews credit James Arnott, who is widely regarded, as the "father of modern cryosurgery" [2,3]. In his own words, Arnott described his cryotherapy technique as "congelation arresting the accompanying inflammation and destroying the vitality of the cancer cell [2]". In addition to treating tumors, Arnott also proposed that cryotherapy could be utilized to treat other dermatologic conditions, including acne vulgaris. Arnott won the prize medal at the Great Exhibition of London of 1851 for his cold equipment that allowed reducing tissue temperature to −20 °C [4] (Figure 1).

From Arnott's early work, the practice of cryotherapy has blossomed into a staple in the practice of modern dermatology [5]. Arnott's idea led to the development of a more practical cryotherapy device consisting of carbon dioxide collector and compressor units, which John Hall-Edwards described in 1911 [6] (Figure 2). In 1925 Giraudeau (cited by [7]) commenced using cryotherapy for acne, with a mixture of solid carbon dioxide (−78.5 °C), acetone, and precipitated sulfur, which was later found out by Dobes et al. [8] to produce better results in papulopustular acne than in nodular lesions. The degree of erythema and desquamation produced by cryotherapy is determined by the time the slush is in contact with the skin [9].

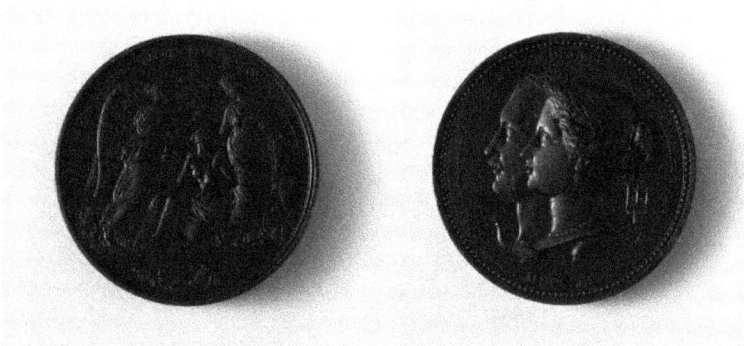

Figure 1. Juror's medal awarded to Dr. James Arnott, Great Exhibition of London, 1851, for his development of cold therapy equipment (reproduced from the Metropolitan Museum of Art, New York City, used under a Creative Commons Attribution 1.0 Universal Public Domain Dedication).

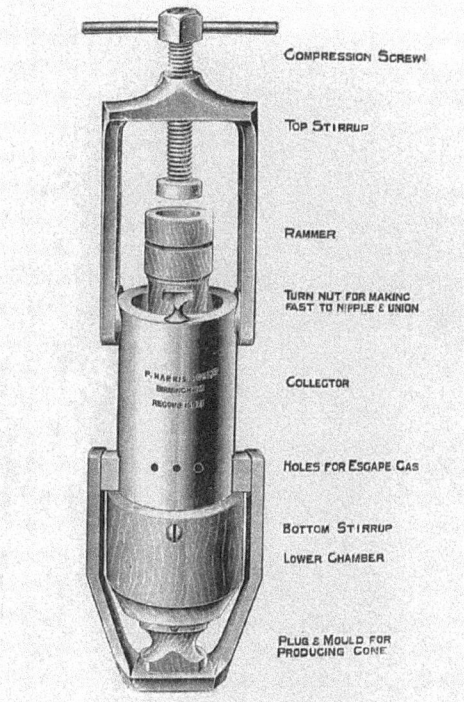

Figure 2. Carbon dioxide snow collector and compressor, as demonstrated by Hall-Edwards 1913 (reproduced from the Wellcome Library, London, used under a Creative Commons Attribution 4.0 International License).

At the end of the 19th century, all the so-called "permanent gases" (oxygen, nitrogen, and hydrogen) were liquefied, and commercial liquefaction of air was established by Carl Von Linde [4,6]. Campbell White used a glass flask that acted as a liquid air sprayer, which became the first portable cryosurgery device (Figure 3) [4]. During the 1920s and 1930s, liquified oxygen ($-182.9\ °C$) was used as a cryogenic agent to treat various skin conditions, including acne [3]. However, liquid oxygen soon became obsolete as a cryogenic agent because of its high combustibility [10].

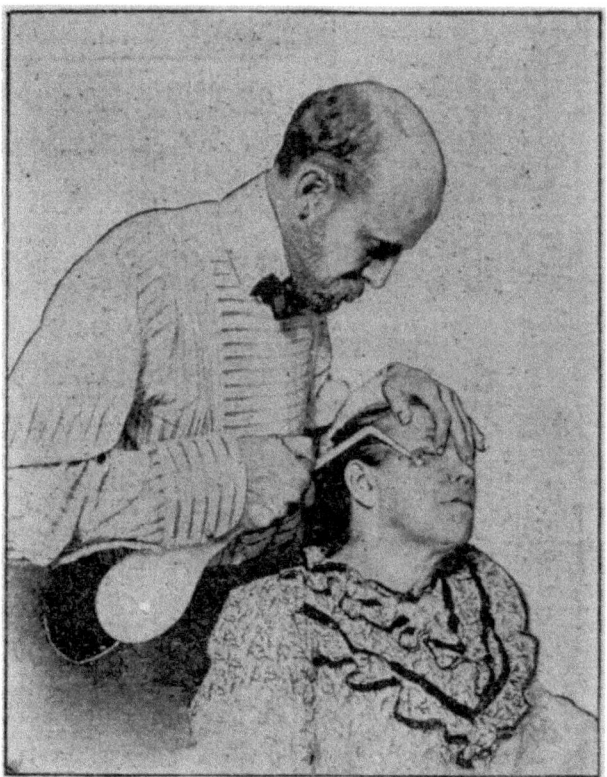

Figure 3. Campbell White treating a skin lesion with sprayed liquid air as it appeared in the New York Tribune in 1900 (reproduced from the Library of Congress, Washington, DC. New York Daily Tribune, October 25, 1900, page 8, image 22. In the public domain).

Liquid nitrogen ($-196\ ^\circ$C) became commercially available and was introduced into clinical practice in 1950 by Herman V. Allington [11], who was the first to publish on the successful use of liquid nitrogen to treat acne. Allington used a cotton swab dipped in liquid nitrogen [4,11]. Later reports in the 1970s mainly used liquid nitrogen as a cryogen source to treat acne. A study of 150 acne patients treated with liquid nitrogen cryotherapy reported excellent results in 95% of cases [12]. In 1973, Goette [13] also reported that liquid nitrogen cryotherapy was effective in treating acne. In 1967, Setrag Zacarian, who brought the term "cryosurgery" into use for the first time, designed a handheld cryosurgical device using liquid nitrogen which gave rise to several models of handheld cryosurgical units [14].

3. Cryotherapy for Acne

Key findings from several clinical studies are summarized in Table 1. Prior to the advent of effective medications, cryotherapy was en vogue in the management of acne patients, however, this approach seems to be regarded as obsolete nowadays, as mentioned by Plewig and Kligman [15]. Modern oral and topical antibiotic regimens and oral isotretinoin have reduced the need for cryosurgical treatments of acne [16]. Although cryosurgery is not a first-line modality of current acne therapy, it can be a helpful alternative when treating patients with acne that cannot be treated either with oral or topical medication, for example, acne during pregnancy [16,17].

3.1. Cystic Acne

For nodulocystic lesions of acne conglobata, a "cryoprobe" method has been applied with acceptable and long-term results [18]. The superficial freezing with liquid nitrogen fastens the resolution of chronic fluctuant nodular lesions and reduces pain [9]. Based on their experience treating more than 2000 patients with cystic or severe acne vulgaris, Wright and Gross [19] observed that cystic acne lesions almost invariably disappear after a few cryotherapy sessions. In a comparative study Cunliffe [20] confirmed the findings of Graham [12] that liquid nitrogen cryotherapy is preferable to intralesional triamcinolone injection when treating cystic acne. Past clinical experiences suggested that cryotherapy may be most effective in treating superficial cystic lesions and least effective against deeper lesions [13]. One hospital-based study from Nepal shows that cryotherapy is still actively used to treat benign conditions including acne cysts, constituting 4% of dermatology patients [21].

3.2. Acne Keloids

Cryotherapy is well described and still frequently used to treat the keloidal type of acne. In 1994, the American Academy of Dermatology's Committee on guidelines of care stated that cryotherapy is an established treatment for keloids and hypertrophic scars [22]. Zouboulis [23] also suggested that cryotherapy could be the treatment of choice for keloids and hypertrophic scars. Röhrs et al. [24] reported that acne keloids showed a 73% improvement or complete regression after multiple cryotherapy sessions in 16 patients. Resistance to the treatment occurred in 12% of the lesions, mostly observed in cases of larger keloids. Excellent and good results were particularly observed in short-duration cases, whereas older keloids showed poor results. Younger patients showed better responses than older patients. The data from a double-blind study by Layton et al. [25] should also be mentioned. The study compared the efficacy and safety of intralesional triamcinolone and cryosurgery for treating acne keloids. The authors demonstrated that by treating early keloids with the latter, 85% showed a moderate to good response regarding lesion flattening. The response to cryosurgery resulted in a significantly better response in early acne keloids characterized by high vascularity. It is recommended that cryotherapy be performed directly before administering intralesional corticosteroid injections [26] because cryotherapy-induced edema facilitates injection into acne nodules and keloids [27].

3.3. Other Subtypes of Acne

The efficacy of cryotherapy in comedonal acne is controversial. Earlier researchers [8,13,15] reported that comedonal acne responded poorly to cryotherapy. A split-face controlled trial study of 25 patients in which liquid nitrogen was applied to acne lesions on one side of the face, and other topical therapies were used on the other side, showed liquid nitrogen to be effective against pustular but not comedonal acne [13]. Plewig and Kligman [15] also noted that although spot cryotherapy is moderately helpful in treating inflammatory lesions such as papules, pustules, and nodules, it does not release comedones. Although some authors suggest that cryotherapy speeds the removal of comedones and promotes acne resolution [28], the advent of effective topical remedies has largely decreased the use of cryosurgery to treat early acne lesions, especially comedones [16]. Cryotherapy is not always very effective for treating deep draining sinuses in acne [29]. According to the author's experience in Korea, a more favorable outcome of cryotherapy tends to be obtained in patients with papulopustular or superficial cystic acne than in patients with comedones, nodules, or deep-seated cysts (Figure 4).

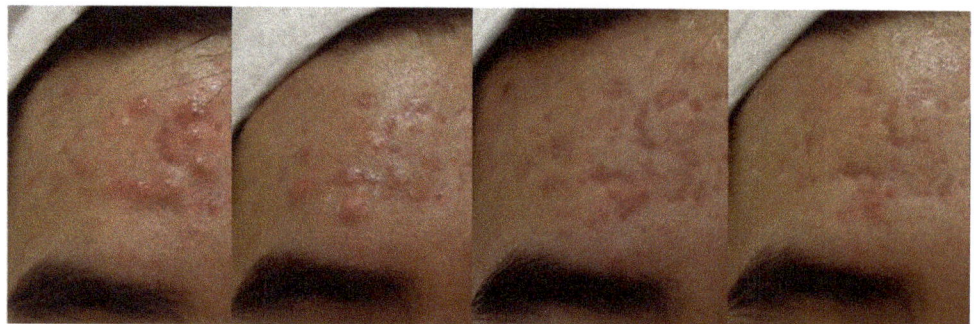

Figure 4. Improvement of inflammatory papules and superficial cysts on the forehead of a Korean adolescent acne patient, after three sessions of local cryotherapy using a temperature-controlled cryotherapy device (TargetCool; RecensMedical, Ulsan, Korea). Permission and consent were given for the use of the photographs.

Table 1. Summary table of the results of clinical studies.

Author, Year	n	Types of Acne	Refrigerant	Delivery Method	Control	Findings
Dobes and Keil, 1940 [8]	115	Papulopustular Nodulocystic Acne scars	Solid carbon dioxide slush	Contact method		Successful results in 70% of papulopustular acne patients Hard nodules respond better than soft cysts Unsatisfactory results in acne scars
Goette, 1973 [13]	25	Comedopapular Papulopustular	Liquid nitrogen	Cotton tip	Topical medications	Cryotherapy-treated pustular acne lesions involuted more rapidly than lesions treated by topical medications
Leyden et al., 1974 [18]	25	Nodulocystic	Carbon dioxide Nitrous oxide Freon	Cryoprobe		Marked flattening or complete resolution of nodulo-cystic lesions in 7–10 days
Layton et al., 1994 [25]	11	Acne keloids	Liquid nitrogen	Spray	Intralesional triamcinolone injection	Cryosurgery proved a significantly better treatment for these more vascular keloids than triamcinolone
Röhrs et al., 1997 [24]	16	Acne keloids	Nitrous oxide Liquid nitrogen	Contact method		Excellent and good results with flattening of the lesions to the skin level or slightly persisting hypertrophy were obtained in 73% of the lesions

3.4. Acne-Induced Hyperpigmentation

Melanocytes are highly susceptible to freezing at temperatures of −4 to −7 °C [30]. Clinically hypopigmentation is one of the most common side effects of cryotherapy [16,26,31,32], which is characterized by an absence of melanosomes in keratinocytes, although melanocytes are preserved [33]. Recently, researchers demonstrated that the pigment-reducing properties of cooling could apply to treat benign skin pigmentation, with a high rate of procedural success and aesthetic improvement at two months post-treatment [34]. In the study, controlled, localized freezing to the epidermis was associated with the least procedural discomfort, social downtime, and minimal risk of postinflammatory hyperpigmentation. This device (Glacial Rx; R2 Technologies, San Ramon, CA, USA) is now FDA-cleared for removing benign skin lesions. A recent study by Kwack et al. [30] further evaluated the effect of a novel temperature-adjustable cryotherapy device on the expression of pigmentation-related biomarkers and found that the expression of tyrosinase, c-kit, melanocortin 1 receptor, and microphthalmia-associated transcription factor showed decreased tendency after local skin cooling under various conditions ($-5\ °C$ to $10\ °C$, for 5, 10, or 20 s). In patients with dark skin, acne shows a tendency to be accompanied by postinflammatory hyperpigmentation [35]. Since acne-induced pigmentation is at least as concerning as the acne lesions themselves and, in many cases, is considered even more troublesome than the acne [35], the use of cryotherapy to treat both acne and postacne hyperpigmentation is worth further investigation.

Brody [28] suggested that cryotherapy is a superlative agent for neurotic excoriations or "acne excoriée," characterized by disfiguring hyperpigmentation of picked lesions. An earlier report by Dobes and Keil [8] also describes that neurotic excoriation of acne lesions can be successfully treated by cryotherapy. A moderate application to excoriated areas will keep the patient's hands off the lesions long enough to heal and inspire the patient not to touch the areas for a variable length of time, with predictable results [28]. There is a report of the successful use of cryotherapy in patients with therapy-resistant prurigo nodularis [36], a neurotic excoriation that shares many features with acne excoriée. Dermatologists found that temperature-controlled cryotherapy effectively blocks itchy sensations [37].

3.5. Hidradenitis Suppurativa

Although hidradenitis suppurativa and acne show little overlap in pathogenesis and clinical features, they often occur together as part of the acne tetrad. They are both characterized by innate inflammation involving interleukin-1 [38]. Bong et al. [39] reported outcomes for ten patients with persistent painful nodules of hidradenitis suppurativa treated with cryotherapy. Cryotherapy was effective in eight of ten patients with limited but persistent painful nodules of hidradenitis suppurativa and was described as a possible treatment for hidradenitis suppurativa [39]. The authors postulated that post-treatment ulceration and healing by secondary intention destroy hair follicles and apocrine glands, which are involved in the pathogenesis of chronic nodule formation [39]. There has been a case report [40] of a modified intralesional cryotherapy technique called "cryoinsufflation" by using an ordinary needle to inject liquid nitrogen directly into the sinus tracts of hidradenitis suppurativa. Cryoinsufflation can also be utilized when planning surgical procedures of hidradenitis suppurativa, including deroofing and limited and radical excision [41].

3.6. Other Inflammatory Dermatoses

The role of cryotherapy in treating other inflammatory skin conditions is worth mentioning since acne vulgaris is regarded as a primary inflammatory disease rather than an infectious condition. Although research on the impact of individual skin characteristics is inconsistent, positive effects on reducing inflammation and oxidative stress have been noted, supported by clinical reports of cryotherapy successfully used in several inflammatory skin conditions [9,37], including atopic dermatitis [42]. Cryotherapy was also reported to be effective in treating psoriasis [43], although many clinicians have hesitated to use cryosurgery in psoriasis since cold injury may induce an isomorphic response (the Koebner phenomenon).

4. Mechanism of Action

4.1. Histologic Studies

Traditionally, freezing-related direct cellular injury is thought to be responsible for the efficacy of cryotherapy in treating acne. Acute inflammation with predominant neutrophils develops 3 to 6 h after liquid nitrogen spraying; 12 to 24 h after, the lymphocytes and macrophages are recruited [44]. Although not fully founded in evidence, it is generally regarded that freezing causes inflammatory lesions to disappear faster than without treatment [15]. This effect may explain cryosurgery's superior efficacy in treating more severe subtypes of acne lesions, i.e., cysts and keloids [31]. As shown in histological observations, cryotherapy produces cold damage to the fibrotic cyst wall, resulting in the chemotaxis of neutrophils, whose proteases will subsequently destroy the cyst wall and allow healing [9,12]. Histological studies also found that cryotherapy eventually causes a reduction in myofibroblasts and mast cells in keloidal lesions, in addition to the normalization of collagen structure and organization [45].

Another histologic finding of cryo-treated acne lesions is vascular disruption. Histologic studies of the refrigerant sprayed on the pig skin showed vascular engorgement with extravasated red blood cells at 15 and 30 s on day zero and normal healing at a subsequent biopsy on day seven [46]. Cryotherapy exhibited significantly better results than intralesional triamcinolone in a randomized study with 11 patients with multiple acne keloids, especially in early vascular lesions [25]. Cryotherapy is effective in treating cystic acne, another subtype characterized by a distinct vascular component. In some patients, pyogenic granuloma-like vascular proliferations form in areas of cystic activity, suggesting that factors unique to cystic acne may play a role in this vascular proliferation [47]. Interestingly, pyogenic granuloma itself responds well to local cryotherapy, which aligns with the findings by Chao et al. [48] that vascular-mediated injury is responsible for the therapeutic efficacy of cryotherapy in microvascular-perfused tissue.

4.2. Possible Mechanisms of Action

Important factors that play a role in the genesis of acne formation include hormones, inflammatory mediators, *Cutibacterium acnes*, and genetics. Testosterone and androgens cause activation and proliferation of keratinocytes, sebaceous cells, and ductal lining cells of the hair follicle, which accumulate in the pilosebaceous unit and result in the formation of pore obstruction and more sebum production. Oxygen availability within the cells can be compromised by the pressure exerted inside the pilosebaceous unit, providing ideal environmental conditions for the growth of *C. acnes* which further promotes acne formation [49].

Several suggested mechanisms of acne cryotherapy include restoration of microflora, improvement of skin microcirculation, normalization of follicular hyperkeratosis, improvement of sebum evacuation, and immunomodulation [50]. Reversal of follicular hyperkeratosis initially has been suggested, based on the findings that cryotherapy induces molecular changes resulting in a decreased expression of Ki-67 [51], an epidermal proliferation marker that is an indicator of ductal hyperproliferation during acne development [52].

A second suggested mechanism is the immunomodulatory action of cryotherapy, which has been also studied in a variety of disorders [42]. Cold has an initial inflammatory effect, but an anti-inflammatory effect becomes evident 24–48 h after freezing the lesion, and faster reabsorption of the lesion occurs [53]. Several reports showed the clinical efficacy of local cooling in the relief of inflammatory acne [7,13,18], producing better results in papulopustular acne than in nodular lesions [8]. It has been noted that cold exposure induces the release of fewer proinflammatory cytokines (IL-2, IL-6, IL-8, IL-9, and TNF-α, among many others) and more anti-inflammatory cytokines (mainly IL-10), in addition, improve humoral and cellular immunity, stimulating B lymphocytes and natural killer lymphocytes (NK cells) [42]. Local cryotherapy has been shown to decrease the level of interleukin-1β, prostaglandin-E2, and nuclear factor-κB, which are known to be elevated in inflammatory acne lesions in vivo [54]. In keloidal lesions treated with cryotherapy, CD163+ M2 macrophages and matrix metalloproteinase-9 were significantly increased, indicating that cryotherapy-recruited macrophages supply matrix metalloproteinase-9, which function in fibrotic resolution in during treatment [55].

Cellular mechanisms governing acne pathogenesis include insulin-stimulated activation of the PI3K-Akt signaling pathways along with mTOR in sebocytes, resulting in increased synthesis of proteins and lipids, cell proliferation, and inflammation [49]. Insulin has been reported to decrease in cold conditions [56], which may imply the possible role of cryotherapy in inhibiting the activation of the signal pathways during acne development.

4.3. Effects on the Sebaceous Gland

Given the preferential susceptibility of lipid-containing cells to cold [57], it might be feasible to hypothesize that controlled local skin cooling causes preferential injury to sebaceous glands. According to a histologic observation by Burge and Dawber [58], a light freezing injury resulted in the shrinkage and degeneration of sebaceous glands. Furthermore, the infiltration of inflammatory cells and partial destruction of sebaceous gland cells have been found 24 h after shallow cryotherapy [59].

Some studies have evaluated in vivo biological effects of cryotherapy on normal sebaceous glands. Ray Jalian et al. [60] investigated the role of controlled local skin cooling in causing preferential injury to sebaceous glands to understand its mechanism in treating acne vulgaris. They observed that cooling-induced damage led to a 20% reduction in sebum output for two weeks, with minimal collateral injury to surrounding tissues. A higher number of freeze–thaw cycles and slower thawing resulted in more significant tissue injury. In mouse ears, peak histologic damage occurred 72 h after treatment; eosinophilic necrotic plugs formed within sebaceous glands, and the number of glands was significantly reduced up to one week after treatment [60]. A significant decrease in sebum secretion has also been reported in patients receiving whole-body cryotherapy [61]. A study using coherent anti-Stokes Raman scattering microscopy has proved a gradual loss of subcellular structures in sebocytes after cold exposure [62], which is consistent with previous findings. The effect of lipid crystallization was demonstrated to have a limited role in causing cellular disruption. Instead, sebocyte loss occurred at temperatures lower than those required for lipid crystallization [62].

Reports of successful treatment of sebaceous hyperplasia using cryotherapy [63–65] may support the concept of "selective cryolysis of sebaceous glands". A recent study involving 40 patients with 517 sebaceous hyperplasia lesions found that six liquid nitrogen cryotherapy sessions at two week intervals resulted in an excellent response [76–100%] in 65.9% of patients, with no recurrence seen at the four month follow-up [66]. The authors concluded that a well-aimed and controlled use of cryosurgery is a cost-effective treatment modality for treating significant cosmetic disfigurement in patients with sebaceous hyperplasia [66]. However, the efficacy of cryotherapy for sebaceous hyperplasia seems to be inferior to electrodessication [65].

Nonetheless, the biological effect of cryotherapy on the sebaceous glands seems to be limited and reversible. Results from a study using a temperature higher than what is used in tumor treatment showed that the sebum output recovered after four weeks [60]. The study further showed that immunohistochemistry-based expression of a proliferative marker (Ki67) and a progenitor basal cell marker (keratin 15) was not disrupted by cooling, which led to the conclusion that cooling-induced damage may be temporary and may occur due to the disruption of cellular architecture, enzymatic activity, and decreased lipid content [60]. Although recovery of most sebaceous glands started 1–2 weeks after treatment, some of the glands never recovered within the experiment, suggesting that some sebaceous glands may be permanently damaged by cooling when the temperature is significantly low [32].

5. Adjunctive Uses of Cryotherapy in Acne Treatment

5.1. Cryotherapy Combined with Intralesional Injections

An alternative to monotherapy with cryotherapy in acne is to use it as an adjuvant treatment. In dermatology practice, cryotherapy has often been combined with intralesional injection therapies [36,67–69]. However, the efficacy of combined cryotherapy and intralesional injections has not been evaluated for acne treatment. Since keloids respond well to combined cryotherapy and intralesional injections, we may assume that keloidal acne could also benefit from combination therapy.

Reports demonstrate that hypertrophic scars and keloids respond rather well to a combination of cryotherapy and intralesional corticosteroid injections. Combined cryotherapy and intralesional steroid injection are often used for small, newly formed acne keloids [70].

Some authors [71] claim that the best treatments for acne keloids are steroid injections plus cryotherapy. Optimal results, with an average of 80% improvement, have been reported with cryosurgery combined with intralesional steroid injection for early acne keloid lesions [15]. Yosipovitch et al. [72] performed a controlled study to evaluate the combined effects of intralesional corticosteroid injections with cryotherapy vs. intralesional corticosteroids or cryotherapy alone and found that the combination treatment was superior to each monotherapy. Therapeutic results may be improved, and scar recurrence reduced when intralesional corticosteroids are combined with cryotherapy [73]. Lesions treated with combination therapy require fewer procedures and have lower recurrence rates [26]. Moreover, it can produce marked flattening of most acne lesions within 48 to 72 h [74,75]. According to a recent survey of 100 dermatology healthcare professionals, the most treated lesions were cysts, followed by inflammatory papules, and pustules [76]. Many dermatologists use the combination because it is inexpensive, quick, simple, and has few side effects [77]. Figure 5 shows an example of the clinical result of combined cryotherapy and triamcinolone injection on cystic acne.

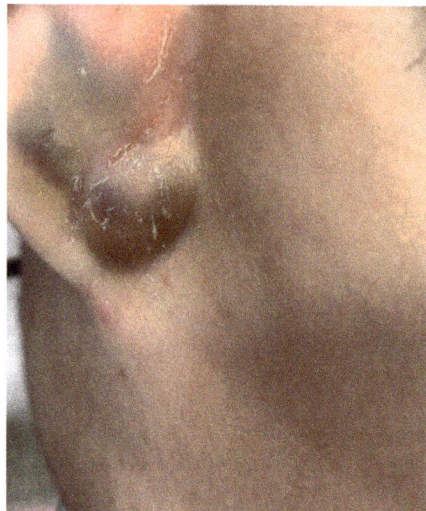 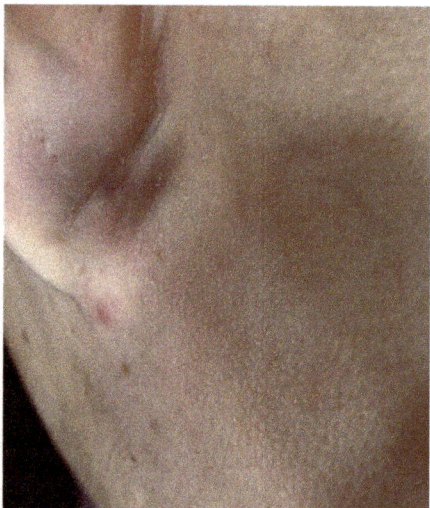

Figure 5. The combined cryotherapy (target temperature at −5 °C, 15 s of spraying) and triamcinolone injection (4.0 mg/mL, 0.2 mL injected intralesionally) yielded a resolution of cystic acne in a 17 year-old Korean male. Before (**left**) and two weeks after combination treatment (**right**). For cryotherapy, a temperature-controlled carbon dioxide spray device (TargetCool; RecensMedical, Ulsan, Korea) was used. Permission and consent were given for the use of the photographs.

5.2. Intralesional Injections in the Treatment of Acne: The Pain Issue

One rationale for the adjuvant use of cryotherapy is that it could effectively reduce the pain of intralesional injection. Injection-related pain is of particular concern when treating pediatric patients, which largely limits the use of intralesional injection in children and adolescents. Pain during injection has not been a major topic in pediatric dermatology, although injections with triamcinolone has been recommended for the fast resolution of nodulocystic lesions in adolescent acne patients [75,78]. Even minor medical procedures such as venipuncture cause significant pain in the pediatric population, compounded by needle phobia in children and adolescents [79]. Nevertheless, interventions to reduce pain and distress are infrequently used [80]. About 3–4% of the world population is estimated to have severe blood injury and injection phobia [81]. Injection phobia was the main reason for 11.5% of the COVID-19 vaccine-hesitant people in the UK [82].

Dermatologists have been using local anesthetics mixed with the suspension of corticosteroids to reduce injection pain. However, although the injectable is prepared with a local anesthetic, patients receiving an intralesional injection with anesthetic experienced no decrease in pain at the time of injection, as demonstrated in a recent double-blind, randomized controlled trial [83]. Several reasons lie behind this phenomenon. First, commonly used local anesthetics, such as lidocaine and bupivacaine, can cause a burning sensation and be a source of significant discomfort due to their acidic pH [84]. Second, intralesional injections may prove challenging because of the high pressures required to deposit an adequate amount of corticosteroid [85], which could result in considerable pain associated with a rapid increase of the pressure inside the lesion. Most of all, mixing local anesthetics with corticosteroids does not diminish the pain associated with the needle puncture itself, the most noxious component of the injection experience [83,86], since the anesthetic effect takes place a few seconds after injection. A recent controlled trial by Zakria et al. [83] counterintuitively revealed that there is even more injection-associated pain when lidocaine with epinephrine is included with the corticosteroid. Based on their findings, the authors recommended diluting the intralesional injection drugs with normal saline rather than lidocaine.

5.3. Local Skin Cooling to Reduce Pain during Intralesional Injection

Pain with intralesional injections is considered a necessary evil, but it can be reduced by simple means, including cooling. Local skin cooling before the procedure can help minimize the pain during intralesional injection [87,88]. Cutaneous cooling for pain relief (cryoanalgesia) has a long history. Its recorded use in surgery was as early as 1807 [88], implying that it could also reduce pain during intralesional injections. Early in 1850, Arnott [2] suggested that the numbing effects of the cold should be further utilized to anesthetize skin before surgery. One of the simplest methods involves cooling the skin using ice packs held in place to be injected, which should be applied for several minutes before injection to get an effective anesthetic effect [88,89]. To achieve a skin surface temperature of 10 °C, the ice pack needs to be applied for about 20 min [90]. The time-consuming nature and the relative lack of good anesthetic effects of ice compression prompted clinicians to use other cryotherapy modalities to get more anesthetic and analgesic effects [91,92]. A recent prospective, open trial involving 21 dermatologic patients who received intralesional triamcinolone injections revealed that the mean pain reduction was 3.4 (a numeric rating scale, 0 to 10) in the liquid nitrogen spray cooling group and 6.9 in the noncooling control group ($p < 0.001$) [92].

While providing a better anesthetic effect than simple ice compression, "surgical cryotherapy" can cause significant cold injury to the skin when used incorrectly [93]. To avoid unwanted side effects such as erythema or blistering, physicians should keep a proper distance and maintain appropriate spray strength and duration [92], making the procedure hard to standardize. Dichlorotetrafluoroethane has also been used to control postsurgical pain and to decrease the pain of injections [94]. One study reported that the anesthetic effects of skin cooling using ethyl chloride spray were comparable to those of a 45 min application of topical lidocaine–prilocaine cream for pain relief during forehead botulinum toxin injections [95]. The literature review found that more research needs to be completed on whether cooling the acne lesion before intralesional injection decreases injection pain.

When treating nodulocystic acne, the author uses a cryotherapy parameter as follows: treatment temperature at −3 °C and spraying time of 9 to 12 s on each lesion. Cryospraying is performed immediately before and during intralesional triamcinolone injections. In practice, the author uses a temperature-controlled cryotherapy unit (TargetCool; Recens-Medical, Ulsan, Korea), which uses pressured carbon dioxide as a refrigerant. This precision cryotherapy device enables users to keep the skin surface temperature constant during spraying with the help of a built-in real-time skin temperature monitoring system.

6. Side Effects

6.1. Pain and Discomfort

Although cooling can reduce the pain sensation, it can also induce pain and discomfort [89]. Cryotherapy is only mildly painful for a brief amount of time. Transient tingling sensation or sensory alteration can develop on the treatment site [66,96,97]. Shortly after freezing erythema and edema are likely to be accompanied by peeling, and this can be unappealing to some patients [31]. In a recent hospital-based study [21], postcryotherapy erythema was seen in 8% of patients. Cryosurgery may cause the temporary crusting of the treated cysts as an undesirable side effect [16].

6.2. Pigmentary Alterations

The most common side effect of cryotherapy is a pigmentary disturbance. Although hyperpigmentation can occur in some patients [26], hypopigmentation is more commonly seen after cryotherapy [30]. Burge et al. [33] have investigated the changes in pigmentation and melanocyte distribution in human skin after a standardized freeze injury. All lesions treated with 5 or 15 s of liquid nitrogen spraying developed hypopigmentation with a peripheral rim of hyperpigmentation. Abnormalities in pigmentation persisted for at least 6 months. The mechanisms underlying melanocyte's sensitivity to cold remain unclear, but some studies have suggested that keratinocytes remain intact while melanocytes undergo different levels of apoptosis at temperatures of −4 to −20 °C for 4 min [32]. On the other hand, a histologic evaluation revealed that liquid nitrogen spraying (5 or 15 s) induced hypopigmentation, which was related to an absence of melanosomes in keratinocytes, although melanocytes were present [33]. These findings suggest that postcryosurgery hypopigmentation is not always synonymous with an absence of melanocytes. A recent study demonstrated that contact cooling of the skin surface causes selective killing and loss of epidermal melanocytes when the tissue temperature is −7.5 °C or cooler, leading to depigmentation [98], and implying that melanocyte damage may be related to the degree of cooling.

After cold-induced skin depigmentation, repigmentation occurs as melanocytes gradually migrate from hair follicles [98]. Although pigmentation changes usually recover within months [96], prolonged freezing for longer than 30 s may result in permanent pigment loss [33]. The risk for pigment abnormalities is related to the duration of freezing [33] and the number of sessions completed [26]. The risk of cryotherapy-induced hypopigmentation should always be considered in dark-skinned patients [16,31]. Cryotherapy for keloids is known to cause hypopigmentation in patients of darker skin types, the same population with a high prevalence of keloidal acne [85].

6.3. Scarring

Scarring is rare after cryotherapy at temperatures of −7.5 °C or warmer [98]. However, aggressive cryotherapy can cause hypertrophic or even atrophic scarring [22,43]. Since atrophic scarring is a long-term consequence of acne vulgaris that can heavily impact the patient's quality of life, aggressive freezing may not be adequate for treating acne.

6.4. Rare Side Effects and Contraindications

Rarely, headaches and syncope can occur after cryotherapy in the forehead or temple area [66]. Cryogen insufflations can occur when spraying after draining the cystic lesion [53]. Cold-induced urticaria can be seen after cryotherapy [89]. Furthermore, physicians should be cautious if a patient has an underlying connective tissue disease, particularly cryoglobulinemia or cryofibrinogenemia [99].

7. Acne Cryotherapy: What Is the Optimal Temperature?

7.1. Therapeutic Temperature Range for Acne

Until now, the most effective and safe temperature and time ranges have not been elucidated when treating acne using cryotherapy, suggesting the need for further investigations. Textbooks say that superficial spraying of liquid nitrogen for 5–7 s for acne treatment is usually enough [53]. A relatively "weak" cooling might be more suitable for the treatment of papules and pustules of acne when we consider the histological findings that a light freezing injury results in changes confined to the hair follicles, whereas a "tumor dose" cryotherapy may destroy hair follicles and result in the necrosis of surrounding tissue [58,59]. In contrast, more aggressive freezing is required when treating more severe acne lesions, such as nodules, cysts, and keloids, since the incomplete resolution of fibrotic nodules or cystic walls may cause worsening of the lesion and may subsequently require surgical treatment [20].

Deep-freezing temperatures of conventional liquid nitrogen cryotherapy [9] are also not required when the cooling aims to reduce the injection pain during acne treatment. A recent study on patients receiving intravitreal injections showed that effective ocular anesthesia could be achieved using a temperature-controlled cryotherapy device at a temperature of $-15\ °C$ [100]. Considering that the cooling rate in the skin layer is much higher than in the vitreous body of the eyeball, the use of an even more ambient temperature is usually enough for skin anesthesia. A weak cooling of around $-3\ °C$ is sufficient in reducing injection pain, as shown in a study by Jung et al. [97].

One of the proposed mechanisms of action showing how cryoanalgesia works are that the lowered temperature slows the neuronal metabolic rate and the speed of neuronal conduction [101]. In this regard, cryosurgery-grade, extremely low temperature is too aggressive when used for pain reduction. The "counterirritant" effect, which occurs when a temperature stimulus overrides a painful stimulus in the same area and causes a reduction in the perception of the painful stimuli [94], may also involve "cooling" rather than "freezing". In contrast to deep freezing, relatively warmer cryotherapy temperatures do not result in permanent nerve damage and cause only temporary blocks of neuronal conduction [102]. The antipruritic effect of local cooling to warmer than the temperature of $-5\ °C$ is regarded to be related to the modulation of the transient receptor potential cation channel subfamily M member 8 (TRPM8) and TRPM8- expressing sensory neurons [37], which is also a target of pain reduction [103].

Recently, Leal-Silva et al. [104] performed a controlled clinical trial to evaluate the safety and efficacy of cryotherapy as a potential treatment for inflammatory acne. In ten patients with inflammatory acne, one side of the face was treated for a maximum period of 5 min at $-15\ °C$, and the other was used as a control. Two treatments, with a four week interval between them, were performed. Incremental significant reductions of the inflammatory lesions of acne were measured in all the subjects at one week and one month after the first treatment, and an even better improvement was recorded one month after the second treatment. Although the number of lesions increased by the third month follow-up visit, all subjects exhibited fewer inflammatory lesions than at the beginning of the study. No significant adverse events were observed. The result of the study imply that a nondestructive temperature setting can be effectively used for acne cryotherapy. This is an important finding since traditional liquid nitrogen cryotherapy has limitations in terms of its safety profile when treating acne.

7.2. Monitoring and Control of Target Temperature during Cryotherapy

With a temperature of around $-10\ °C$, cooling damages sebaceous glands, disrupts some enzymatic activities, and reduces sebum output for two weeks, with minimal injury to surrounding tissues [60]. These findings suggest that treatment of sebaceous gland disorders may be achievable through brief, noninvasive skin cooling, implying less aggressive cryotherapy as an effective treatment of acne vulgaris using controlled cooling. Unfortunately, conventional cryotherapy has been used at a fixed temperature for each cryogen under various time conditions and freeze–thaw cycles [30,105]. Since the traditional cryotherapy technique is empirical and largely dependent upon the physician's experience, it is very hard to standardize the clinical practice. The proper technique, involving proper distance from the skin surface, spraying time, and controlling the white frosting degree of the skin [93], is crucial to use conventional liquid nitrogen cryotherapy safely. As yet, a consensus on the parameters of liquid nitrogen cryotherapy for acne treatment has not been reached.

One of the important technological innovations in dermatologic cryosurgery is the incorporation of the temperature sensor unit in the device (Cry-Ac Tracker Cam; Brymill Cryogenic Systems, Ellington, CT; Figure 6). Using a real-time temperature monitoring, this liquid nitrogen cryotherapy device facilitated the controlled timely destruction of the target tissue [106]. The infrared light sensor continuously and safely monitors skin temperature, along with the indicators showing how fast skin temperature decreases [107], while still lacking a free adjustment of the desired temperature.

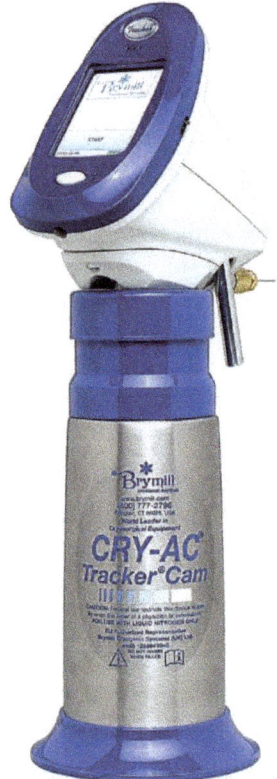

Figure 6. An updated cryotherapy device (Cry-Ac Tracker Cam) that measures the skin temperature when spraying liquid nitrogen on the selected skin lesion using an infrared sensor. The operator can set the device to indicate when a predetermined freeze temperature has been achieved at the lesion (courtesy of Brymill Cryogenic Systems, Ellington, CT).

The limited ability to adjust target temperature highlighted the need for accurate control of the target temperature during cooling and prompted the development of a "precision cryotherapy" device. Precise control of target temperature is based on an enhanced understanding of nozzle design and cryogen spray characteristics, such as mean droplet size, velocity, temperature, evaporation rates, and their relation to the heat extraction rate from the skin surface [108]. An example of such a precision cryotherapy device (TargetCool; Figure 7) features a unique capability of regulating the thermodynamic state (temperature and pressure) of cryogenic substances (e.g., carbon dioxide) by applying heat to cryogenic substances. A real-time temperature reading by an infrared sensor is used to measure the error between the set cooling temperature and the target temperature, and a feedback controller is used to calculate the heat required to achieve a desired thermodynamic state of cryogen substance, leading to rapid and precision cooling at the target area [30]. This technology has been reported to be an effective and safe modality to provide cooling anesthesia to the eye as local anesthesia for intravitreal injections [100]. It has been shown to help reduce pain during laser tattoo removal [97]. Another recent study shows the clinical efficacy of a contact-type cryolipolysis device (CoolSculpting System; ZELTIQ Aesthetics, Pleasanton, CA, USA) in treating inflammatory acne [104]. Using temperature control during the treatment, these devices are expected to be helpful in training other physicians to perform cryotherapy reliably [107].

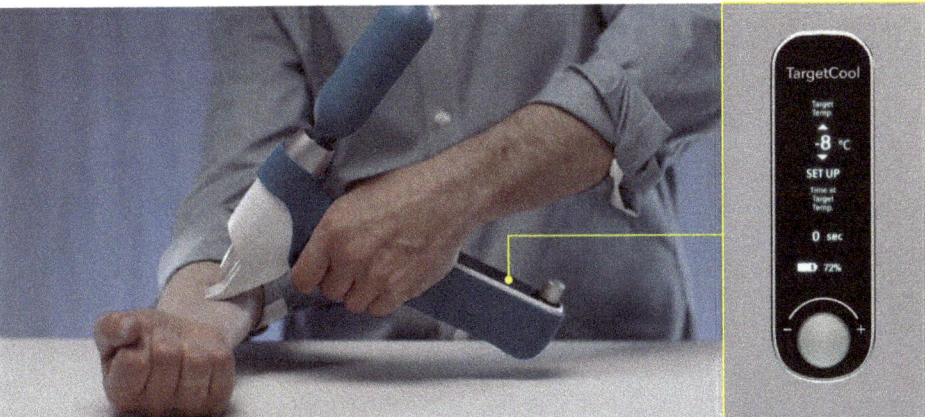

Figure 7. A novel cryotherapy device (TargetCool) developed to provide precise, controlled tissue cooling to reduce pain and inflammation of local procedures. This device uses pressurized carbon dioxide as a cryogen and can actively monitor and maintain the target temperature at a preset temperature (courtesy of RecensMedical, Ulsan, Korea).

8. Conclusions

After nearly two centuries, cryotherapy is still gaining interest in several fields of medicine, including dermatologic surgery. Dermatological cryotherapy has long been used to treat various types of acne, especially nodulocystic and keloidal subtypes. Additionally, it is a convenient, instant, and effective local anesthesia in acne patients anxious about intralesional injection-associated procedural pain. With the development of advanced cryotherapy devices, it is now possible to monitor and precisely control the target temperature, enabling physicians to standardize the protocol and minimize the adverse effects of local cryotherapy. Advances in technology are expected to promote acne cryotherapy and make it widely applicable. However, further controlled trials with larger sample sizes are needed to confirm the efficacy and provide the scientific basis for cryotherapy in acne treatment.

Funding: This research received no external funding.

Institutional Review Board Statement: Not applicable due to the nature of this article (review).

Informed Consent Statement: Written informed consent has been obtained for patient photographs appearing in this article.

Data Availability Statement: Not applicable.

Conflicts of Interest: The author declares no conflict of interest.

References

1. Taub, A.F. Procedural treatments for acne vulgaris. *Dermatol. Surg.* **2007**, *33*, 1005–1026. [CrossRef] [PubMed]
2. Arnott, J. Practical illustrations of the remedial efficacy of a very low or anaesthetic temperature. I. In cancer. *Lancet* **1850**, *56*, 257–259. [CrossRef]
3. Cooper, S.M.; Dawber, R.P.R. The history of cryosurgery. *J. R. Soc. Med.* **2001**, *94*, 196–201. [CrossRef] [PubMed]
4. Awad, S.M.I. The story behind cryosurgery. *J. Surg. Dermatol.* **2017**, *2*, 191–193. [CrossRef]
5. Crain, C.; Gibbons, J.A.; Marion, T. The father of modern cryotherapy. *SKIN J. Cutan Med.* **2019**, *3*, 283. [CrossRef]
6. Hall-Edwards, J.F. *Carbon Dioxide Snow: Its Therapeutic Uses, Methods of Collection and Application*; Simpkin, Marshall, Hamilton, Kent: London, UK, 1913.
7. Karp, F.L.; Nieman, H.A.; Lerner, C. Cryotherapy for acne and its scars. *Arch. Derm. Syphilol.* **1939**, *39*, 995. [CrossRef]
8. Dobes, W.L.; Keil, H. Treatment of acne vulgaris by cryotherapy (slush method). *Arch. Derm. Syphilol.* **1940**, *42*, 547–558. [CrossRef]
9. Kaminsky, A. Less common methods to treat acne. *Dermatology* **2003**, *206*, 68–73. [CrossRef]
10. Pasquali, P. A short history of cryosurgery. In *Cryosurgery*; Springer: Berlin/Heidelberg, Germany, 2015; pp. 3–17. [CrossRef]
11. Allington, H.V. Liquid nitrogen in the treatment of skin diseases. *Calif Med.* **1950**, *72*, 153–155.
12. Graham, G.F. Cryotherapy against acne vulgaris yields "good to excellent results". *Dermatol. Pract.* **1972**, *5*, 13–15.
13. Goette, D.K. Liquid nitrogen in the treatment of acne vulgaris: A comparative study. *S. Med. J.* **1973**, *66*, 1131–1132. [CrossRef] [PubMed]
14. Zacarian, S.A. Cryosurgery in dermatologic disorders and in the treatment of skin cancer. *J. Cryosurg.* **1968**, *1*, 70–75.
15. Plewig, G.; Kligman, A.M. Physical therapy. In *Acne and Rosacea*, 3rd ed.; Plewig, G., Kligman, A.M., Eds.; Springer: Berlin/Heidelberg, Germany, 2000; pp. 697–705. [CrossRef]
16. Usatine, R.P.; Stulberg, D.L.; Colver, G.B. *Cutaneous Cryosurgery*, 4th ed.; CRC Press: Boca Raton, FL, USA, 2014. [CrossRef]
17. Pasquali, P. Cryosurgery. In *Surgery of the Skin: Procedural Dermatology*, 2nd ed.; Robinson, J.K., Hanke, C.W., Siegel, D.M., Fratila, A., Eds.; Elsevier: Amsterdam, The Netherlands, 2010; pp. 153–166.
18. Leyden, J.J.; Mills, O.H.; Kligman, A.M. Cryoprobe treatment of acne conglobata. *Br. J. Dermatol.* **1974**, *90*, 335–341. [CrossRef] [PubMed]
19. Wright, C.S.; Gross, E.R. Solid carbon dioxide therapy for cystic acne. *Arch. Dermatol.* **1949**, *59*, 664. [CrossRef]
20. Cunliffe, W.J. Treatment of acne. In *Acne*; Cunliffe, W.J., Ed.; Martin Dunitz: London, UK, 1989; pp. 252–287.
21. Thapa, D.P.; Jha, A.K.; Shrestha, S.; Joshi, S. Cryosurgery in a dermatology setup: A hospital based study. *Our Dermatol. Online* **2018**, *9*, 137–139. [CrossRef]
22. Committee on Guidelines of Care, Task Force on Cryosurgery. Guidelines of care for cryosurgery. American Academy of Dermatology Committee on Guidelines of Care. *J. Am. Acad. Dermatol.* **1994**, *31*, 648–653.
23. Zouboulis, C.C. Principles of cutaneous cryosurgery: An update. *Dermatology* **1999**, *198*, 111–117. [CrossRef]
24. Röhrs, H.; Orfanos, C.E.; Zouboulis, C.C. Cryosurgical treatment of acne keloids. *J. Investig. Dermatol.* **1997**, *108*, 396.
25. Layton, A.M.; Yip, J.; Cunliffe, W.J. A comparison of intralesional triamcinolone and cryosurgery in the treatment of acne keloids. *Br. J. Dermatol.* **1994**, *130*, 498–501. [CrossRef]
26. Binic, I. Keloids and hypertrophic scars. In *European Handbook of Dermatological Treatments*, 3rd ed.; Springer: Berlin/Heidelberg, Germany, 2015; pp. 455–464. [CrossRef]
27. Dilworth, G.R. Acne surgery. *Can. Fam. Physician* **1983**, *29*, 955–958.
28. Brody, H.J. Solid carbon dioxide: Usage in slush or block form as therapeutic agent in dermatology. In *Dermatological Cryosurgery and Cryotherapy*; Springer: London, UK, 2016; pp. 201–206. [CrossRef]
29. Jansen, T.; Lindner, A.; Plewig, G. Draining sinus in acne and rosacea: A clinical, histopathologic and experimental study. *Hautarzt* **1995**, *46*, 417–420. [CrossRef] [PubMed]
30. Kwack, M.H.; Lee, S.; Lee, E.H.; Ha, G.U.; Kim, G.H.; Lee, W.J. Effect of a precision cryotherapy device with temperature adjustability on pigmentation. *Indian J. Dermatol.* **2022**, *67*, 204. [CrossRef] [PubMed]
31. Graham, G.F.; Tuchayi, S.M. Acne. In *Dermatological Cryosurgery and Cryotherapy*; Springer: London, UK, 2016; pp. 319–323. [CrossRef]
32. Gage, A.A.; Meenaghan, M.A.; Natiella, J.R.; Greene, G.W. Sensitivity of pigmented mucosa and skin to freezing injury. *Cryobiology* **1979**, *16*, 348–361. [CrossRef] [PubMed]
33. Burge, S.M.; Bristol, M.; Millard, P.R.; Dawber, R.P.R. Pigment changes in human skin after cryotherapy. *Cryobiology* **1986**, *23*, 422–432. [CrossRef]
34. Munavalli, G.S.; Boey, G.; Bowes, L.E.; Kilmer, S.L.; LaTowsky, B.C.; Zelickson, B.D. Multi-center study of a novel, intelligent device delivering controlled, epidermal freezing for the treatment of benign pigmented lesions. *Lasers Surg. Med.* **2019**, *51*, S27. [CrossRef]
35. Elbuluk, N.; Grimes, P.; Chien, A.; Hamzavi, I.; Alexis, A.; Taylor, S.; Gonzalez, N.; Weiss, J.; Desai, S.R.; Kang, S. The pathogenesis and management of acne-induced post-inflammatory hyperpigmentation. *Am. J. Clin. Dermatol.* **2021**, *22*, 829–836. [CrossRef]
36. Stoll, D.M.; Fields, J.P.; King, L.E. Treatment of prurigo nodularis: Use of cryosurgery and intralesional steroids plus lidocaine. *J. Dermatol. Surg. Oncol.* **1983**, *9*, 922–924. [CrossRef]

37. Lee, E.H.; Lee, H.J.; Park, K.D.; Lee, W.J. Effect of a new cryotherapy device on an itchy sensation in patients with mild atopic dermatitis. *J. Cosmet. Dermatol.* **2021**, *20*, 2906–2910. [CrossRef]
38. Pink, A.; Anzengruber, F.; Navarini, A.A. Acne and hidradenitis suppurativa. *Br. J. Dermatol.* **2018**, *178*, 619–631. [CrossRef]
39. Bong, J.L.; Shalders, K.; Saihan, E. Treatment of persistent painful nodules of hidradenitis suppurativa with cryotherapy. *Clin. Exp. Dermatol.* **2003**, *28*, 241–244. [CrossRef]
40. Pagliarello, C.; Fabrizi, G.; Feliciani, C.; di Nuzzo, S. Cryoinsufflation for Hurley stage II hidradenitis suppurativa: A useful treatment option when systemic therapies should be avoided. *JAMA Dermatol.* **2014**, *150*, 765. [CrossRef] [PubMed]
41. Daveluy, S. Cryoinsufflation in the presurgical assessment of hidradenitis suppurativa. *J. Am. Acad. Dermatol.* **2020**, *82*, e127. [CrossRef] [PubMed]
42. Dzidek and Piotrowska. The use of cryotherapy in cosmetology and the influence of cryogenic temperatures on selected skin parameters: A review of the literature. *Cosmetics* **2022**, *9*, 100. [CrossRef]
43. Nouri, K.; Chartier, T.K.; Eaglstein, W.H.; Fla, M.; Taylor, J.R. Cryotherapy for psoriasis. *Arch. Dermatol.* **1997**, *133*, 1608. [CrossRef]
44. de Souza, R.C.A.; Cunha, J.M.; Ferreira, S.H.; Cunha, F.Q.; Lima, H.C. Different inflammatory mediators induce inflammation and pain after application of liquid nitrogen to the skin. *Cryobiology* **2006**, *53*, 319–329. [CrossRef] [PubMed]
45. Har-Shai, Y.; Amar, M.; Sabo, E. Intralesional cryotherapy for enhancing the involution of hypertrophic scars and keloids. *Plast. Reconstr. Surg.* **2003**, *111*, 1841–1852. [CrossRef]
46. Dzubow, L.M. Histologic and temperature alterations induced by skin refrigerants. *J. Am. Acad. Dermatol.* **1985**, *12*, 796–810. [CrossRef]
47. Rosenthal, J.M.; Mann, R.E.; Cohen, S.R. Identical twins presenting with pyogenic granuloma-like vascular proliferations during isotretinoin therapy. *JAAD Case Rep.* **2020**, *6*, 378–380. [CrossRef]
48. Chao, B.H.; He, X.; Bischof, J.C. Pre-treatment inflammation induced by TNF-α augments cryosurgical injury on human prostate cancer. *Cryobiology* **2004**, *49*, 10–27. [CrossRef]
49. Lalrengpuii, J.; Raza, K.; Mishra, A.; Shukla, R. Retinoid nanoparticles: Approachable gateway for acne treatment. *Health Sci. Rev.* **2022**, *4*, 100042. [CrossRef]
50. Kotova, T.G.; Tsybusov, S.N.; Kochenov, V.I.; Tcyganov, M.I. Application of cryogenic methods in skin diseases of different etiology. In *Dermatologic Surgery and Procedures*; InTech: London, UK, 2018. [CrossRef]
51. Kim, J.H.; Uh, J.A.; Lee, J.H.; Lee, S.K.; Kim, M.S.; Lee, U.H. A study of clinical, histopathologic, and immunohistochemical changes after cryotherapy in actinic keratosis. *J. Am. Acad. Dermatol.* **2022**, *87*, AB133. [CrossRef]
52. Knaggs, H.E.; Holland, D.B.; Morris, C.; Wood, E.J.; Cunliffe, W.J. Quantification of cellular proliferation in acne using the monoclonal antibody Ki-67. *J. Investig. Dermatol.* **1994**, *102*, 89–92. [CrossRef] [PubMed]
53. Blanco, M.A.L.; Panagiotopoulos, A.; Pasquali, P. Cryosurgery for common benign lesions. In *Cryosurgery*; Springer: Berlin/Heidelberg, Germany, 2015; pp. 93–105. [CrossRef]
54. Guillot, X.; Tordi, N.; Laheurte, C.; Pazart, L.; Prati, C.; Saas, P.; Wendling, D. Local ice cryotherapy decreases synovial interleukin 6, interleukin 1β, vascular endothelial growth factor, prostaglandin-E2, and nuclear factor kappa B p65 in human knee arthritis: A controlled study. *Arthritis Res. Ther.* **2019**, *21*, 180. [CrossRef] [PubMed]
55. Lee, Y.; Kim, S.; Kim, J.; Kim, J.; Song, S.; Lee, W.; Lee, J.H. Tissue-remodelling M2 macrophages cecruits matrix metalloproteinase-9 for cryotherapy-induced fibrotic resolution during keloid treatment. *Acta Derm. Venereol.* **2020**, *100*, 1–8. [CrossRef] [PubMed]
56. Tikuisis, P.; Ducharme, M.B.; Moroz, D.; Jacobs, I. Physiological responses of exercised-fatigued individuals exposed to wet-cold conditions. *J. Appl. Physiol.* **1999**, *86*, 1319–1328. [CrossRef]
57. Garibyan, L.; Cornelissen, L.; Sipprell, W.; Pruessner, J.; Elmariah, S.; Luo, T.; Lerner, E.A.; Jung, Y.; Evans, C.; Zurakowski, D.; et al. Transient alterations of cutaneous sensory nerve function by noninvasive cryolipolysis. *J. Investig. Dermatol.* **2015**, *135*, 2623–2631. [CrossRef]
58. Burge, S.M.; Dawber, R.P.R. Hair follicle destruction and regeneration in guinea pig skin after cutaneous freeze injury. *Cryobiology* **1990**, *27*, 153–163. [CrossRef]
59. Ma, J.; Yu, X.; Lv, J.; Lin, D.; Lin, J.; Bai, Y.; Wang, Y.; Li, X.; Dong, J. Cryotherapy mediates histopathological and microstructural changes during the treatment of skin and subcutaneous tumors in dogs. *Cryobiology* **2021**, *98*, 164–171. [CrossRef]
60. Ray Jalian, H.; Tam, J.; Vuong, L.N.; Fisher, J.; Garibyan, L.; Mihm, M.C.; Zurakowski, D.; Evans, C.L.; Anderson, R.R. Selective cryolysis of sebaceous glands. *J. Investig. Dermatol.* **2015**, *135*, 2173–2180. [CrossRef]
61. Anna, M.; Magdalena, S.K. Evaluation of the influence of whole-body cryotherapy on selected skin parameters in healthy individuals: Pilot study. *Cryobiology* **2021**, *100*, 77–80. [CrossRef]
62. Jung, Y.; Tam, J.; Ray Jalian, H.; Rox Anderson, R.; Evans, C.L. Longitudinal, 3D in vivo imaging of sebaceous glands by coherent anti-stokes Raman scattering microscopy: Normal function and response to cryotherapy. *J. Investig. Dermatol.* **2015**, *135*, 39–44. [CrossRef] [PubMed]
63. Wheeland, R.G.; Wiley, M.D. Q-tip cryosurgery for the treatment of senile sebaceous hyperplasia. *J. Dermatol. Surg. Oncol.* **1987**, *13*, 729–730. [CrossRef] [PubMed]
64. Pakula, A.; Garden, J. Sebaceous hyperplasia and basal cell carcinoma in a renal transplant patient receiving cyclosporine. *J. Am. Acad. Dermatol.* **1992**, *26*, 139–140. [CrossRef] [PubMed]
65. Hussein, L.; Perrett, C.M. Treatment of sebaceous gland hyperplasia: A review of the literature. *J. Dermatolog. Treat.* **2021**, *32*, 866–877. [CrossRef] [PubMed]

66. Ataş, H.; Gönül, M. Evaluation of the efficacy of cryosurgery in patients with sebaceous hyperplasia of the face. *J. Cutan Med. Surg.* **2017**, *21*, 202–206. [CrossRef]
67. el Darouti, M.A.; al Rubaie, S.M. Cutaneous leishmaniasis: Treatment with combined cryotherapy and intralesional stibogluconate injection. *Int. J. Dermatol.* **1990**, *29*, 56–59. [CrossRef]
68. Dowlati, B.; Firooz, A.; Dowlati, Y. Granuloma faciale: Successful treatment of nine cases with a combination of cryotherapy and intralesional corticosteroid injection. *Int. J. Dermatol.* **1997**, *36*, 548–551. [CrossRef]
69. Ibrahim, H.; el Taieb, M.; Nada, E.; Kamal, E.; Hegazy, E. Combined intralesional injection of tuberculin purified protein derivative plus cryotherapy versus each alone in the treatment of multiple common warts. *Dermatol. Ther.* **2022**, *35*, e15350. [CrossRef]
70. Emad, M.; Omidvari, S.; Dastgheib, L.; Mortazavi, A.; Ghaem, H. Surgical excision and immediate postoperative radiotherapy versus cryotherapy and intralesional steroids in the management of keloids: A prospective clinical trial. *Med. Princ. Pract.* **2010**, *19*, 402–405. [CrossRef]
71. Rusciani, A.; Ricci, F.; Curinga, G. Acne scar treatment. In *European Handbook of Dermatological Treatments*, 3rd ed.; Springer: Berlin/Heidelberg, Germany, 2015; pp. 1073–1080. [CrossRef]
72. Yosipovitch, G.; Sugeng, M.W.; Goon, A.; Chan, Y.; Goh, C. A comparison of the combined effect of cryotherapy and corticosteroid injections versus corticosteroids and cryotherapy alone on keloids: A controlled study. *J. Dermatolog. Treat.* **2001**, *12*, 87–90. [CrossRef]
73. Boutli-Kasapidou, F.; Tsakiri, A.; Anagnostou, E.; Mourellou, O. Hypertrophic and keloidal scars: An approach to polytherapy. *Int. J. Dermatol.* **2005**, *44*, 324–327. [CrossRef] [PubMed]
74. Song, Y.; Guo, Y. Granulomatous reaction to intralesional Kenalog (triamcinolone) injection in acne: A case report. *Am. J. Dermatopathol.* **2019**, *41*, 652–654. [CrossRef] [PubMed]
75. Levine, R.M.; Rasmussen, J.E. Intralesional corticosteroids in the treatment of nodulocystic acne. *Arch. Dermatol.* **1983**, *119*, 480–481. [CrossRef] [PubMed]
76. Gallagher, T.; Taliercio, M.; Nia, J.K.; Hashim, P.W.; Zeichner, J.A. Dermatologist use of intralesional triamcinolone in the treatment of acne. *J. Clin. Aesthet. Dermatol.* **2020**, *13*, 41–43.
77. Leeming, J.A. Intralesional triamcinolone in the treatment of cystic acne. *S. Afr. Med. J.* **1965**, *39*, 567–571.
78. Young, K.D. Pediatric procedural pain. *Ann. Emerg. Med.* **2005**, *45*, 160–171. [CrossRef]
79. Lim, K. Painless steroid injections for hypertrophic scars and keloids. *Br. J. Plast. Surg.* **2004**, *57*, 475–477. [CrossRef]
80. Humphrey, G.B.; Boon, C.M.J.; van Linden van den Heuvell, G.F.E.C.; van de Wiel, H.B.M. The occurrence of high levels of acute behavioral distress in children and adolescents undergoing routine venipunctures. *Pediatrics* **1992**, *90*, 87–91. [CrossRef]
81. Wani, A.L.; Ara, A.; Bhat, S.A. Blood injury and injection phobia: The neglected one. *Behav. Neurol.* **2014**, *2014*, 471340. [CrossRef]
82. Freeman, D.; Lambe, S.; Yu, L.M.; Freeman, J.; Chadwick, A.; Vaccari, C.; Waite, F.; Rosebrock, L.; Petit, A.; Vanderslott, S.; et al. Injection fears and COVID-19 vaccine hesitancy. *Psychol. Med.* **2021**, 1–11. [CrossRef]
83. Zakria, D.; Patrinely, J.R.; Dewan, A.K.; Albers, S.E.; Wheless, L.E.; Simmons, A.N.; Drolet, B.C. Intralesional corticosteroid injections are less painful without local anesthetic: A double-blind, randomized controlled trial. *J. Dermatolog. Treat.* **2022**, *33*, 2034–2037. [CrossRef] [PubMed]
84. Strazar, R.; Lalonde, D. Minimizing injection pain in local anesthesia. *CMAJ* **2012**, *184*, 2016. [CrossRef] [PubMed]
85. Chuang, G.S.; Rogers, G.S.; Zeltser, R. Poiseuille's law and large-bore needles: Insights into the delivery of corticosteroid injections in the treatment of keloids. *J. Am. Acad. Dermatol.* **2008**, *59*, 167–168. [CrossRef] [PubMed]
86. Verbov, J. The place of intralesional steroid therapy in dermatology. *Br. J. Dermatol.* **1976**, *94*, 51–57. [CrossRef] [PubMed]
87. Goldman, L. Reactions following intralesional and sublesional injections of corticosteroids. *JAMA* **1962**, *182*, 613–616. [CrossRef]
88. Nduka, C.; van Dam, H.; Davis, K.; Shibu, M. Painless steroid injections for hypertrophic scars and keloids. *Br. J. Plast. Surg.* **2003**, *56*, 842. [CrossRef]
89. Alsantali, A. A comparative trial of ice application versus EMLA cream in alleviation of pain during botulinum toxin injections for palmar hyperhidrosis. *Clin. Cosmet. Investig. Dermatol.* **2018**, *11*, 137–140. [CrossRef] [PubMed]
90. Kanlayanaphotporn, R.; Janwantanakul, P. Comparison of skin surface temperature during the application of various cryotherapy modalities. *Arch. Phys. Med. Rehabil.* **2005**, *86*, 1411–1415. [CrossRef] [PubMed]
91. Trescot, A.M. Cryoanalgesia in interventional pain management. *Pain Physician* **2003**, *6*, 345–360. [CrossRef]
92. Lee, J.H.; Lee, R.W.; Eun, S.H.; Jung, H.M.; Kim, G.M.; Bae, J.M. Liquid nitrogen spray cooling for reducing injection pain: A pilot study. *Ann. Dermatol.* **2022**, *34*, 144. [CrossRef]
93. Plotkin, S. Clinical comparison of preinjection anesthetics. *J. Am. Podiatr. Med. Assoc.* **1998**, *88*, 73–79. [CrossRef] [PubMed]
94. Baumann, L.; Frankel, S.; Welsh, E.; Halem, M. Cryoanalgesia with dichlorotetrafluoroethane lessens the pain of botulinum toxin injections for the treatment of palmar hyperhidrosis. *Dermatol. Surg.* **2003**, *29*, 1057–1060. [CrossRef] [PubMed]
95. Irkoren, S.; Ozkan, H.S.; Karaca, H. A clinical comparison of EMLA cream and ethyl chloride spray application for pain relief of forehead botulinum toxin injection. *Ann. Plast. Surg.* **2015**, *75*, 272–274. [CrossRef] [PubMed]
96. Graham, G.F. Cryosurgical treatment of acne. *Cutis* **1975**, *16*, 509–513.
97. Jung, S.; Yoo, K.H.; Na, S.; Kim, J. Efficacy of a new cryotherapy device on pain relief during the laser tattoo removal. *Med. Lasers* **2022**, *11*, 173–177. [CrossRef]
98. Chuang, G.S.; Farinelli, W.; Anderson, R.R. Selective cryolysis of melanocytes: Critical temperature and exposure time to induce selective pigmentary loss in Yucatan pig skin. *Lasers Surg Med.* **2021**, *53*, 978–985. [CrossRef] [PubMed]

99. Stewart, R.H.; Graham, G.F. A complication of cryosurgery in a patient with cryofibrinogenemia. *J. Dermatol. Surg. Oncol.* **1978**, *4*, 743–744. [CrossRef]
100. Chao, D.L.; Rinella, N.T.; Khanani, A.M.; Wykoff, C.C.; Kim, G.H. Cooling anesthesia for intravitreal injection: Results of the prospective open-label, dose-ranging COOL-1 trial. *Clin. Ophthalmol.* **2021**, *15*, 4659–4666. [CrossRef]
101. Ernst, E.; Fialka, V. Ice freezes pain? A review of the clinical effectiveness of analgesic cold therapy. *J. Pain Symptom Manag.* **1994**, *9*, 56–59. [CrossRef]
102. Zhou, L.; Kambin, P.; Casey, K.F.; Bonner, F.J.; O'Brien, E.; Shao, Z.; Ou, S. Mechanism research of cryoanalgesia. *Neurol. Res.* **1995**, *17*, 307–311. [CrossRef]
103. De Caro, C.; Cristiano, C.; Avagliano, C.; Bertamino, A.; Ostacolo, C.; Campiglia, P.; Gómez-Monterrey, I.; La Rana, G.; Gualillo, O.; Calignano, A.; et al. Characterization of new TRPM8 modulators in pain perception. *Int. J. Mol. Sci.* **2019**, *20*, 5544. [CrossRef] [PubMed]
104. Leal-Silva, H.; Carmona-Hernández, E.; Grijalva-Vázquez, M.; Padilla-Ascencio, B. Crioterapia en acné inflamatorio. *Dermatol. Rev. Mex.* **2018**, *62*, 461–468.
105. Cunliffe, W.J. Acne. In *European Handbook of Dermatological Treatments*, 2nd ed.; Springer: Berlin/Heidelberg, Germany, 2003; pp. 3–9. [CrossRef]
106. Krunic, A.L.; Marini, L.G. Cryosurgery. In *European Handbook of Dermatological Treatments*, 3rd ed.; Katsambas, A.D., Lotti, T.M., Dessinioti, C., Massimiliano D'Erme, A., Eds.; Springer: Berlin/Heidelberg, Germany, 2015; pp. 1139–1149. [CrossRef]
107. Abramovits, W. Tissue temperature monitors. In *Dermatological Cryosurgery and Cryotherapy*; Abramovits, W., Graham, G., Har-Shai, Y., Strumia, R., Eds.; Springer: London, UK, 2016; pp. 135–136. [CrossRef]
108. Aguilar, G.; Majaron, B.; Verkruysse, W.; Zhou, Y.; Nelson, J.S.; Lavernia, E.J. Theoretical and experimental analysis of droplet diameter, temperature, and evaporation rate evolution in cryogenic sprays. *Int. J. Heat Mass Transf.* **2001**, *44*, 3201–3211. [CrossRef]

Disclaimer/Publisher's Note: The statements, opinions and data contained in all publications are solely those of the individual author(s) and contributor(s) and not of MDPI and/or the editor(s). MDPI and/or the editor(s) disclaim responsibility for any injury to people or property resulting from any ideas, methods, instructions or products referred to in the content.

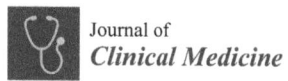

Review

Skincare in Rosacea from the Cosmetologist's Perspective: A Narrative Review

Danuta Nowicka [1,*], Karolina Chilicka [2], Iwona Dzieńdziora-Urbińska [2] and Renata Szyguła [2]

[1] Department of Dermatology, Venereology and Allergology, Wrocław Medical University, 50-368 Wrocław, Poland
[2] Faculty of Health Sciences, University of Opole, 45-060 Opole, Poland
* Correspondence: danuta.nowicka@umed.wroc.pl

Abstract: Rosacea is a common skin disease that affects about 5% of the general population. Its symptoms include telangiectasia, persistent erythema, burning/stinging sensation, dry skin sensation, and pruritus. It is characterized by a chronic course with frequent exacerbation. It often coexists with anxiety and depression, reducing the quality of life of affected patients. The etiopathogenesis of rosacea is complex and not fully elucidated; hence, there is no causative effective treatment. In this review, we highlight the role of a cosmetologist in the treatment of rosacea and the maintenance of remission. As part of medical treatment, patients are advised to introduce lifestyle changes and use proper skin care; a cosmetologist can help educate patients affected with rosacea, create effective home care programs for skin care, and support them with treatments in beauty salons. Proper skin care is essential, including the use of dermocosmetics, cleansing of the skin, and frequent visits to beauty salons for tailored apparatus procedures. A cosmetologist is more accessible to patients and can help implement healthy daily habits, including skin care and eating habits, as well as support and mediate good communication between the patient and the patient's treating physician, thereby improving compliance and ensuring long-term satisfactory outcomes.

Keywords: rosacea; cosmetics; cosmetology; professional treatment; patient education

Citation: Nowicka, D.; Chilicka, K.; Dzieńdziora-Urbińska, I.; Szyguła, R. Skincare in Rosacea from the Cosmetologist's Perspective: A Narrative Review. *J. Clin. Med.* **2023**, *12*, 115. https://doi.org/10.3390/jcm12010115

Academic Editor: Hei Sung Kim

Received: 27 November 2022
Revised: 17 December 2022
Accepted: 20 December 2022
Published: 23 December 2022

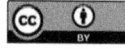

Copyright: © 2022 by the authors. Licensee MDPI, Basel, Switzerland. This article is an open access article distributed under the terms and conditions of the Creative Commons Attribution (CC BY) license (https://creativecommons.org/licenses/by/4.0/).

1. Introduction

Rosacea is a common skin disease with characteristic symptoms such as telangiectasia, persistent erythema, burning/stinging sensation, dry skin sensation, and pruritus [1]. It can be accompanied by the presence of small pus-filled bumps. Asymptomatic periods are interrupted by frequent exacerbations that can last from a couple of weeks to months. Rosacea can be mistaken for acne, other skin problems, or natural ruddiness [2]. Rosacea can affect anyone. A meta-analysis showed that the prevalence of rosacea is 5.46% in the general population and 2.39% in dermatological outpatients [3]. This skin condition affects women slightly more frequently than men and decreases with age. The prevalence reaches 13.5% in people aged 18–25 years, 9.6% in people aged 26–54 years, and only 1.0% in people aged 55 years and older. The occurrence of unpleasant and uncomfortable skin sensations is more frequent in women than in men (26% vs. 18.3%) [4]. Data on incidence are limited. A systematic review on incidence of rosacea identified only one study from the UK reporting the incidence of 1.65 per 1000 person-years [3]. Previously, rosacea was classified according to subtypes; however, the current guidelines recommend a phenotype approach that is believed to more accurately address patient characteristics and help better choose personalized treatment [5,6]. Until now, no causative treatment for rosacea has been developed; however, currently available treatments can help control the disease and reduce its signs and symptoms [2]. This condition is not life-threatening; however, due to the chronic course, the signs visible on patient's face, and the lack of effective treatment, it is often accompanied by anxiety and depression, which is a burden for affected patients [1,7,8].

The care of rosacea skin is a challenge for a cosmetologist. This chronic inflammatory disease has multifactorial etiopathogenesis, including the involvement of the immune and neurovascular systems. In addition, an interplay of risk factors and clinical symptoms can reduce patient quality of life, which, in turn, can worsen the course of the disease and affect patient functioning [2]. For the treatment of rosacea, it is important to build a good relationship and trust between the treating physician/cosmetologist and the patients. This is because symptoms can be triggered by some environmental factors or lifestyle habits. Patients can modify their lifestyles and avoid harmful factors if they have a good knowledge of risk factors and are motivated to do so.

2. Methods

We conducted a review of the literature to provide an up-to-date overview of the research on rosacea and the treatment of rosacea from the cosmetologist's perspective. Such a perspective is often overlooked in the scientific literature; however, proper skin care and lifestyle are part of a successful approach to rosacea. The results are presented in the form of a topical review in which the selection of the content is based on the authors' experience.

3. Food Items and Other Triggering Factors for Flares of Rosacea

In 2022, the National Rosacea Society conducted a survey and collected responses from 1066 patients with rosacea [9]. The aim of this survey was to investigate which factors can trigger or aggravate the symptoms of the disease. The most important factors were sun exposure, emotional stress, and hot water. The survey pointed out the importance of diet and a wide variety of substances that can cause flares such as alcohol, spicy foods, certain fruits and vegetables, marinated meats, and dairy products. The evidence on food items that are responsible for disease flares comes from small studies or case reports [10]. Food triggers include figs, bananas, plums, chocolate, cheese, yoghurts, cream, soy sauce, eggplant, spinach, beans, peas, and broad beans. Regarding drinks, strong and hot coffee or tea, alcohol, and sweeteners added to drinks can act by activating transient receptor potential ion channels leading to functional impairment of the skin barrier. Although some patients with rosacea indicate that coffee has the potential to worsen symptoms, a large study provided opposite conclusions. The study by Li et al. found that 82,737 women with rosacea who consumed more caffeine had a lower risk of incident rosacea, highlighting its possible protective effect [11]. Nevertheless, patients should be informed that the temperature of the beverage and byproducts are equally important for flares as the main ingredients. Furthermore, the consumption of histamine-rich foods and sugary foods can also lead to rosacea exacerbations [12].

Food items and diet can also have a positive impact on the rosacea course. Daily supplementation of omega-3 acids contributes to a reduction in inflammation and the prevention of telangiectasia [13,14]. In addition, the diet should be easily digestible, alkaline, and rich in products containing fiber, as well as vitamins C, PP, and B2 [15]. Lastly, patients with rosacea often suffer from gastrointestinal diseases. Supporting a healthy gut microbiome can translate into improving general functioning in this group of patients [12].

4. Role of Microorganisms in the Development of Rosacea

The importance of microbes in the pathogenesis of rosacea is still controversial. A constant interaction among the skin, microorganisms, and the environment leads to a disturbed balance of the microflora, which in turn leads to the development of dermatoses. Pathogens such as *Demodex folliculorum*, *Bacillus oleronius*, *Helicobacter pylori*, *Staphylococcus epidermidis*, and *Chlamydophila pneumoniae* play the greatest role in the development of rosacea [16,17]. Many of the abovementioned microorganisms belong to the human physiological flora; therefore, it is difficult to define their role in the development of the disease. Microorganisms residing on the surface of human skin interact closely with the immune system and protect the host against the attack of infectious agents.

The composition of the skin microbiome depends on various factors such as sex, age, and comorbidities, as well as the environmental conditions of the skin, pH, humidity, or lipid composition [18,19]. Human skin microorganisms show the presence of receptor ligands for keratinocytes. Toll-like receptor 2 (TLR2) and NALP3 receptor trigger the inflammatory cascade [20,21]. Stimulation of keratinocytes leads to the release of inflammatory factors such as cytokines and chemokines, as well as the stimulation of angiogenesis through the production of vascular growth factors and cathelicidin stimulated by serine protease [22,23]. Changes in the environmental conditions on the skin and the inflammation present there cause quantitative and qualitative changes in the human microbiome. These conditions favor the multiplication of *Demodex* spp. and cutaneous staphylococci (*S. epidermidis*). However, it should be mentioned that new microorganisms inhabiting the skin still stimulate the immune system, leading to dilation of blood vessels, intensification of chemotaxis, and, as a result, a change in the erythematous form of rosacea to a maculopapular form [17].

D. folicullorum, which belongs to the mite species, is believed to play an important role in the pathogenesis of rosacea. This mite is mainly associated with maculopapular and ocular forms [24]. It is considered to be a commensal microorganism; however, in some cases, it can activate inflammation and, thus, alter functions of the immune system. Chitin released from *D. folicullorum* has been shown to stimulate TLR2 in keratinocytes, which in turn leads to the development of inflammatory and erythematous changes and disorders of the sebaceous glands [25]. Research has shown that anti-*Demodex* antibodies occur mainly in people affected by rosacea. In addition, *D. folicullorum* is considered a cofactor of the inflammatory reaction in the body because the number of mites correlates with the level of activation of the immune system [21,25]. Moreover, the presence of *D. folicullorum* is found in the secretions from the sebaceous unit in a large percentage of patients with rosacea, while, in healthy subjects, this percentage is much lower. Overall, a higher concentration of the pathogen in hair-sebaceous units correlates with the occurrence of rosacea, such a relationship is not observed in healthy people [21,26]. Human *Demodex* spp. also has its own microbes, which consist of several to several dozen species of bacteria. The greatest amount of DNA of various bacterial strains was isolated from *D. folicullorum* bottling in patients with the maculopapular form of rosacea; it was slightly lower in patients with the erythematous form, while it was almost absent in healthy people. The most numerous bacteria living in the microbiota of *Demodex* mites are *Firmicutes*, *Proteobacteriae*, and *Actinobacteriae*, as well as *Bartonella quintana*. The last one was isolated from a patient with the erythematous form and is the etiological factor of root fever and endocarditis. *B. quintana* is transmitted by human lice, and it is believed that various species of mites, including *D. folicullorum*, may be a vector for the transmission of infection, but there is no evidence that *B. quintana* influences the development of rosacea [27,28]. However, one of the *Demodex*-inhabiting species, *Bacillus oleronius*, is believed to play a role in the pathogenesis of rosacea. *B. oleronius* antigens have been shown to initiate inflammation, and two peptides, 83 and 62 kDa, are highly immunogenic [29]. Bacterial proteins have the ability to activate neutrophils, release metalloproteinases, and synthesize cathelicidin. Proinflammatory cytokines are released, e.g., tumor necrosis factor (TNF)-α and interleukin (IL)-8, stimulating the development of inflammation around the hair follicle [30]. Additionally, bacterial liposaccharides cause the destruction of the hair follicle wall, negatively affecting the migration of epidermal cells, and, in the case of eyelash involvement in the eye form, they damage the corneal epithelium [16,29]. A positive correlation was also demonstrated between serum reactivity to *B. oleronius* antigens and the erythematosus-vascular form of rosacea [31]. A number of scientific studies also indicate the role of *S. epidermidis* in rosacea [32]. In the maculopapular form of rosacea, bacteria have been observed to grow and secrete proteins that stimulate the immune system, which has not been observed in the *S. epidermidis* strains that are found in healthy people. This is a consequence of the exacerbation of inflammation in rosacea [33].

Pathogenic bacteria that infect internal organs can also contribute to the development or exacerbation of skin diseases. There are reports on the role of *H. pylori* in the pathogenesis of skin diseases, including rosacea [34,35]. Stimulation of gastrin secretion by *H. pylori* contributes to paroxysmal erythema, which is part of the clinical picture of rosacea. After *H. pylori* eradication, it was found that the skin condition of patients with rosacea improved significantly; therefore, it is assumed that the Cag A cytotoxin characteristic of this bacterium may be a factor that exacerbates the course of rosacea [36]. Research shows that the Cag A gene was present in 67% of patients with rosacea and that reactive antibodies to the CagA cytotoxin were detected in 75% of patients with rosacea. However, at present, the role of *H. pylori* infection in rosacea is rather negated [34]. Chronic infection by *Chlamydia pneumoniae* may also play a role in the pathogenesis of rosacea. *C. pneumoniae* antigens were found in 40% of skin biopsies in patients with rosacea, and reactive antibodies against *C. pneumoniae* were present in the blood in 90% of cases [37].

5. Microbiome and Its Role in Rosacea

The term microbiome denotes the collection of genomes of all microorganisms that inhabit the human body. Microbiota is a collection of microorganisms as cells, while microflora is an old term denoting the total of living microorganisms in a given environment. Currently, it is used for the population of bacteria itself (bacterial microflora) [38]. For many years, research has been conducted on the human microbiome, demonstrating that it plays an important role in maintaining systemic homeostasis through the ability to metabolize food substances, increase the absorption of minerals, produce B and K vitamins, prevent intestinal colonization by pathogenic bacteria, reduce inflammatory processes, inactivate toxins and carcinogens, and stimulate of the maturation of cells of the immune system. Intestinal dysbiosis leads to the development of many lifestyle diseases, including acne and rosacea [38]. The compositions of skin microbiota can change with age and during the course of the disease. An imbalance in skin microbiota can also contribute to skin pathologies [39]. The human microbiome consists of approximately 30 trillion microorganisms and 3.3 million microbial genes, which are responsible for the proper functioning of the human immune system [40]. The intestinal microbiome comprises about 90% of bacteria belonging to *Bacteroidetes* and *Firmicutes*, with the remainder comprising *Actinobacteria*, *Proteobacteria*, and *Verrucomicrobia* [38]. The results of the conducted research emphasize the diversity of the microbiome in patients with rosacea (Table 1).

Table 1. Selected studies on the composition of microflora in people with rosacea.

Study	Study Conclusions
Chen et al. [41]	Using next-generation sequencing, a decrease in the colon microbiome was observed in patients and a simultaneous increase in colonization by *Rabdochlamydia*, *Bifidobacterium*, *Sarcina*, and *Ruminococcus* and a decrease in colonization by *Lactobacillus*, *Megasphaera*, *Acidaminococcus*, *Haemophilus*, *Roseburia*, and *Clostridium*.
Nam et al. [42]	The study showed increased colonization by *Acidaminococcus*, *Megasphaera*, and *Lactobacillus*.
Agnoletti et al. [43]	The study showed a relationship between the maculopapular form of rosacea, SIBO syndrome, *Helicobacter pylori* infection, and the presence of the erythematous phase of acne.
Yun et al. [44]	The study indicated the possibility of altering the blood microbiome in the course of rosacea and other dermatological diseases. The presence of *Chromatiaceae*, *Fusobacteriaceae*, and *Rheinheimer* was demonstrated in patients with rosacea.
Thompson et al. [45]	The skin analysis in the course of rosacea showed an increased amount of *Actinobacteria*, including *Serratia marcescens* and *Cutibacterium acnes* compared to patients with acne vulgaris.
O'Reilly et al. [46]	In people with the presence of erythematous changes with telangiectasias and maculopapulars, an increased amount of *Demodex folliculorum* was found.
Dahl et al. [47]	High levels of *Staphylococcus epidermidis* were found in patients with rosacea. This microorganism is able to produce proteins at higher temperatures in patients with rosacea, which influences its pathogenic role.

6. Skin Care in Rosacea

The use of dermocosmetics is of great importance in the daily care of skin with rosacea. These are preparations intended for a specific type of skin, and their main purpose is to prevent and reduce skin ailments. They combine the properties of a drug and a cosmetic.

Patients with rosacea often experience problems with tolerance to cosmetics; therefore, it is important that the selected cosmetic is intended for rosacea skin. Otherwise, there is a high risk of exacerbation of the disease [48]. The case–control survey on skin care habits compared the skin care patterns of 1245 people with rosacea with 1538 people without skin problems [49]. The survey found factors that contributed to the development of rosacea. These were using foaming cleansers, makeup more than six times a week, facial masks more than four times per week, facial treatments in beauty salons more than once per week, and beauty salon products. Moisturizing products and sunscreen creams had protective effects.

The composition of dermocosmetics is of great importance, as selected active substances and vehicle types can either heal skin lesions or contribute to the exacerbation of skin problems [50]. Vitamin C plays a key role because it has a protective and antioxidant effect, and it neutralizes free radicals. Additional advantages include brightening and antiaging properties, as well as strengthening blood vessels and reducing redness [51,52]. Vitamin K has a sealing effect on blood vessels and reduces erythema. The main action of vitamin PP is the inhibition of histamine secretion, which is responsible for the dilation of blood vessels and the intensification of erythema. It also reduces inflammatory processes and has an anti-swelling effect. Its advantage is that it can be used in light emulsions because it dissolves well in water. Allantoin and D-panthenol are very often used in dermocosmetics because they have a soothing and healing effect. Bioflavonoids are responsible for the regeneration of blood vessels, and they have astringent, anti-inflammatory, and anti-swelling properties. The use of flavonoid licochalcone has been shown to reduce erythema in patients with pre-rosacea and rosacea [53]. Essential unsaturated fatty acids are responsible for regulating the permeability of the stratum corneum, thus reducing inflammatory processes. Using them in daily care increases the elasticity of the skin, thus enhancing its protective functions against various negative factors [15]. Ceramides play a very important role in keeping the skin at a constant temperature, which is a very desirable effect. One should not forget about acids, which are used in various skin problems; however, in the case of rosacea, we use polyhydroxy acids (gluconolactone) and bionic acids (lactobionic, maltobionic, and cellobionic). Acids not only improve the functioning of the epidermal barrier, but also protect the skin against ultraviolet rays and free radicals, as well as smooth the surface of the skin. Retinaldehyde is a substance that improves the thickness of the epidermis, reduces erythema and the amount of telangiectasia, and reduces inflammation. In color cosmetics, silicon dioxide is very often used, which, thanks to its green color, is used as a preparation that camouflages telangiectasia. Tissue metalloproteinase inhibitors (TIMPS) are present in algae extracts. Their main action is to prevent skin thinning, prevent blood vessels expansion, and positively influence the inhibition of inflammatory processes.

A variety of factors should be avoided in skincare. The patient with rosacea should avoid using soaps, cosmetic preparations with alcohol, skin-drying preparations, and fine and coarse peelings. Sunscreens are recommended to protect the skin against UV radiation which is one of the most important factors responsible for triggering factors for flares of rosacea; however, chemical filters are not recommended because they can irritate the surface of the epidermis and aggravate the disease. Instead, mineral filters are recommended that do not irritate the skin and contain titanium and zinc oxide and dioxide. Furthermore, physical filters have the advantage of being colored to mask erythema and other skin eruptions [51]. Cosmetics used should aim to protect the skin against triggering factors such as ultraviolet radiation from the sun, wind, and pollutants, as well as cold and hot temperatures [2].

For skin care at home, not only is the composition of cosmetics important, but so is the frequency of using them. The skin should be cleansed every day to remove triggering molecules from the environment. However, for everyday face care and cleansing, dermocosmetics for sensitive skin are recommended, containing moisturizing and softening substances that do not destroy the protective lipid layer [54].

7. Cosmetology Treatments

Patients with rosacea are common clients of many beauty and cosmetology salons. For this reason, procedures should be in place on how to proceed with patients affected by this skin condition. In the first step, the patient must go through a cosmetic interview, determining the indications and contraindications for treatments and the frequency of treatments [49]. Furthermore, various treatment techniques can be combined to diversify and enhance the effects; however, some combinations are not recommended in the treatment of rosacea [48].

Several types of light and laser treatment have been proven to be effective in the treatment of rosacea symptoms; however, their effectiveness and safety profile differ depending on the characteristics of the patient. Intense pulsed light (IPL) therapy with a wavelength of 560 nm is indicated to reduce telangiectasia and erythema, as well as papules and pustules. The treatment alleviates inflammation, itching, swelling, burning, and pain. Hemoglobin is the chromophore, and the action of IPL is based on photothermolysis or thermal damage to the vessels, which provides the effect of intravascular coagulation [2,55]. The use of a single IPL treatment in combination with a topical skin care regimen can produce a significant, long-term reduction in overall facial redness. More than 80% of patients undergoing IPL claim to be satisfied or very satisfied with treatment. The procedure is safe; however, transient burning may occur after the procedure [56]. Although good results can be achieved after a single treatment, experts recommend multiple sessions at intervals of 1–3 weeks [2]. Other types of light therapy are also effective. Pulsed dye laser (PDL) with a wavelength of 595 nm is indicated in the occurrence of telangiectasia and erythema. The use of longer pulses reduces discoloration, as well as produces longer periods without exacerbations [57]. The use of a neodymium:yttrium–aluminum–garnet laser (Nd-YAG) with a wavelength of 1064 nm shows effectiveness in the treatment of papules and pustules and in reducing telangiectasia. It is the best choice of other light-based therapies for patients with rosacea with large and deep telangiectasias and is considered to be a good option for patients with dark skin. Longer pulses of this laser deliver equivalent energy at a slower rate uniformly and gently in comparison to short pulse durations; thus, Nd-YAG is also a good option for patients suffering from easy bruising [58]. It was also found that using the "in motion" technique diminishes side-effects in patients with rosacea [59]. Potassium titanyl phosphate (KTP) with a wavelength of 532 nm is the most suitable for patients with superficial and thin telangiectasias. This laser is the best option for people with fragile capillaries who easily develop bruises. On the other hand, it is not recommended for skins with higher phototypes, as there is a risk of skin discoloration [58,60]. Pro-yellow laser with a wavelength of 577 nm laser is a novel treatment with little evidence. The application of this treatment resulted in a reduction in symptoms of erythematotelangiectatic rosacea. In addition, the treatment was very well tolerated [61]. Furthermore, a pro-yellow laser was shown to reduce the density of *D. folliculorum* and *D. brevis* on the skin of patients with rosacea [62]. A light-emitting diode (LED) modifies cellular activity, which results in the anti-inflammatory effect by producing low-intensity nonthermal irradiation. This type of treatment is indicated in erythematous and inflammatory lesions [2]. Its effectiveness was explained in an experimental model that reported that LED downregulates cathelicidin, kallikrein, and TLR2 expressions in keratinocytes and rosacea-like mouse skin [63]. Although light and laser therapy is safe and can be used in many patients when chosen carefully, it has some contraindications such as active skin inflammation, cardiovascular failure, venous thrombosis, treatment with photosensitizing drugs, cancer, pregnancy, lactation, implanted pacemaker, autoimmune diseases, skin photoallergies, herpes simplex infection, a fresh tan (at least 8 weeks waiting period from the last sunbathing is recommended), and tuberculosis [61,64,65].

Low-density micro-focused ultrasound can reduce signs of erythematotelangiectatic rosacea [66]. After a single treatment, over 90% of the patients reported improvement that was maintained for up to 1 year. The procedure is generally safe; however, transient side-effects such as bruising, tenderness, and redness develop in one-third of treated patients.

Some researchers attempted to introduce active substances through the skin in order to reduce the symptoms of rosacea. A variety of techniques can be used for this purpose such as intradermal microinjections (mesotherapy), microneedling, sonophoresis, and ultrasound. These treatments increase the penetration of active substances into the skin. Several substances have been investigated so far, including antifibrinolytic agents (tranexamic acid), antioxidants and angioprotectors (vitamin C), organic silica, amino acids, and hyaluronic acid [2,67].

Although many treatments bring good results, some other technologies should be avoided in patients with rosacea. These include treatments that use increased temperature, e.g., with the use of masks or apparatus treatments, such as manual facial cleansing with wapozon, diamond microdermabrasion, and dermapen. Any procedures that may intensify erythema or increase the temperature of tissues are contraindicated. Generally, strong massages should be avoided, but lymphatic drainage and gentle stroking movements are acceptable.

Cosmetologists should propose skincare that has a soothing effect on erythema and aims to constrict blood vessels. The cosmetics used in the treatments should be non-irritating and have a low degree of fragrance. Apparatus treatments are to ensure the proper penetration of active ingredients into the skin, as well as provide a protective and filmogenic effect. The ingredients contained in cosmetics should also rebuild the lipid barrier. Recommended ingredients can include extracts of sweet almonds, wheat germ, oils (avocado and evening primrose), and jojoba. A soothing effect can be obtained using soy extract, d-panthenol, allantoin, or peptides. The anti-inflammatory effect can be ensured by using hops, cornflower, green tea, linseed, and chamomile. Cosmetics with probiotics, prebiotics, and synbiotics are new to the market, but have been proven to stimulate the growth of natural microflora, as well as smooth and nourish the skin [48,56,68,69].

The limitation of this research is the nonsystematic nature of this review. The selection of the articles included was based on the author's professional experience gained in the treatment of rosacea. For this reason, bias cannot be excluded, and gaps in the current knowledge were not identified.

8. Conclusions

Treatment of rosacea poses challenges for the treating physician and patients; therefore, the role a cosmetologist plays in the treatment of rosacea is of high importance. The implementation of appropriate treatment and proper office and home care are the basis for obtaining good outcomes. A cosmetologist is more accessible to patients and can help to implement healthy daily habits, including skin care and eating habits, as well as support and mediate good communication between the patient and patient's treating physician, thereby improving compliance and ensuring long-term satisfactory outcomes.

Author Contributions: Conceptualization, K.C.; methodology, K.C.; software, K.C.; validation, K.C.; formal analysis, I.D.-U.; investigation D.N.; resources, K.C. and R.S.; data curation, D.N. and I.D.-U.; writing—original draft preparation, K.C., R.S., I.D.-U. and D.N.; writing—review and editing D.N.; visualization D.N.; supervision D.N.; project administration, K.C. funding acquisition, D.N. All authors have read and agreed to the published version of the manuscript.

Funding: This research received no external funding.

Institutional Review Board Statement: Not applicable.

Informed Consent Statement: Not applicable.

Data Availability Statement: Not applicable.

Conflicts of Interest: The authors declare no conflict of interest.

References

1. Yang, F.; Wang, L.; Shucheng, H.; Jiang, X. Differences in clinical characteristics of rosacea across age groups: A retrospective study of 840 female patients. *J. Cosmet. Dermatol.* **2022**. [CrossRef] [PubMed]
2. Oliveira, C.M.M.; Almeida, L.M.C.; Bonamigo, R.R.; Lima, C.W.G.; Bagatin, E. Consensus on the therapeutic management of rosacea-Brazilian Society of Dermatology. *An. Bras. Dermatol.* **2020**, *95* (Suppl. S1), 53–69. [CrossRef]
3. Gether, L.; Overgaard, L.K.; Egeberg, A.; Thyssen, J.P. Incidence and prevalence of rosacea: A systematic review and meta-analysis. *Br. J. Dermatol.* **2018**, *179*, 282–289. [CrossRef] [PubMed]
4. Richard, M.A.; Paul, C.; Nijsten, T.; Gisondi, P.; Salavastru, C.; Taieb, C.; Trakatelli, M.; Puig, L.; Stratigos, A. Prevalence of most common skin diseases in Europe: A population-based study. *J. Eur. Acad. Dermatol. Venereol.* **2022**, *36*, 1088–1096. [CrossRef] [PubMed]
5. Kang, C.N.; Shah, M.; Tan, J. Rosacea: An Update in Diagnosis, Classification and Management. *Ski. Ther. Lett.* **2021**, *26*, 1–8.
6. Schaller, M.; Almeida, L.M.C.; Bewley, A.; Cribier, B.; Del Rosso, J.; Dlova, N.C.; Gallo, R.L.; Granstein, R.D.; Kautz, G.; Mannis, M.J.; et al. Recommendations for rosacea diagnosis, classification and management: Update from the global ROSacea COnsensus 2019 panel. *Br. J. Dermatol.* **2020**, *182*, 1269–1276. [CrossRef]
7. Baldwin, H.E.; Harper, J.; Baradaran, S.; Patel, V. Erythema of Rosacea Affects Health-Related Quality of Life: Results of a Survey Conducted in Collaboration with the National Rosacea Society. *Dermatol. Ther.* **2019**, *9*, 725–734. [CrossRef]
8. Tan, J.; Steinhoff, M.; Bewley, A.; Gieler, U.; Rives, V. Characterizing high-burden rosacea subjects: A multivariate risk factor analysis from a global survey. *J. Dermatol. Treat.* **2020**, *31*, 168–174. [CrossRef]
9. New Survey Pinpoints Leading Factors That Trigger Symptoms. Available online: http://www.rosacea.org/rosacea-review/2002/summer/new-survey-pinpoints-leading-factors-that-trigger-symptoms (accessed on 10 November 2022).
10. Searle, T.; Ali, F.R.; Carolides, S.; Al-Niaimi, F. Rosacea and Diet: What is New in 2021? *J. Clin. Aesthetic Dermatol.* **2021**, *14*, 49–54.
11. Li, S.; Chen, M.L.; Drucker, A.M.; Cho, E.; Geng, H.; Qureshi, A.A.; Li, W.Q. Association of Caffeine Intake and Caffeinated Coffee Consumption With Risk of Incident Rosacea in Women. *JAMA Dermatol.* **2018**, *154*, 1394–1400. [CrossRef]
12. Weiss, E.; Katta, R. Diet and rosacea: The role of dietary change in the management of rosacea. *Dermatol. Pract. Concept.* **2017**, *7*, 31–37. [CrossRef] [PubMed]
13. Bhargava, R.; Kumar, P.; Kumar, M.; Mehra, N.; Mishra, A. A randomized controlled trial of omega-3 fatty acids in dry eye syndrome. *Int. J. Ophthalmol.* **2013**, *6*, 811–816. [CrossRef] [PubMed]
14. Shen, S.; Yan, G.; Cao, Y.; Zeng, Q.; Zhao, J.; Wang, X.; Wang, P. Dietary supplementation of n-3 PUFAs ameliorates LL37-induced rosacea-like skin inflammation via inhibition of TLR2/MyD88/NF-κB pathway. *Biomed. Pharmacother.* **2023**, *157*, 114091. [CrossRef]
15. Yuan, X.; Huang, X.; Wang, B.; Huang, Y.X.; Zhang, Y.Y.; Tang, Y.; Yang, J.Y.; Chen, Q.; Jian, D.; Xie, H.F.; et al. Relationship between rosacea and dietary factors: A multicenter retrospective case-control survey. *J. Dermatol.* **2019**, *46*, 219–225. [CrossRef]
16. Mehrholz, D.M.; Nowicki, R.; Barańska-Rybak, W.M. Infectious agents in the pathogenesis of rosacea. *Dermatol. Rev./Przegląd Dermatol.* **2016**, *103*, 323–329. [CrossRef]
17. Holmes, A.D. Potential role of microorganisms in the pathogenesis of rosacea. *J. Am. Acad. Dermatol.* **2013**, *69*, 1025–1032. [CrossRef] [PubMed]
18. Chen, Y.E.; Tsao, H. The skin microbiome: Current perspectives and future challenges. *J. Am. Acad. Dermatol.* **2013**, *69*, 143–155. [CrossRef] [PubMed]
19. Grice, E.A.; Segre, J.A. The skin microbiome. *Nat. Rev. Microbiol.* **2011**, *9*, 244–253. [CrossRef]
20. Yamasaki, K.; Kanada, K.; Macleod, D.T.; Borkowski, A.W.; Morizane, S.; Nakatsuji, T.; Cogen, A.L.; Gallo, R.L. TLR2 expression is increased in rosacea and stimulates enhanced serine protease production by keratinocytes. *J. Investig. Dermatol.* **2011**, *131*, 688–697. [CrossRef]
21. Casas, C.; Paul, C.; Lahfa, M.; Livideanu, B.; Lejeune, O.; Alvarez-Georges, S.; Saint-Martory, C.; Degouy, A.; Mengeaud, V.; Ginisty, H.; et al. Quantification of Demodex folliculorum by PCR in rosacea and its relationship to skin innate immune activation. *Exp. Dermatol.* **2012**, *21*, 906–910. [CrossRef]
22. Yamasaki, K.; Gallo, R.L. Rosacea as a disease of cathelicidins and skin innate immunity. *J. Investig. Dermatol. Symp. Proc.* **2011**, *15*, 12–15. [CrossRef] [PubMed]
23. Ewa Robak, E.; Kulczycka, L. Trądzik różowaty-współczesne poglądy na patomechanizm i terapię. *Postep. Hig. Med. Dosw. (Online)* **2010**, *64*, 439–450.
24. Powell, F.C. Rosacea and the pilosebaceous follicle. *Cutis* **2004**, *74*, 9–12.
25. Koller, B.; Müller-Wiefel, A.S.; Rupec, R.; Korting, H.C.; Ruzicka, T. Chitin modulates innate immune responses of keratinocytes. *PLoS ONE* **2011**, *6*, e16594. [CrossRef] [PubMed]
26. Lazaridou, E.; Fotiadou, C.; Ziakas, N.G.; Giannopoulou, C.; Apalla, Z.; Ioannides, D. Clinical and laboratory study of ocular rosacea in northern Greece. *J. Eur. Acad. Dermatol. Venereol.* **2011**, *25*, 1428–1431. [CrossRef]
27. Murillo, N.; Mediannikov, O.; Aubert, J.; Raoult, D. Bartonella quintana detection in Demodex from erythematotelangiectatic rosacea patients. *Int. J. Infect. Dis.* **2014**, *29*, 176–177. [CrossRef] [PubMed]
28. Murillo, N.; Aubert, J.; Raoult, D. Microbiota of Demodex mites from rosacea patients and controls. *Microb. Pathog.* **2014**, *71–72*, 37–40. [CrossRef]

29. Lacey, N.; Delaney, S.; Kavanagh, K.; Powell, F.C. Mite-related bacterial antigens stimulate inflammatory cells in rosacea. *Br. J. Dermatol.* **2007**, *157*, 474–481. [CrossRef]
30. McMahon, F.; Banville, N.; Bergin, D.A.; Smedman, C.; Paulie, S.; Reeves, E.; Kavanagh, K. Activation of Neutrophils via IP3 Pathway Following Exposure to Demodex-Associated Bacterial Proteins. *Inflammation* **2016**, *39*, 425–433. [CrossRef]
31. O'Reilly, N.; Menezes, N.; Kavanagh, K. Positive correlation between serum immunoreactivity to Demodex-associated Bacillus proteins and erythematotelangiectatic rosacea. *Br. J. Dermatol.* **2012**, *167*, 1032–1036. [CrossRef]
32. Whitfeld, M.; Gunasingam, N.; Leow, L.J.; Shirato, K.; Preda, V. Staphylococcus epidermidis: A possible role in the pustules of rosacea. *J. Am. Acad. Dermatol.* **2011**, *64*, 49–52. [CrossRef] [PubMed]
33. Cheung, G.Y.; Duong, A.C.; Otto, M. Direct and synergistic hemolysis caused by Staphylococcus phenol-soluble modulins: Implications for diagnosis and pathogenesis. *Microbes Infect.* **2012**, *14*, 380–386. [CrossRef] [PubMed]
34. Argenziano, G.; Donnarumma, G.; Iovene, M.R.; Arnese, P.; Baldassarre, M.A.; Baroni, A. Incidence of anti-Helicobacter pylori and anti-CagA antibodies in rosacea patients. *Int. J. Dermatol.* **2003**, *42*, 601–604. [CrossRef] [PubMed]
35. Shiotani, A.; Okada, K.; Yanaoka, K.; Itoh, H.; Nishioka, S.; Sakurane, M.; Matsunaka, M. Beneficial effect of Helicobacter pylori eradication in dermatologic diseases. *Helicobacter* **2001**, *6*, 60–65. [CrossRef] [PubMed]
36. Utaş, S.; Ozbakir, O.; Turasan, A.; Utaş, C. Helicobacter pylori eradication treatment reduces the severity of rosacea. *J. Am. Acad. Dermatol.* **1999**, *40*, 433–435. [CrossRef]
37. Fernandez-Obregon, A.; Patton, D.L. The role of *Chlamydia pneumoniae* in the etiology of acne rosacea: Response to the use of oral azithromycin. *Cutis* **2007**, *79*, 163–167. [CrossRef]
38. Woźniacka, A.; Czuwara, J.; Krasowska, D.; Chlebus, E.; Wąsik, G.; Wojas-Pelc, A.; Rudnicka, L.; Narbutt, J.; Adamski, Z.; Batycka-Baran, A.; et al. Rosacea. Diagnostic and therapeutic recommendations of the Polish Dermatological Society. Part 1. Epidemiology, classification and clinical presentation. *Dermatol. Rev./Przegląd Dermatol.* **2022**, *109*, 101–121. [CrossRef]
39. Condrò, G.; Guerini, M.; Castello, M.; Perugini, P. Acne Vulgaris, Atopic Dermatitis and Rosacea: The Role of the Skin Microbiota-A Review. *Biomedicines* **2022**, *10*, 2523. [CrossRef]
40. Polkowska-Pruszyńska, B.; Gerkowicz, A.; Krasowska, D. The gut microbiome alterations in allergic and inflammatory skin diseases—An update. *J. Eur. Acad. Dermatol. Venereol.* **2020**, *34*, 455–464. [CrossRef]
41. Chen, Y.J.; Lee, W.H.; Ho, H.J.; Tseng, C.H.; Wu, C.Y. An altered fecal microbial profiling in rosacea patients compared to matched controls. *J. Formos. Med. Assoc.* **2021**, *120*, 256–264. [CrossRef]
42. Nam, J.H.; Yun, Y.; Kim, H.S.; Kim, H.N.; Jung, H.J.; Chang, Y.; Ryu, S.; Shin, H.; Kim, H.L.; Kim, W.S. Rosacea and its association with enteral microbiota in Korean females. *Exp. Dermatol.* **2018**, *27*, 37–42. [CrossRef] [PubMed]
43. Agnoletti, A.F.; Parodi, A.; Schiavetti, I.; Savarino, V.; Rebora, A.; Paolino, S.; Cozzani, E.; Drago, F. Etiopathogenesis of rosacea: A prospective study with a three-year follow-up. *G. Ital. Dermatol. Venereol.* **2017**, *152*, 418–423. [CrossRef] [PubMed]
44. Yun, Y.; Kim, H.N.; Chang, Y.; Lee, Y.; Ryu, S.; Shin, H.; Kim, W.S.; Kim, H.L.; Nam, J.H. Characterization of the Blood Microbiota in Korean Females with Rosacea. *Dermatology* **2019**, *235*, 255–259. [CrossRef] [PubMed]
45. Thompson, K.G.; Rainer, B.M.; Antonescu, C.; Florea, L.; Mongodin, E.F.; Kang, S.; Chien, A.L. Comparison of the skin microbiota in acne and rosacea. *Exp. Dermatol.* **2021**, *30*, 1375–1380. [CrossRef]
46. O'Reilly, N.; Bergin, D.; Reeves, E.P.; McElvaney, N.G.; Kavanagh, K. Demodex-associated bacterial proteins induce neutrophil activation. *Br. J. Dermatol.* **2012**, *166*, 753–760. [CrossRef]
47. Dahl, M.V.; Ross, A.J.; Schlievert, P.M. Temperature regulates bacterial protein production: Possible role in rosacea. *J. Am. Acad. Dermatol.* **2004**, *50*, 266–272. [CrossRef]
48. Torok, H.M. Rosacea skin care. *Cutis* **2000**, *66*, 14–16.
49. Huang, Y.X.; Li, J.; Zhao, Z.X.; Zheng, B.L.; Deng, Y.X.; Shi, W.; Steinhoff, M.; Xie, H.F. Effects of skin care habits on the development of rosacea: A multi-center retrospective case-control survey in Chinese population. *PLoS ONE* **2020**, *15*, e0231078. [CrossRef]
50. Draelos, Z.D. Vehicle Effects on the Rosacea Skin Barrier. *J. Drugs Dermatol.* **2021**, *20*, 630–632. [CrossRef]
51. Zegarska, B.; Placek, W. Zasady pielęgnacji skóry w przebiegu trądziku różowatego. *Dermatol. Estet.* **2004**, *6*, 281–284.
52. Kallis, P.J.; Price, A.; Dosal, J.R.; Nichols, A.J.; Keri, J. A Biologically Based Approach to Acne and Rosacea. *J. Drugs Dermatol.* **2018**, *17*, 611–617. [PubMed]
53. Broniarczyk-Dyła, G.; Prusińska-Bratoś, M.; Kmieć, M.L. Original paperAssessment of the influence of licochalcone on selected functional skin parameters in patients with impaired vasomotor disorders and rosacea. *Adv. Dermatol. Allergol./Postępy Dermatol. Alergol.* **2011**, *28*, 241–247.
54. Goh, C.L.; Wu, Y.; Welsh, B.; Abad-Casintahan, M.F.; Tseng, C.J.; Sharad, J.; Jung, S.; Rojanamatin, J.; Sitohang, I.B.S.; Chan, H.N.K. Expert consensus on holistic skin care routine: Focus on acne, rosacea, atopic dermatitis, and sensitive skin syndrome. *J. Cosmet. Dermatol.* **2022**. [CrossRef] [PubMed]
55. Juliandri, J.; Wang, X.; Liu, Z.; Zhang, J.; Xu, Y.; Yuan, C. Global rosacea treatment guidelines and expert consensus points: The differences. *J. Cosmet. Dermatol.* **2019**, *18*, 960–965. [CrossRef]
56. Deaver Peterson, J.; Katz, T.M. Open-label study assessing the efficacy and tolerability of topical skin care and sun protection alone and in combination with intense pulsed light therapy. *J. Cosmet. Dermatol.* **2019**, *18*, 1758–1764. [CrossRef]
57. Kennedy Carney, C.; Cantrell, W.; Elewski, B.E. Rosacea: A review of current topical, systemic and light-based therapies. *G. Ital. Dermatol. Venereol.* **2009**, *144*, 673–688.

58. Husein-ElAhmed, H.; Steinhoff, M. Light-based therapies in the management of rosacea: A systematic review with meta-analysis. *Int. J. Dermatol.* **2022**, *61*, 216–225. [CrossRef]
59. Piccolo, D.; Zalaudek, I.; Genovesi, C.; Dianzani, C.; Crisman, G.; Fusco, I.; Conforti, C. Long-pulsed Nd:YAG laser using an "in motion" setting to treat telangiectatic rosacea. *Ann. Dermatol. Venereol.* **2022**, *in press*. [CrossRef]
60. Uebelhoer, N.S.; Bogle, M.A.; Stewart, B.; Arndt, K.A.; Dover, J.S. A split-face comparison study of pulsed 532-nm KTP laser and 595-nm pulsed dye laser in the treatment of facial telangiectasias and diffuse telangiectatic facial erythema. *Dermatol. Surg.* **2007**, *33*, 441–448. [CrossRef]
61. Kapicioglu, Y.; Sarac, G.; Cenk, H. Treatment of erythematotelangiectatic rosacea, facial erythema, and facial telangiectasia with a 577-nm pro-yellow laser: A case series. *Lasers Med. Sci.* **2019**, *34*, 93–98. [CrossRef]
62. Temiz, S.A.; Durmaz, K.; Işık, B.; Ataseven, A.; Dursun, R. The effect of 577-nm pro-yellow laser on demodex density in patients with rosacea. *J. Cosmet. Dermatol.* **2022**, *21*, 242–246. [CrossRef] [PubMed]
63. Lee, J.B.; Bae, S.H.; Moon, K.R.; Na, E.Y.; Yun, S.J.; Lee, S.C. Light-emitting diodes downregulate cathelicidin, kallikrein and toll-like receptor 2 expressions in keratinocytes and rosacea-like mouse skin. *Exp. Dermatol.* **2016**, *25*, 956–961. [CrossRef]
64. Lee, J.H.; Kim, M.; Bae, J.M.; Cho, B.K.; Park, H.J. Efficacy of the long-pulsed 1064-nm neodymium:yttrium-aluminum-garnet laser (LPND) (rejuvenation mode) in the treatment of papulopustular rosacea (PPR): A pilot study of clinical outcomes and patient satisfaction in 30 cases. *J. Am. Acad. Dermatol.* **2015**, *73*, 333–336. [CrossRef] [PubMed]
65. Ablon, G. Phototherapy with Light Emitting Diodes: Treating a Broad Range of Medical and Aesthetic Conditions in Dermatology. *J. Clin. Aesthetic Dermatol.* **2018**, *11*, 21–27.
66. Schlessinger, J.; Lupin, M.; McDaniel, D.; George, R. Safety and Effectiveness of Microfocused Ultrasound for Treating Erythematotelangiectatic Rosacea. *J. Drugs Dermatol.* **2019**, *18*, 522.
67. Daadaa, N.; Litaiem, N.; Karray, M.; Bacha, T.; Jones, M.; Belajouza Noueiri, C.; Goucha, S.; Zeglaoui, F. Intradermal tranexamic acid microinjections: A novel treatment option for erythematotelangiectatic rosacea. *J. Cosmet. Dermatol.* **2021**, *20*, 3324–3329. [CrossRef]
68. Del Rosso, J.Q.; Tanghetti, E.; Webster, G.; Stein Gold, L.; Thiboutot, D.; Gallo, R.L. Update on the Management of Rosacea from the American Acne & Rosacea Society (AARS). *J. Clin. Aesthetic Dermatol.* **2019**, *12*, 17–24.
69. Musthaq, S.; Mazuy, A.; Jakus, J. The microbiome in dermatology. *Clin. Dermatol.* **2018**, *36*, 390–398. [CrossRef]

Disclaimer/Publisher's Note: The statements, opinions and data contained in all publications are solely those of the individual author(s) and contributor(s) and not of MDPI and/or the editor(s). MDPI and/or the editor(s) disclaim responsibility for any injury to people or property resulting from any ideas, methods, instructions or products referred to in the content.

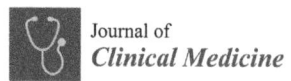

Article

Prospective Evaluation of a Topical Botanical Skin Care Regimen on Mild to Moderate Facial and Truncal Acne and Mood

Yvonne Nong [1,2], Nimrit Gahoonia [1,3], Julianne Rizzo [1,4], Waqas Burney [1], Raja K. Sivamani [1,5,6,*] and Jessica Maloh [1,*]

1. Integrative Skin Science and Research, Sacramento, CA 95815, USA
2. College of Human Medicine, Michigan State University, East Lansing, MI 48824, USA
3. College of Osteopathic Medicine, Touro University, Vallejo, CA 94592, USA
4. School of Medicine, University of California Davis, Sacramento, CA 95817, USA
5. Pacific Skin Institute, Sacramento, CA 95815, USA
6. Department of Dermatology, University of California Davis, Davis, CA 95816, USA
* Correspondence: raja.sivamani.md@gmail.com (R.K.S.); jessica@integrativeskinresearch.com (J.M.)

Abstract: Acne vulgaris is a common inflammatory condition that can be associated with profound psychosocial impacts. Conventional treatment includes topical retinoids, benzoyl peroxide, and antimicrobials, and some may cause irritation and skin dryness. In this 8-week open-label study, we examined the effects of a botanical skin care regimen (Codex Labs Shaant Balancing regimen) on mild to moderate facial and truncal acne. Twenty-four male and female subjects between the ages of 12 and 45 years were assessed for eligibility, 20 were enrolled, and 15 completed all study visits. Facial and truncal acne lesion counts, skin hydration, sebum excretion rate, and mood were assessed at baseline, week 4, and week 8. Total facial lesion counts (inflammatory and non-inflammatory lesions) decreased by 20.5% at week 4 ($p = 0.06$) and by 25.2% at week 8 ($p < 0.05$). Inflammatory lesion counts on the trunk were found to decrease at week 8 relative to baseline by 48% ($p < 0.05$). Forehead sebum excretion rate decreased by 40% at week 4 ($p = 0.07$) and 22% at week 8 ($p = 0.08$), and cheek skin hydration increased by 27.6% at week 4 ($p = 0.14$) and 65% at week 8 ($p = 0.10$). Participants also experienced significant improvement in components of a positive effect, such as feeling "strong" and "inspired", and a decrease in negative effects, such as feeling "irritable." Overall, the botanical skin care regimen was found to be well-tolerated. Our study suggests that a botanical skin care regimen may reduce facial and truncal acne lesion counts, increase skin hydration, reduce sebum production, and augment positive effects and moods in those with mild to moderate facial and truncal acne.

Keywords: botanical; acne vulgaris; topical; regimen; skincare

1. Introduction

Acne vulgaris is one of the most common dermatologic conditions, affecting over 85% of adolescents and young adults, and it can have major impacts on both physical and mental health [1]. The pathogenesis of acne is multifaceted; prime contributors include the colonization with *Cutibacterium acnes* (*C. acnes*), overactive sebum production, follicular hyperkeratinization, and inflammation [2]. Acne is typically present on the face, shoulders, chest, and back with inflammatory lesions such as papules and pustules, along with non-inflammatory lesions such as open or closed comedones [3,4]. As many of these lesions heal, they can leave behind post-inflammatory hyperpigmentation and scarring [5]. Acne is associated with feelings of low self-esteem, decreased confidence, depression, and anxiety, with a quality of life that is impacted negatively overall [6,7].

Common first line treatment options for acne include topical retinoids and topical antimicrobial products [8]. One of the side effects of retinoids is skin irritation [9]. Topical antimicrobials include benzoyl peroxide, clindamycin, and erythromycin [10]. Antibiotics can lead to the development of drug-resistant bacteria [11,12], and the regular use of benzoyl

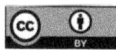

peroxide to reduce the development of drug-resistant bacteria may cause drying and scaling, which can lead to discomfort and irritation [13]. Given these undesirable effects, combination therapy or alternative therapies for acne that include naturally derived ingredients have garnered public interest. While there is a sentiment that botanicals and naturally derived products may not be as efficacious, there is growing evidence that botanicals and naturally derived ingredients can be efficacious in the treatment of acne [14–16].

One of the primary drivers for the natural skin care market is the growing awareness about the benefits of botanically derived ingredients [17]. For example, *Centella asiatica* has been found to offer anti-inflammatory effects in acne, while also improving skin dryness and irritation [18]. Bakuchiol is a plant-derived phytochemical that was found to have comparable effects to topical retinoids in improving wrinkles and hyperpigmentation but with less facial irritation than retinoids [19]. Extracts from biotech amplified *Tetraselmis* algae have well-characterized antioxidant properties [20]. Additionally, natural ingredients with absorbent properties such as bentonite may be helpful for managing excess sebum production and have demonstrated anti-inflammatory and skin regenerative effects [21]. Based on these findings, we investigated the impact of a botanical-based regimen that contained *Centella asiatica*, *Tetraselmis chui*, and bakuchiol on its effect on mild-to-moderate acne and its influence on mood.

2. Methods

2.1. Subjects

This study was conducted between March 2022 and December 2022 as an 8-week open-label study. Institutional Review Board approval was received on 5 March 2022 by Allendale, and the study was listed on clinicaltrials.gov (NCT05271487). Written informed consent was received from all participants prior to enrollment. Subjects from the greater Sacramento region were recruited. Inclusion criteria included males and females between the ages of 12 and 45 years old, with mild-to-moderate acne classified by an investigator global assessment (IGA) of 2 or 3, along with the presence of at least 10 inflammatory lesions and at least 15 total acne lesions. Subjects who had more than two nodules were excluded. Those with severe acne (IGA ≥ 4), women who were pregnant or breastfeeding, those who were current smokers or had a smoking history of >10 pack-years, those unwilling to discontinue facial products except for what is provided in the study, and those who changed their hormonal-based contraception within 3 months prior to enrollment were excluded from the study. Those who had isotretinoin use within the 3 months prior to joining the study and those who were unable to discontinue oral antibiotic, probiotic, topical antibiotics, and topical benzoyl peroxide use were also excluded from the study. Patients were advised to not seek any cosmetic treatments during the study or other medicated acne products.

2.2. Investigational Products

The skin care regimen consisted of a cleanser, oil control cream, exfoliator, toner, spot treatment, clay mask, and body scrub, commercially available as the Shaant collection (Codex Labs, Menlo Park, CA, USA). Compliance was assessed using a product log where participants were asked to make note of each time they used a product on a given day. Participant instructions for product use are outlined in Table 1.

2.3. Study Visits and Procedures

Written consent and assent were obtained prior to enrollment. Subjects were asked to undergo a 2-week washout from topical antibiotics or benzoyl peroxide use or a 4-week washout for oral probiotic supplements or oral antibiotic use. The study consisted of a total of 4 visits (a screening visit, a baseline visit, a visit after 4 weeks of product use, and a visit after 8 weeks of product use).

Table 1. Products used.

Products
Shaant Balancing Foam Cleanser
Shaant Balancing Refining Toner
Shaant Balancing Oil Control Cream
Shaant Balancing Exfoliating Facial Scrub
Shaant Balancing Clay Mask
Shaant Balancing Spot Treatment
Shaant Balancing Body Scrub

At baseline, week 4, and week 8, facial and truncal lesion count for inflammatory and non-inflammatory lesions was performed by a trained doctor or board-certified dermatologist. During these visits, biophysical features such as stratum corneum hydration and sebum excretion rate were obtained using the MoisturemeterSC® (Delfin Technologies, Kuopio, Finland) and the Sebumeter® (Courage+Khazaka electronic GmbH, Köln, Germany), respectively. Facial photographs were also captured at baseline, week 4, and week 8 using BTBP 3D Clarity Pro® Facial Modeling and Analysis System (Brigh-Tex BioPhotonics, San Jose, CA, USA).

Mood was assessed at baseline, week 4, and week 8 using the validated Positive and Negative Affect Schedule (PANAS) questionnaire. This 20-item survey asked respondents to rate how often they felt each adjective in the prior week using the following 5-point Likert-type scale: 1 = "very slightly or not at all", 2 = "a little", 3 = "moderately", 4 = "quite a bit", and 5 = "extremely".

At week 4 and week 8 visits, tolerability was evaluated using an 11-question survey inquiring about potential symptoms (i.e., itching, burning, stinging, scaling, redness, hypo- or hyperpigmentation) experienced with the product use. Participants were asked to rate these symptoms on a 3-point scale, with "0" indicating none, "1" as mild, "2" as moderate, and "3" as severe.

3. Results

Out of 24 eligible participants, 4 did not enroll after screening, and 20 enrolled into the study. A total of 15 completed all visits per-protocol, 2 withdrew due to inability to meet time commitment, and 3 were lost to follow up (Figure 1). The majority of participants were female (23/24), and the mean age was 24.4 ± 7.3 years. The mean IGA severity at enrollment was 2.7.

3.1. Facial and Trunk Lesion Counts

Lesion counts improved from baseline at both week 4 and week 8 in Figure 2. For facial acne (Figure 2A), the number of non-inflammatory lesions decreased by 14.2% at week 4 ($p = 0.10$) and by 14.8% at week 8 ($p = 0.07$) relative to baseline. Inflammatory lesions decreased by 10.5% at week 4 ($p = 0.44$) and by 25.2% at week 8 ($p = 0.16$). Total lesion counts (inflammatory and non-inflammatory lesions) decreased by 20.5% at week 4 ($p = 0.06$) and significantly by 25.2% at week 8 ($p < 0.05$) relative to baseline.

With regards to truncal acne (Figure 2B), there was also an 8.4% reduction in inflammatory lesions at week 4 relative to baseline ($p = 0.39$) and a 48.9% reduction at week 8 ($p < 0.05$) relative to baseline.

Representative photo of the results is shown in Figure 3.

3.2. Sebum Excretion Rate

The sebum excretion rate was found to have a decreasing trend on the forehead at both follow-up visits relative to baseline (Figure 4). From baseline to week 4, the average percent change was nearly a 40% reduction on the forehead ($p = 0.07$) and nearly a 35% reduction on the cheeks ($p = 0.08$). At week 8, there was a decrease in sebum excretion of about 22% on the forehead ($p = 0.08$).

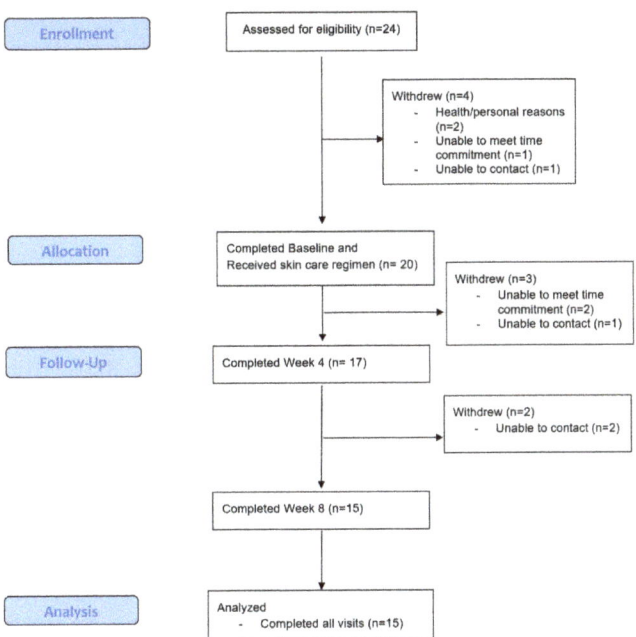

Figure 1. CONSORT (Consolidated Standards of Reporting Trials) flow diagram.

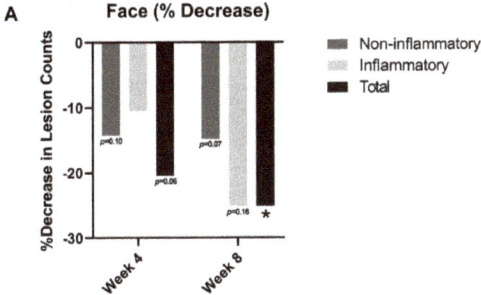

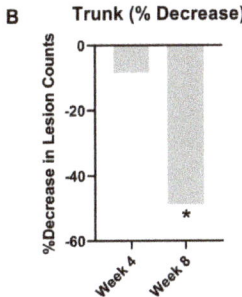

Figure 2. (**A**) Facial acne lesion counts and truncal lesion counts; (**B**) truncal acne inflammatory lesion counts at week 4 and week 8 relative to baseline. * = $p < 0.05$.

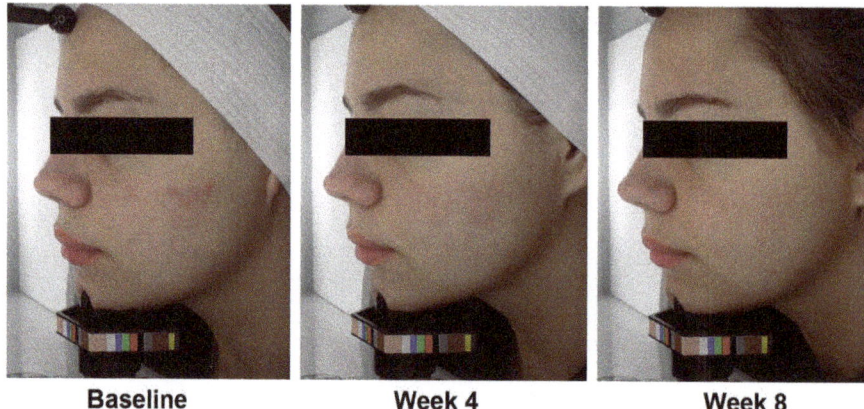

Figure 3. Acne photographs from a representative participant at baseline, week 4, and week 8.

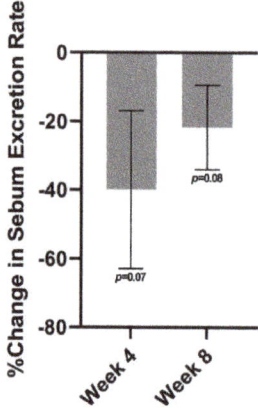

Figure 4. The sebum excretion rate at week 4 and at week 8 relative to baseline on the forehead.

3.3. Skin Hydration

Skin hydration trended towards an increase at both follow-up visits relative to baseline (Figure 5). By week 4, there was an average increase in skin hydration of 19.1% on the forehead ($p = 0.19$) and an increase of 27.6% on the cheeks ($p = 0.14$). At week 8, a 41.1% increase in skin hydration was found on the forehead ($p = 0.14$), and a 65% increase was found on the cheek ($p = 0.10$).

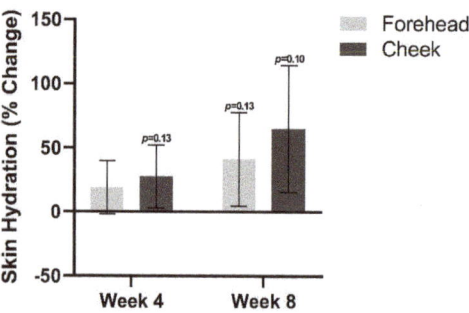

Figure 5. Skin hydration at week 4 and week 8 relative to baseline.

3.4. Mood and Affect Score

After 8 weeks of use, the acne regimen was found to improve components of positive and negative effects (Figure 6). Overall, participants had an average 0.73 point increase in feeling "strong" ($p \leq 0.05$) and a 0.53 increase in feeling "inspired" ($p < 0.05$). Additionally, at week 8, negative effects decreased, such as feeling "scared" was found to decrease by 0.46 ($p = 0.06$), while feeling "irritable" decreased by 1 point ($p < 0.05$).

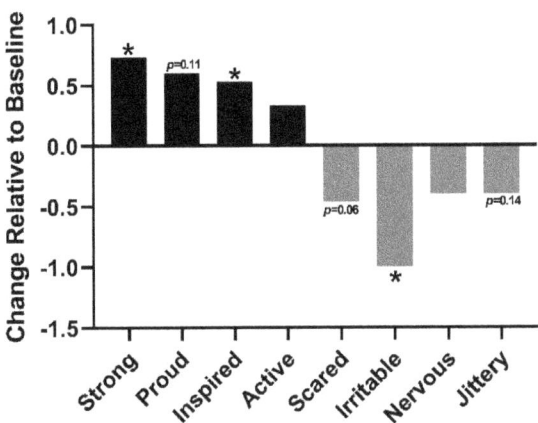

Figure 6. Components of positive effects (strong, proud, inspired, active) and negative effects (scared, irritable, nervous, jittery) at week 8 relative to baseline. * = $p < 0.05$.

3.5. Tolerability

Overall, the products were found to be well-tolerated (Figure 7). On average, after 8 weeks of product use, participants rated symptoms of itching, burning, and stinging at 0.16, 0.16, and 0.25, respectively, on a 3.0 scale where 0 = no symptoms and 3 = severe. Scaling, erythema, hypopigmentation, and hyperpigmentation were almost never observed, on average, while using the product. No adverse effects were reported.

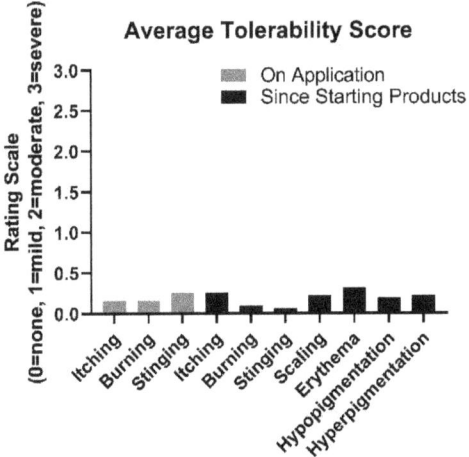

Figure 7. Average tolerability ratings from participants at week 8.

4. Discussion

There is a growing interest in natural, plant-based products for acne, yet few studies have sought to understand the effects of botanical compounds to help prevent and treat this common skin condition. Most clinical trials have focused on individual ingredients rather than a formulation or skincare regimen. This study examined the effect of a combination of botanical products intended to target various components of acne pathophysiology such as inflammation, *C. acnes* colonization, oil production, and follicular hyperkeratinization.

In this open-label clinical trial, a botanical-based skin care regimen improved the lesion count in those with mild-to-moderate acne. Both non-inflammatory and inflammation improved with this regimen, showing that both the comedones and papules of acne may improve with treatment. Moreover, there was a trend towards increased skin hydration and a trend towards decreased sebum excretion rate, which suggests that these products may help to control acne for oily skin types without drying the skin. This trend contrasts that of benzoyl peroxide, which generates free radicals in the skin and may damage the cutaneous barrier [22]. A study found that benzoyl peroxide-induced oxidative stress was attenuated when mice were pre-treated with spearmint extracted from the *Mentha spicata* plant [23]. This suggests that plant-based ingredients, especially those with antioxidant and anti-inflammatory properties, may help to counteract unwanted side effects associated with mainstay treatment options for acne. Although benzoyl peroxide was not tested in this particular regimen, it would be interesting to see if this regimen may allow for benzoyl peroxide to be used along with this regimen.

Many plant-based ingredients have been shown to synergistically target multiple pathways contributing to acne development and help explain the improvement in both the inflammatory and non-inflammatory lesions noted in this study. Tannins, such as those found in *Hamamelis virginiana* (or witch hazel), which is in the study toner product, act as an astringent with anti-inflammatory properties and have been shown to inhibit *C. acnes*-induced inflammation [24]. In addition, bakuchiol, derived from the leaves and seeds of the *Psoralea corylifolia* plant, is found in the balancing oil control cream and targets the inflammatory pathways in acne while also reducing skin discoloration [25]. For example, one study found that a cream containing 0.5% bakuchiol reduced the number of inflammatory lesions while improving existing post-inflammatory hyperpigmentation in a cohort of subjects with Fitzpatrick skin types III-VI with mild-to-moderate acne [25]. Because bakuchiol may have retinoid-like properties [26], it may target follicular hyperkeratinization as well. Bakuchiol is typically well tolerated at doses of 1%, as used in the botanical regimen studied here. The botanical regimen also utilizes *Tetraselmis chui*, which is an algae that has been reported to reduce sebum production on the face [27].

Another important aspect of the study regimen and study results worth highlighting is the Shaant Balancing Body Scrub, which was applied to the back, chest, and shoulders. Studies suggest that, while approximately 50% of facial acne patients also experience truncal acne, the trunk region tends to be overlooked in clinical trials [28,29]. The standard treatment option for truncal acne has been topical benzoyl peroxide, but there may be concern around the risk of bleaching clothes and the tendency toward skin irritation [29,30]. The results here suggest another option for those that are seeking treatment for truncal acne without an oral or systemic treatment.

With regards to the spot treatment, one of the main ingredients is sulfur. This can sometimes be found in combination with sodium sulfacetamide or may also be used alone. Mainly used in formulations for its anti-inflammatory benefits, research has shown that a sodium sulfacetamide/sulfur emollient foam can markedly reduce the *C. acnes* colony count in vitro [31].

Additionally, an ingredient commonly found in all of the products is patchouli extract from the *Pogostemon cablin* plant [32]. Aside from its pleasant smell, patchouli has many therapeutic potentials. Commonly used in aromatherapy, patchouli has been shown to exert antidepressant-like activity by decreasing cortisol and increasing dopamine and serotonin, and it may be a potential contributing mechanism by which positive and negative effects and mood were improved in this study [33]. The effect of aromatherapy on mood also points to another potential advantage of incorporating botanical ingredients in topical formulations. Given that acne is associated with feelings of low self-esteem, embarrassment, and limitations on daily activities of living and social interactions, more research should be conducted to understand how the scent offered by botanicals in topical products may impact the skin–brain axis [33,34].

Of note, this was an open-label study and there was no comparator group. A placebo control is not possible with a regimen as utilized here. While there was no way to assess their individual effects, their various effects have potential to be synergistic. This allows for targeting multiple pathways of a condition simultaneously that may include the skin directly as well as the mind–body connection. However, study results warrant future studies that may utilize a head-to-head design against other regimens/therapies or as an adjuvant to pharmaceutical therapies.

There are several limitations to this study. This study was a pilot study, and the results found here should be investigated with a larger sample size. The study duration was 8 weeks, which allowed us to assess early changes in acne; however, future studies could utilize the results here to justify a longer trial of 12 weeks or longer. Since the products were utilized as a regimen, we can only comment on the effect of the regimen as a whole and not the individual products' effects. The majority of participants were female. Nevertheless, the efficacy results warrant further study with expansion of the study population to include more males. While this study did not assess the prevalence of depression or anxiety, we were still able to measure statistically significant shifts in mood based on positive and negative effect scores over study duration.

5. Conclusions

The use of a botanical skin care regimen (Codex Labs Shaant Balancing regimen) may help to improve the lesion count on the face and trunk in individuals with mild-to-moderate acne, while also improving various aspects of mood. Additional factors such as skin hydration and sebum production may also improve or stabilize during treatment. Further research with larger sample sizes is needed to better understand the benefits and mechanisms of botanical skincare regimens in the prevention and treatment of mild-to-moderate acne.

Author Contributions: Conceptualization, R.K.S. and J.M.; methodology, J.M. and R.K.S.; formal analysis, Y.N., W.B. and R.K.S.; investigation, Y.N., N.G. and J.M.; resources, R.K.S.; data curation, Y.N., N.G. and J.M.; writing—original draft preparation, Y.N., N.G., J.R. and J.M.; writing—review and editing, R.K.S. and J.M.; visualization, W.B., Y.N., R.K.S. and J.M.; supervision, R.K.S. and J.M.; project administration, Y.N., N.G., R.K.S. and J.M.; funding acquisition, R.K.S. All authors have read and agreed to the published version of the manuscript.

Funding: Codex Labs Corp. The source of funding had no role in design of the study, drafting of the manuscript, or the decision to submit for publication.

Institutional Review Board Statement: The Allendale IRB reviewed this protocol (CB_Acne_01) on 5 March 2022. All participants provided written consent or assent in the cases of minors with written consent from their parent/guardian.

Informed Consent Statement: Written informed consent and assent where applicable were obtained from all subjects involved in the study.

Data Availability Statement: No publicly archived datasets.

Conflicts of Interest: J.M. serves as a consultant to Codex Labs Corp. R.K.S. serves as a scientific advisor for LearnHealth, Codex Labs Corp, and Arbonne and as a consultant to Burt's Bees, Novozymes, Nutrafol, Incyte, Fotona, Biogena, Bristol Myer Squibb, Novartis, Element Apothec, Abbvie, Leo, UCB, Sun, Sanofi, Regeneron Pharmaceuticals.

References

1. Bhate, K.; Williams, H.C. Epidemiology of acne vulgaris. *Br. J. Dermatol.* **2013**, *168*, 474–485. [CrossRef] [PubMed]
2. Zaenglein, A.L.; Pathy, A.L.; Schlosser, B.J.; Alikhan, A.; Baldwin, H.E.; Berson, D.S.; Bowe, W.P.; Graber, E.M.; Harper, J.C.; Kang, S.; et al. Guidelines of care for the management of acne vulgaris. *J. Am. Acad. Dermatol.* **2016**, *74*, 945–973.e933. [CrossRef] [PubMed]
3. Tan, A.U.; Schlosser, B.J.; Paller, A.S. A review of diagnosis and treatment of acne in adult female patients. *Int. J. Womens Dermatol.* **2018**, *4*, 56–71. [CrossRef] [PubMed]
4. Masterson, K.N. Acne Basics: Pathophysiology, Assessment, and Standard Treatment Options. *J. Dermatol. Nurses Assoc.* **2018**, *10*, S2–S10. [CrossRef]
5. Connolly, D.; Vu, H.L.; Mariwalla, K.; Saedi, N. Acne Scarring-Pathogenesis, Evaluation, and Treatment Options. *J. Clin. Aesthet. Dermatol.* **2017**, *10*, 12–23.
6. Gorelick, J.; Daniels, S.R.; Kawata, A.K.; Degboe, A.; Wilcox, T.K.; Burk, C.T.; Douse-Dean, T. Acne-Related Quality of Life among Female Adults of Different Races/Ethnicities. *J. Dermatol. Nurses Assoc.* **2015**, *7*, 154–162. [CrossRef]
7. Sood, S.; Jafferany, M.; Vinaya Kumar, S. Depression, psychiatric comorbidities, and psychosocial implications associated with acne vulgaris. *J. Cosmet. Dermatol.* **2020**, *19*, 3177–3182. [CrossRef]
8. Hauk, L. Acne Vulgaris: Treatment Guidelines from the AAD. *Am. Fam. Physician.* **2017**, *95*, 740–741.
9. Thielitz, A.; Abdel-Naser, M.B.; Fluhr, J.W.; Zouboulis, C.C.; Gollnick, H. Topical retinoids in acne–an evidence-based overview. *J. Dtsch. Dermatol. Ges.* **2008**, *6*, 1023–1031. [CrossRef]
10. Kraft, J.; Freiman, A. Management of acne. *CMAJ* **2011**, *183*, E430–E435. [CrossRef]
11. Cunliffe, W.J.; Holland, K.T.; Bojar, R.; Levy, S.F. A randomized, double-blind comparison of a clindamycin phosphate/benzoyl peroxide gel formulation and a matching clindamycin gel with respect to microbiologic activity and clinical efficacy in the topical treatment of acne vulgaris. *Clin. Ther.* **2002**, *24*, 1117–1133. [CrossRef]
12. Simonart, T.; Dramaix, M. Treatment of acne with topical antibiotics: Lessons from clinical studies. *Br. J. Dermatol.* **2005**, *153*, 395–403. [CrossRef]
13. Sevimli Dikicier, B. Topical treatment of acne vulgaris: Efficiency, side effects, and adherence rate. *J. Int. Med. Res.* **2019**, *47*, 2987–2992. [CrossRef]
14. Fisk, W.A.; Lev-Tov, H.A.; Sivamani, R.K. Botanical and phytochemical therapy of acne: A systematic review. *Phytother. Res.* **2014**, *28*, 1137–1152. [CrossRef] [PubMed]
15. Chilicka, K.; Rusztowicz, M.; Rogowska, A.M.; Szygula, R.; Asanova, B.; Nowicka, D. Efficacy of Hydrogen Purification and Cosmetic Acids in the Treatment of Acne Vulgaris: A Preliminary Report. *J. Clin. Med.* **2022**, *11*, 6269. [CrossRef]
16. Chilicka, K.; Rogowska, A.M.; Szygula, R.; Taradaj, J. Examining Quality of Life After Treatment with Azelaic and Pyruvic Acid Peels in Women with Acne Vulgaris. *Clin. Cosmet. Investig. Dermatol.* **2020**, *13*, 469–477. [CrossRef] [PubMed]
17. Natural Skin Care Products Market Size, Share & Trends Analysis Report By Type (Mass, Premium), By Product (Facial Care, Body Care), By End-Use (Men, Women), By Distribution Channel, By Region, And Segment Forecasts, 2022–2030. Available online: https://www.grandviewresearch.com/industry-analysis/natural-skin-care-products-market (accessed on 3 February 2023).
18. Park, K.S. Pharmacological Effects of Centella asiatica on Skin Diseases: Evidence and Possible Mechanisms. *Evid. Based Complement. Alternat. Med.* **2021**, *2021*, 5462633. [CrossRef] [PubMed]
19. Dhaliwal, S.; Rybak, I.; Ellis, S.R.; Notay, M.; Trivedi, M.; Burney, W.; Vaughn, A.R.; Nguyen, M.; Reiter, P.; Bosanac, S.; et al. Prospective, randomized, double-blind assessment of topical bakuchiol and retinol for facial photoageing. *Br. J. Dermatol.* **2019**, *180*, 289–296. [CrossRef]
20. Jo, W.S.; Yang, K.M.; Park, H.S.; Kim, G.Y.; Nam, B.H.; Jeong, M.H.; Choi, Y.J. Effect of Microalgal Extracts of Tetraselmis suecica against UVB-Induced Photoaging in Human Skin Fibroblasts. *Toxicol. Res.* **2012**, *28*, 241–248. [CrossRef]
21. Lee, J.Y.; Suh, H.N.; Choi, K.Y.; Song, C.W.; Hwang, J.H. Regenerative and anti-inflammatory effect of a novel bentonite complex on burn wounds. *Vet. Med. Sci.* **2022**, *8*, 2422–2433. [CrossRef]
22. Slaga, T.J.; Klein-Szanto, A.J.P.; Triplett, L.L.; Yotti, L.P. Skin Tumor-Promoting Activity of Benzoyl Peroxide, a Widely Used Free Radical-Generating Compound. *Science* **1981**, *213*, 1023–1025. [CrossRef]
23. Saleem, M.; Alam, A.; Sultana, S. Attenuation of benzoyl peroxide-mediated cutaneous oxidative stress and hyperproliferative response by the prophylactic treatment of mice with spearmint (Mentha spicata). *Food Chem. Toxicol.* **2000**, *38*, 939–948. [CrossRef] [PubMed]
24. Piazza, S.; Martinelli, G.; Vrhovsek, U.; Masuero, D.; Fumagalli, M.; Magnavacca, A.; Pozzoli, C.; Canilli, L.; Terno, M.; Angarano, M.; et al. Anti-Inflammatory and Anti-Acne Effects of Hamamelis virginiana Bark in Human Keratinocytes. *Antioxidants* **2022**, *11*, 1119. [CrossRef] [PubMed]
25. Brownell, L.; Geen, S.; Lee, W.L. A Clinical Study Evaluating the Efficacy of Topical Bakuchiol (UP256) Cream on Facial Acne. *J. Drugs. Dermatol.* **2021**, *20*, 307–310. [CrossRef] [PubMed]
26. Chaudhuri, R.K.; Bojanowski, K. Bakuchiol: A retinol-like functional compound revealed by gene expression profiling and clinically proven to have anti-aging effects. *Int. J. Cosmet. Sci.* **2014**, *36*, 221–230. [CrossRef]
27. Herrmann, M.; Gaebler, S.; Stuhlmann, D.; Welsoh, A.-C.; Meyer, I. Tetraselmis Extract. February 27 2019. Available online: https://patents.google.com/patent/WO2019166520A1/fr (accessed on 3 February 2023).

28. Del Rosso, J.Q.; Bikowski, J.B.; Baum, E.; Smith, J.; Hawkes, S.; Benes, V.; Bhatia, N. A closer look at truncal acne vulgaris: Prevalence, severity, and clinical significance. *J. Drugs Dermatol.* **2007**, *6*, 597–600. [PubMed]
29. Tan, J.K.L.; Dirschka, T. A New Era for Truncal Acne: Emerging from a Legacy of Neglect. *Dermatol. Ther.* **2021**, *11*, 665–668. [CrossRef] [PubMed]
30. Yang, Z.; Zhang, Y.; Lazic Mosler, E.; Hu, J.; Li, H.; Zhang, Y.; Liu, J.; Zhang, Q. Topical benzoyl peroxide for acne. *Cochrane. Database. Syst. Rev.* **2020**, *3*, Cd011154. [CrossRef]
31. Del Rosso, J.Q. The use of sodium sulfacetamide 10%-sulfur 5% emollient foam in the treatment of acne vulgaris. *J. Clin. Aesthet. Dermatol.* **2009**, *2*, 26–29.
32. Muhammad, S.; H.P.S., A.K.; Abd Hamid, S.; Danish, M.; Marwan, M.; Yunardi, Y.; Abdullah, C.K.; Faisal, M.; Yahya, E.B. Characterization of Bioactive Compounds from Patchouli Extracted via Supercritical Carbon Dioxide (SC-CO$_2$) Extraction. *Molecules* **2022**, *27*, 6025. [CrossRef]
33. Astuti, P.; Khairan, K.; Marthoenis, M.; Hasballah, K. Antidepressant-like Activity of Patchouli Oil var. Tapak Tuan (Pogostemon cablin Benth) via Elevated Dopamine Level: A Study Using Rat Model. *Pharmaceuticals* **2022**, *15*, 608. [CrossRef] [PubMed]
34. Hazarika, N.; Archana, M. The Psychosocial Impact of Acne Vulgaris. *Indian. J. Dermatol.* **2016**, *61*, 515–520. [CrossRef] [PubMed]

Disclaimer/Publisher's Note: The statements, opinions and data contained in all publications are solely those of the individual author(s) and contributor(s) and not of MDPI and/or the editor(s). MDPI and/or the editor(s) disclaim responsibility for any injury to people or property resulting from any ideas, methods, instructions or products referred to in the content.

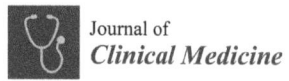

Article

Satisfaction with Life and Coping Strategies among Patients with Hidradenitis Suppurativa: A Cross-Sectional Study

Julia E. Rymaszewska *, Piotr K. Krajewski, Łukasz Matusiak, Joanna Maj and Jacek C. Szepietowski *

Department and Clinic of Dermatology, Allergology and Venerology, Wroclaw Medical University, 50-367 Wroclaw, Poland
* Correspondence: julia.rymaszewska@student.umw.edu.pl (J.E.R.); jacek.szepietowski@umw.edu.pl (J.C.S.)

Abstract: Introduction: Hidradenitis suppurativa (HS) is a chronic recurrent inflammatory dermatosis with vast psychosocial burden. The objective of this study is to thoroughly analyze satisfaction with life (SWL) and coping strategies of HS patients in relation to the clinical and psychosocial factors. Methods: 114 HS patients (53.1% females; mean age 36.6 ± 13.1 years) were enrolled. Severity of the disease was measured using Hurley staging and International HS Score System (IHS4). Instruments utilized: Satisfaction with Life Scale (SWLS); Coping-Orientation to Problems-Experienced Inventory (Brief COPE); HS Quality of Life Scale (HiSQoL); Patient Health Questionnaire-9 (PHQ-9); Generalized Anxiety Disorder-7 (GAD-7); General Health Questionnaire (GHQ-28). Results: SWL was low in 31.6% of HS patients. No relation was found between SWL and Hurley staging and IHS4. SWL correlated with GHQ-28 (r = −0.579 $p < 0.001$), PHQ-9 (r = −0.603 $p < 0.001$), GAD-7 (r = −0.579 $p < 0.001$), and HiSQoL (r = −0.449 $p < 0.001$). Problem-focused coping strategies were most commonly used, followed by emotion-focused coping and avoiding coping strategies. Significant differences were found between the following coping strategies and SWL: self-distraction ($p = 0.013$), behavioral-disengagement ($p = 0.001$), denial ($p = 0.003$), venting ($p = 0.019$), and self-blame ($p = 0.001$). Conclusions: HS patients present low SWL which correlates with psychosocial burden. Reducing anxiety–depression comorbidity and encouraging optimal coping strategies may be of great importance in holistic approach to HS patients.

Keywords: hidradenitis suppurativa; acne inversa; satisfaction with life; coping; coping mechanisms

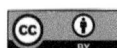

1. Introduction

Hidradenitis suppurativa (HS) is a disease of skin appendages and belongs to the spectrum of chronic inflammatory skin disorders. The condition presents itself in puberty with severely inflamed nodules, abscesses and draining tunnels, oozing skin lesions and intense scarring, which are localized in the armpits, under the breasts in women and in the anogenital area [1,2]. Aggravating, burdensome pain and itching as well as a malodourous discharge are the leading symptoms among patients with HS [3–5]. Up until now, the topic of the etiopathogenesis of this disease is being studied, although research on the main origin leans towards an autoinflammatory and genetic as well as a suspected hormonal background [6–8]. Additionally, HS patients usually present with other comorbidities such as, obesity and metabolic syndrome [9,10].

In the light of the above-described clinical manifestations, HS is likely to cause notable psychological distress [11–15]. Moreover, our recent study suggested that reasonable number of HS patients suffered from mental disorders, namely, depression and anxiety [16]. This in turn may lead to difficulties related to satisfaction with life (SWL), and utilization of different types of coping strategies [17]. However, the literature on the above-mentioned topics in HS patients is scarce [17].

Hence, the objective of the present study was to thoroughly analyze the satisfaction with life and coping strategies used in our cohort of HS patients.

2. Materials and Methods

2.1. Participants and Study Design

Our study enrolled 114 consecutive patients suffering from HS. This cross-sectional study included 61 (53.3%) females and 53 (46.5%) males. The mean patients' age was 36.6 ± 13.1 years (Table 1). Demographic and clinical data concerning the HS were collected. Moreover, the severity of HS was assessed by experienced dermatologists. Then, enrolled patients filled out the below given set of questionnaires in validated Polish language versions.

Table 1. Demographic and clinical characteristics of HS patients.

Characteristics	Whole Group (n = 114)	Females (n = 61)	Males (n = 53)	p
Sex, number of participants (%)				
Males	53 (46.5)	NA	NA	NA
Females	61 (53.5)			
Age Mean ± SD (years)	36.56 ± 13.10	37.47 ± 13.63	39.92 ± 12.5	NS
Duration of the disease Mean ± SD (years)	9.76 ± 8.20	10.9 ± 7.99	8.57 ± 8.38	0.028
Number of hospitalizations, Mean ± SD (years)	1.7 ± 2.63	1.86 ± 3.23	1.51 ± 1.66	NS
Hurley stages, n (%)				
I	28 (24.6)	17 (27.9)	11 (20.8)	NS
II	76 (66.7)	41 (67.2)	35 (66.0)	NS
III	10 (8.8)	3 (4.9)	7 (13.2)	NS
IHS4 severity stage, n (%)				
Mild	26 (22.8)	15 (24.6)	11 (20.8)	NS
Moderate	40 (35.1)	21 (34.4)	19 (35.8)	NS
Severe	48 (42.1)	25 (41.0)	23 (43.4)	NS

n—number of patients; SD—standard deviations; NA—not applicable; NS—not significant; IHS4—International Hidradenitis Suppurativa Score System.

This study received approval from the Wroclaw Medical University Ethics Committee (KB-901/2022). The data were collected from two different regions of Poland (southwest and southeast Poland) between September 2020 and September 2021.

2.2. Assessments

2.2.1. HS Severity

Hurley staging [18] and International Hidradenitis Suppurativa Severity Score System (IHS4) [19] were utilized in assessing staging and clinical severity of HS. Hurley staging is a widely used grading system to characterize the extend of HS lesions. It categorizes HS patients into 3 groups based on the presence and extend of lesions, scaring and sinus tracts. Hurley stage I presents as inflammatory nodule or abscess formation, single or multiple without scaring and sinus tracts. Hurley stage II groups with recurrent abscesses or nodules with sinus tract formation and scaring. Typically, multiple separated lesions are present. Hurley stage III presents as diffuse involvement with multiple interconnected sinus tracts, scaring and abscesses covering entire area [18]. IHS4 is a validated tool to assess clinical severity of HS calculated with the following formula: IHS4 (points) = (number of nodules multiplied by 1) + (number of abscesses multiplied by 2) + (number of draining tunnels multiplied by 4) [19]. The following cut-off points of IHS4 were used to classify the patients into different severity groups: up to 3 points—mild HS; 4–10 points—moderate HS; and above 10 points—severe HS [18,19].

2.2.2. Satisfaction with Life

Satisfaction with life was assessed using the Satisfaction with life Scale (SWLS) [20]. SWLS is a 5-item scale, where a patient estimates to what extent each of them relates to his/her life so far, rated on a 7-point scale from 1 point—"I completely disagree" to 7 points—"I completely agree". The overall score is the sum of all grades. The range of results ranges from 5 to 35 points, the higher the score, the greater the sense of SWL. In order to determine the sense of SWL, the values were converted to a sten scale. In the interpretation of the results, the values in the range from 1 to 4 points are presented as low, the results in the range of 5 to 6 points are presented as average, and those in the range from 7 to 10 points are presented as high SWL [20].

2.2.3. Coping Strategies

A shortened version of the Coping Orientation to Problems Experienced Inventory, Brief COPE was employed [21]. It is a tool for measuring coping strategies, assessing typical ways of reacting and feeling in situations of experiencing severe stress. It involves 28 statements that are included in 14 coping strategies (2 statements in each strategy). The following strategies are analyzed: active coping (items 2, 7), planning (items 14, 25), positive reframing (items 12, 17), acceptance (items 20, 24), sense of humor (items 18, 28), turning to religion (items 22, 27), seeking emotional support (items 5, 15), seeking informational support (items 10, 23), self-distraction (items 1, 19), denial (items 3, 8), venting (items 9, 21), substance use (items 4, 11), behavioral disengagement (items 6, 16) and self-blame (items 13, 26). For each statement, the respondent marks 1 out of 4 possible answers, which are scored: "I almost never do this" (0 points), "I rarely do this" (1 point), "I often do this" (2 points) and " I almost always do that "(3 points). Each of the 14 coping strategies is assessed separately by adding together the points for the answers to the two statements that make it up and dividing the sum by 2. Out of 14 strategies, 3 main domains of strategies were distinguished as subscales: problem-focused coping (active coping, seeking informational support, positive reframing and planning), emotion-focused coping (seeking emotional support, venting, sense of humor, acceptance, turning to religion and self-blame) and avoidant coping (self-distraction, denial, substance use and behavioral disengagement). The higher the score, the more often the test person uses a given strategy [22].

2.2.4. Psychopathological Symptoms

The General Health Questionnaire (GHQ-28) [23] is a 28-item scale utilized for screening of minor psychiatric and non-psychotic disorders. It is divided into 4 subscales: somatic symptoms (items 1–7); anxiety/insomnia (items 8–14); social dysfunction (items 15–21); and severe depression (items 22–28). The GHQ-28 can be scored from 0 to 3 points for each response (total possible score on the ranging from 0 to 84 points) [23].

Mental status of the participants in the last 14 days was additionally assessed with Patient Health Questionnaire-9 (PHQ-9) [24] and the Generalized Anxiety Disorder-7 (GAD-7) [25]. Each item of both scales can be scored from 0 to 3 points (0 points—not at all, 1 point—several days, 2 points—more than half days, 3 points—nearly every day). The PHQ-9 scale includes 9 items about feeling sad, depressed, or hopeless, sleep disturbance, lack of energy, appetite changes, problems with focusing on certain tasks and thoughts about hurting oneself or death. The PHQ-9 total score ranges between 0 and 27 points. The GAD-7 has 7 questions to evaluate the sense of anxiety, tension, nervousness, the ability to control these feelings, the ease with which they appear and problems with relaxing. The GAD-7 total score ranges between 0 and 21 points. The higher the scores for both scales the higher risk for the development of depression (PHQ-9) and anxiety (GAD-7) [24,25].

2.2.5. Quality of Life

HS-specific quality of life was measured with Hidradenitis Suppurativa Quality of Life Scale, HiSQoL [26]. HISQoL is 17-item scale evaluating HS patients' quality of life within the last 7 days. It contains a 5-point item tool which consolidates responses such as "extremely", "very much", "moderately", "slightly" and "not at all" with answers scored 4, 3, 2, 1 and 0 points, respectively [17]. Additionally, subsidiary items such as "unable to do, due to my HS" (score 4 points) and/or "I do not normally do this, HS did not influence" (score 0 points) were given. Moreover, this questionnaire was divided into three subscales: activities–adaptations, psychosocial and symptoms [27]. The higher the score of the questionnaire, the greater the decreased quality of life of HS patients.

2.3. Statistical Analysis

The statistical analysis of the obtained results was performed using IBM SPSS Statistics v. 26 (SPSS INC., Chicago, IL, USA) software. All the data were assessed for normal or non-normal distribution. The minimum, maximum, mean, standard deviation, median and quartiles were calculated. Analyzed quantitative variables were evaluated depending on the normality using the T-student or Mann–Whitney U test. The correlations between variables were assessed with Spearman or Pearson correlations. The Chi2 test was used for the comparison of qualitative data. Differences in coping strategies between different HS severity stages (assessed with Hurley and IHS4), as well as for the different levels of satisfaction with life were assessed using Kruskal-Wallis's 1-way analysis of variance on ranks with the post hoc analysis according to the Bonferroni correction. A 2-sided p value ≤ 0.05 was considered to be statistically significant.

3. Results

3.1. Clinical HS Severity

According to Hurley staging the majority of our patients, 75 subjects (65.8%) presented with Hurley stage II, 25 patients (21.9%) patients were diagnosed with Hurley stage I and the remaining 14 (12.3%) with Hurley stage III. The mean clinical severity of the disease assessed with IHS4 among our study group was 14.6 ± 17.0 points. In relation to cut-off points of IHS4, 26 patients (22.8%) suffered from mild HS, 42 (36.8%) from moderate HS and 46 subjects (40.4%) had severe disease. Mean duration of HS was 9.76 ± 8.20 years (Table 1).

3.2. Satisfaction with Life

Among our group of HS patients, 36 subjects (31.6%) reported low SWL. Average SWL was found in 48 patients (42.1%) and the remaining ones—30 patients (26.3%)—showed high SWL.

Results presented in Table 2 show that SWL of both female and male subjects with HS were practically the same. No statistically significant difference was found in SWL between different HS severity groups (both Hurley and IHS4). Additionally, there was no correlation between SWLS and IHS4 scores. Moreover, SWLS did not correlate with patients' age, number of hospitalizations due to HS and the duration of the disease.

Table 2. Satisfaction with life among patients with hidradenitis suppurativa.

SWLS	Whole Group ($n = 114$)	Females ($n = 61$)	Males ($n = 53$)	p
Total score, mean $\pm$ SD	19.8 ± 5.7	19.53 ± 5.94	19.7 ± 5.7	NS
SWL, n (%)				
• Low	36 (31.6)	21 (34.4)	15 (28.3)	
• Intermediate	48 (42.1)	24 (39.4)	24 (45.3)	NS
• High	30 (26.3)	16 (26.2)	14 (26.4)	

n—number of patients; SD—standard deviations; NA—not applicable; NS—not significant; SWL—satisfaction with life; SWLS—Satisfaction with Life Scale.

There was a moderate negative correlation ($r = -0.579\ p < 0.001$) between SWLS and psychopathological symptoms, measured by the GHQ-28. A strong negative correlation ($r = -0.603\ p < 0.001$) between SWLS and depressive symptoms (PHQ-9) among our HS patients was also found. Moreover, a moderate negative correlation ($r = -0.579\ p < 0.001$) was demonstrated between SWLS and anxiety symptoms (GAD-7) in HS subjects. Additionally, SWL significantly moderately negatively correlated (r = −0.449 p < 0.001) with HS-specific quality of life measured by HiSQoL (Figure 1).

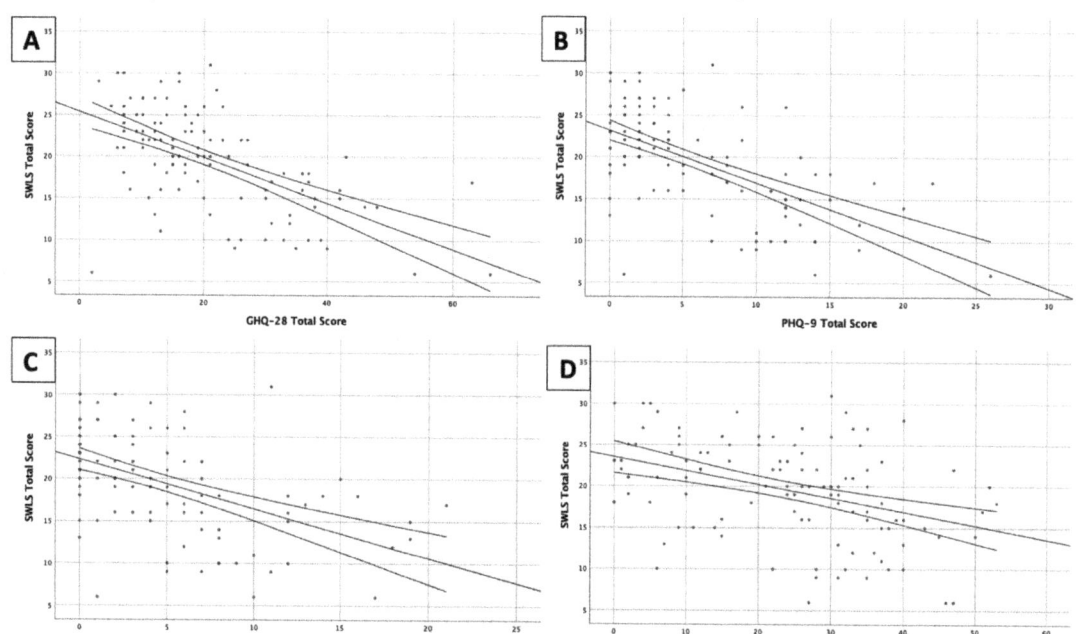

Figure 1. Correlations between satisfaction with life and (**A**) GHQ-28, (**B**) PHQ-9, (**C**) GAD-7 and (**D**) HiSQoL. Each dot represents each patient's questionnaire score.

Taking into consideration different domains of HiSQoL, there was a moderate significant negative correlation (r = −0.478, p < 0.001) between SWLS and psychosocial part of HiSQoL questionnaire. SWL of our HS subjects also correlated negatively weakly with the remaining domains of HiSQoL: activities–adaptation and symptoms (r = −0.366 p < 0.001 and r = −0.331, p = 0.011, respectively). The same above correlations were observed separately for female and male HS patients (Table 3).

Table 3. Correlations of satisfaction with life with different psychosocial aspects.

SWLS Total Score	GHQ-28	PHQ-9	GAD-7	HiSQoL Total Score	HiSQoL Activities–Adaptations	HiSQoL Symptoms	HiSQoL Psychosocial
Whole group (n = 114)	r = −0.579 p < 0.001	r = −0.603 p < 0.001	r = −0.579 p < 0.001	r = −0.449 p < 0.001	r = −0.366 p < 0.001	r = −0.331 p = 0.011	r = −0.478 p < 0.001
Females (n = 61)	r = −0.533 p < 0.001	r = −0.699 p < 0.001	r = −0.624 p < 0.001	r = −0.455 p < 0.001	r = −0.364 p = 0.005	r = −0.455 p < 0.001	r = −0.458 p < 0.001
Males (n = 53)	r = −0.636 p < 0.001	r = −0.507 p < 0.001	r = −0.549 p < 0.001	r = −0.483 p < 0.001	r = −0.406 p = 0.003	r = −0.305 p = 0.026	r = −0.497 p < 0.001

SWLS—Satisfaction with Life Scale; GHQ-28—General Health Questionnaire 28; PHQ-9—Patient Health Questionnaire 9; GAD-7—Generalized Anxiety Disorder 7; HiSQoL—Hidradenitis Suppurativa Quality of Life; n—number of patients.

3.3. Coping Strategies

Among HS patients studied, patients' problem-focused coping strategies were most commonly used, followed by emotion-focused coping and avoiding coping strategies (Table 4). There was no difference in the use of main domains of coping strategies between females and males (Figure 2). Concerning particular coping strategies active coping, planning, acceptance, seeking emotional support and seeking informational support were most frequently used by the entire group of patients (Table 4). After stratifying the results according to gender, seeking informational support ($p = 0.039$) and self-distraction ($p = 0.028$) were strategies utilized more frequently by females than males (Table 4). There were significant differences in utilizing emotion-focused coping and avoidant coping mechanisms among patients with different Hurley staging groups ($p = 0.027$ and $p = 0.034$), respectively. Patients with Hurley I used both above-mentioned strategies more often than the Hurley II patients ($p = 0.022$ and $p = 0.028$, respectively) and Hurley III subjects (differences not significant) (Figure 3). Moreover, additional differences were disclosed in particular coping strategies between patients with different HS severities. Turning to religion tended to be most frequently used in patients with the most severe disease ($p = 0.036$ for Hurley staging and $p = 0.034$ for IHS4). Self-distraction and venting appeared to be more commonly implemented among patients with Hurley I disease ($p = 0.026$ and $p = 0.037$, respectively). No other significant difference in types of coping mechanisms and disease severities were found (Figure 3).

Table 4. Differences in coping strategies among patients with hidradenitis suppurativa.

Coping Strategies Mean ± SD	Whole Group (n = 114)	Females (n = 61)	Males (n = 53)	p
Problem-focused coping	1.75 ± 0.65	1.82 ± 0.63	1.68 ± 0.68	NS
• Active coping	1.96 ± 0.85	1.98 ± 0.85	1.92 ± 0.87	NS
• Planning	1.93 ± 0.88	1.95 ± 0.87	1.92 ± 0.9	NS
• Positive reframing	1.52 ± 0.76	1.58 ± 0.74	1.44 ± 0.79	NS
• Seeking informational support	1.61 ± 0.84	1.76 ± 0.83	1.6 ± 0.87	0.039
Emotion-focused coping	1.17 ± 0.65	1.25 ± 0.38	1.08 ± 0.47	NS
• Acceptance	1.84 ± 0.8	1.97 ± 0.73	1.7 ± 0.86	NS
• Sense of humor	0.89 ± 0.63	0.87 ± 0.64	0.91 ± 0.62	NS
• Turning to religion	0.54 ± 0.79	0.59 ± 0.85	0.47 ± 0.7	NS
• Seeking emotional support	1.76 ± 0.8	1.89 ± 0.72	1.61 ± 0.87	NS
• Venting	1.01 ± 0.75	1.12 ± 0.71	0.88 ± 0.77	NS
• Self-blame	0.98 ± 0.82	1.07 ± 0.92	0.89 ± 0.68	NS
Avoidant coping	0.83 ± 0.46	0.91 ± 0.45	0.75 ± 0.47	NS
• Self-distraction	1.53 ± 0.85	1.71 ± 0.8	1.33 ± 0.88	0.028
• Denial	0.66 ± 0.7	0.68 ± 0.8	0.64 ± 0.57	NS
• Substance use	0.46 ± 0.74	0.52 ± 0.83	0.39 ± 0.63	NS
• Behavioral disengagement	0.68 ± 0.7	0.73 ± 0.71	0.63 ± 0.7	NS

SD—standard deviation; n—number of patients; NS—not significant.

3.4. Relationship between Satisfaction with Life and Coping Strategies

We identified the significant differences between SWL and the following coping strategies: self-distraction ($p = 0.013$), behavioral disengagement ($p = 0.001$), denial ($p = 0.003$), venting ($p = 0.019$) and self-blame ($p = 0.001$) (Figure 4). Thus, patients with high SWL tended to utilize self-distraction less frequently ($p = 0.012$) than patients with low SWL. Subjects with intermediate and high SWL used behavioral disengagement more sporadically than patients with low SWL ($p = 0.004$ and $p = 0.002$, respectively). Moreover, HS patients with low SWL utilized denial more often ($p = 0.002$) in comparison to subjects with high SWL. Consequently, HS subjects with low SWL made use of the whole coping domain, i.e., avoidant coping, more often than those with intermediate and high SWL ($p = 0.002$ and $p < 0.001$, respectively). Furthermore, venting was used more often ($p = 0.036$) amid participants with low SWL than with high SWL. Additionally, HS patients with low SWL tended to employ self-blame more often than subjects with intermediate and high SWL ($p = 0.043$ and $p = 0.001$, respectively).

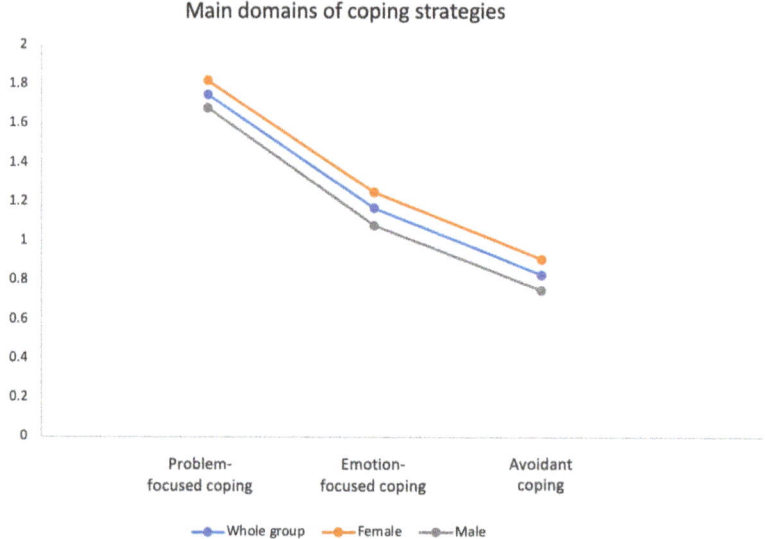

Figure 2. Frequency of utilizing of main domains of coping strategies.

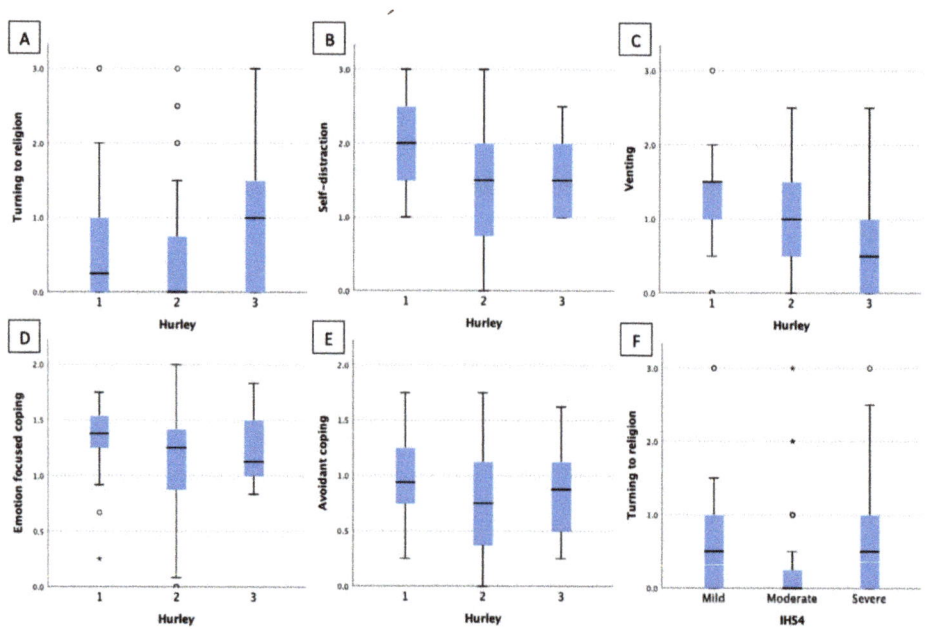

Figure 3. Coping strategies in different HS severity. (**A**) turning to religion/Hurley; (**B**) self-distraction/Hurley; (**C**) venting/Hurley; (**D**) emotion focused coping/Hurley; (**E**) avoidant coping/Hurley; (**F**) turning to religion/IHS4. Each dot represents each patient's questionnaire score, while asterisks represent outlier data.

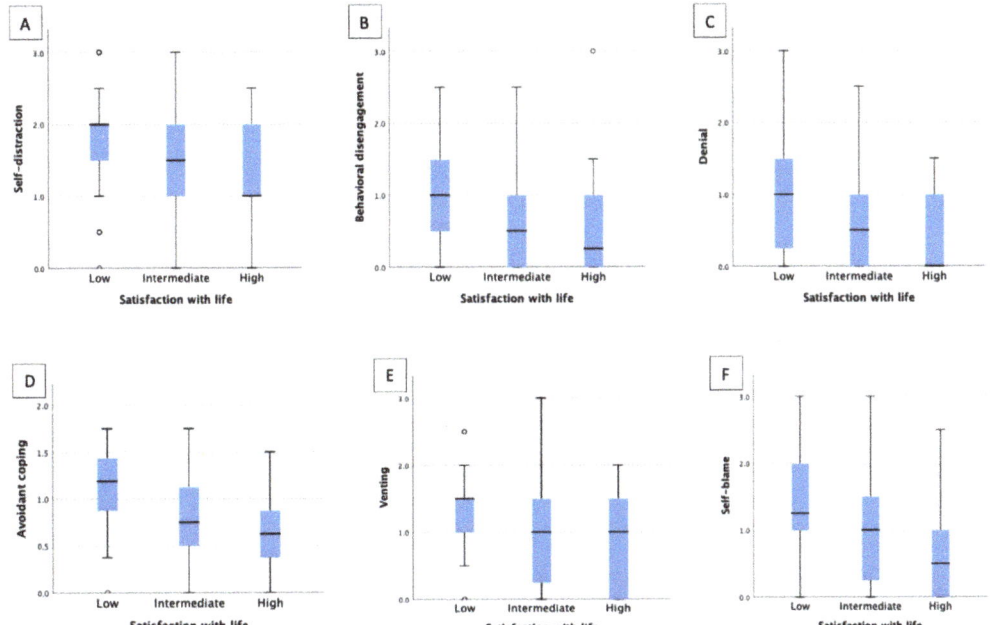

Figure 4. Coping strategies in HS patients with various satisfaction with life. (**A**) self-distraction/SWL; (**B**) behavioral disengagement/SWL; (**C**) denial/SWL; (**D**) avoidant coping/SWL; (**E**) venting/SWL1 (**F**) self-blame/SWL. Each dot represents each patient's questionnaire score.

4. Discussion

In our study, we focused on assessing factors like satisfaction with life and coping strategies in a group of HS patients in southwest and southeast Poland. The newest research shows that in Europe, HS prevalence ranges from 0.001 to 1.4% [28]. Perhaps these big discrepancies are related to a growing awareness of the disease. An example can be an Italian study by Bettoli et al. [29]. They presented an investigation of potential differences between two successive Italian HS patient registries 2009–2013 vs. 2015–2019 and came to the conclusion that the illness frequency estimations were growing from 5:10,000 to 4:100 people, respectively [29].

Despite the importance of SWL and coping mechanisms, these elements seem to have attracted insufficient attention in the scientific literature [17]. To handle the emotional pressures experienced by individuals with chronic illnesses, patients must learn to regulate their emotions, which involves experiencing, processing and modifying their emotional reactions. The resources required for daily self-care management of chronic disease are depleted by overwhelming emotional demands, which has a negative impact on health outcomes [30]. The diagnosis of HS is known to have a major negative impact on mental health, leading to long-term psychological suffering characterized, among other psychopathological variables, by depressive or anxiety symptoms [14,31]. To our knowledge, this is the first study to identify how demographic and clinical characteristics relate to the chronic disease, as well as how coping mechanisms relate to the overall life satisfaction of patients with HS.

A paper conducted by Matusiak et al. [13], utilizing a different tool which included satisfaction of life (Quality of Life Enjoyment and Satisfaction Questionnaire Short Form O-LES-Q-SF) among HS patients, demonstrated no significant correlation between questionnaire-related scores and patient's gender and duration of the HS disease, similar to our investigation. Their results showed that the patients with the most severe HS (Hurley III) had significantly lower O-LES-Q-SF scores [13]. They could be considered different from our findings;

however, Matusiak et al. [13] evaluated a complex Quality of Life paradigm, so it is difficult to compare these results directly. Additionally, it is noteworthy that Matusiak et al. [13] results may differ to ours since their study with a lower sample size consisted of significantly more HS patients with Hurley stage III (22.2% in comparison to ours 8.8%). A similar study on SWL in chronic dermatoses was conducted by Soliman et al. [32] on psoriatic patients. Their results (based on the same Satisfaction with Life Scale, SWLS) showed a quite similar average SWL in psoriatic patients in comparison to our HS group (mean: 21.2 points and 19.8 points, respectively). Moreover, the results of our study are in agreement with Soliman et al.'s [32] findings concerning lack of influence of gender, severity and duration of the disease on SWL [32].

The high rate (appr. 1/3 of respondents) of low SWL among our HS patients is worrying. Investigation of the possible reasons for this outcome should be crucial. Our research shows that factors other than sociodemographic factors related to the disease and its severity are important for the determination of the level of SWL. Additionally, taking into account the structure of the SWLS, which contains general questions regarding the assessment of SWL, skin disease does not seem to be the main or the most significant factor influencing the SWL. Many causes can be possible, including psychological ones, personality traits and social relations in private and work life, which were not analyzed in our study. In our research, we took into account a very important factor, one that is directly influencing the assessment of SWL, which is the mental state of the respondents at the time of filling out the questionnaires. Our study revealed that lower SWL was directly affected by the higher severity of mental symptoms such as anxiety and depression among our respondents.

Kowalewska et al. [33] conducted a study on psoriatic patients and assessed relationships between the acceptance of illness, quality of life and SWL [33]. The respondents evaluated their SWL as low (37%), where our results yielded 31.6% of low SWL in the group of our HS patients. Additionally, Kowalewska et al. [33] showed that levels of SWL in both genders slightly differ. In our paper, we found no significant differences among SWL between patients of both genders. In comparison to Kowalewska et al. [33], where only 18.13% of females had moderate SWL, our group presented 39.4% patients with intermediate SWL. Further, high SWL in our male group was only 26.4%; in Kowalewska et al.'s [33] study, it was 48.48%.

When comparing the level of SWL in two chronic diseases assessed based on our study and that of Kowalewska et al. [33], we can posit that the differences in SWL outcomes can be justified by the fact that the age of both measured groups was slightly different, as well as the different number of patients analyzed (psoriasis N = 366 and HS N = 114) [33].

A high percentage (62%) of patients with low SWL suffering from systemic lupus erythematosus was found by Kulczycka et al. [34] This result is almost twice as high as in our study (31.6%). They utilized the same SWLS [34]. In both studies, the number of participants and their age groups were similar. Kulczycka et al. [34] also found a lack of significant correlation between the severity of systemic lupus erythematosus symptoms and SWL. This leads us to hypothesize that the type of a chronic disease, especially the ones which manifest themselves not only dermatologically but also systemically, influences the level of life satisfaction of the patients.

The findings of our study provide a significant contribution to our understanding of patient SWL and coping mechanisms. The outcomes concerning the coping strategies of the population are supported by other research on other chronic diseases, not only those of a dermatological nature. Coping strategies are a relatively stable feature for an individual, not very susceptible to fluctuations and changes over time. Many individuals rely not only on one coping strategy, but on several different ones over their lifetime [35].

Among our group of patients, the most often utilized coping strategies were active coping, planning and acceptance. The findings of this study are in accordance with the paper by Richards et al. [36]. They analyzed coping strategies in a different disease of a dermatological nature—polymorphic light eruption. Their results, based also on the

Brief-COPE questionnaire, demonstrated that the most often used adaptive strategies were: acceptance (76%), active coping (67%) and planning (60%) [36].

Our current study concerning coping strategies may find further explanation in a previous study by Finzi et al. [22]. They aimed to define the prevalence of psychopathological distress and coping mechanisms among patients with psoriasis. They utilized the same Brief-COPE scale and a shortened version of GHQ-28 scale—GHQ-12. Their results showed that the highest scores were obtained in two main strategies: planning and active coping. Additionally, in a cohort analyzed by Finzi et al. [22], men had notably higher scores than women in strategies such as self-distraction, venting, religion, use of emotional support and denial [22]. It is noteworthy that our study on a different chronic and debilitating dermatosis—namely, HS—yielded similar results concerning the general group of HS patients. However, in our paper, after stratifying the results according to gender, we established that seeking informational support and self-distraction were strategies utilized more frequently by women than men.

Researchers have also evaluated coping mechanisms with the help of the Brief-COPE scale among patients with inflammatory bowel disease. The pattern revealed that emotion-focused coping was the predominantly utilized mechanism [37]. This is partially in agreement with our clinical sample. We established that certain coping strategies, belonging to two different strategies (problem-focused and emotional-focused coping), were most frequently used by the entire group of our HS patients. Problem-focused coping includes strategies that aim to alter or remove a stressor. However, emotion-focused coping incorporates dealing with the stressor while utilizing one's emotional responses [38]. Therefore, we hypothesize that choosing certain coping strategies by HS patients can be influenced by current circumstances and common HS symptoms, such as odor, sourness and the visibility of lesions.

Our current study identified significant differences between SWL and certain coping strategies. Self-distraction was therefore used by patients with high SWL less frequently in comparison to those with low SWL. In contrast to patients with low SWL, subjects with intermediate and high SWL sporadically employed the behavioral disengagement strategy in comparison to patients with low SWL. Denial was also used more frequently by HS patients with low SWL compared to participants with high SWL. HS individuals with low SWL used the avoidant coping domain more frequently than those with moderate and high SWL. A study by Ziarko et al. [39] measured the role of coping and life satisfaction among patients with a different chronic disease such as rheumatoid arthritis. They established that strategies such as turning to religion, seeking emotional support and denial were the primary determinants of the level of their life satisfaction. Yet another relevant outcome of our study is that the patients who utilize denial as a coping mechanism were less satisfied with their lives. Ziarko et al. [39], however, presented results stating that the patients adopting active coping strategies and self-distraction are more satisfied with their lives [39].

Among patients suffering from multiple sclerosis, a chronic and debilitating neurological disease, acceptance, planning and positive reframing strategies were shown to moderate the distress caused by the disease. It was suspected by the authors that a certain way of perceiving coping with the disease by patients with multiple sclerosis might be due to the fact that the main additional burden was the COVID-19 pandemic [40].

Furthermore, interesting findings regarding SWL and coping strategies were established by Blaževi et al. [41]. In their paper, patients suffering from chronic urticaria were less satisfied with their lives in comparison to ones with acute urticaria. Additionally, patients with acute urticaria used turning to religion, seeking emotional support and denial strategies to a greater degree compared to patients with chronic urticaria. Numerous research has shown that the purpose of emotion-focused coping is to lessen or ease the emotional arousal brought on by a stressful circumstance, in this case—acute urticaria [42]. We hypothesize that among these patients, choosing more emotional strategies indicates high emotionality, which, in turn, can lead to an acute urticaria appearing in a more stressful situation. In chronic urticaria, patients might choose emotional strategies less often, which suggests that in chronic urticaria, the emotional response to stress may be less important in the chronic course of illness.

We are aware of the limitations of our study. HS is rare condition, and we ran the study only in two regions of our country. It will be worth confirming our findings in the multicenter study involving more HS patients in the future. Moreover, the data were collected only by utilizing self-reported questionnaires. The screening of the mental status was not confirmed with detailed psychiatric examination. Moreover, the data were collected only in two centers. We are unable to determine the exact reason for the lower SWL of the surveyed patients. We have not analyzed SWL in relation to location of the HS lesions, including the anogenital region. It is probably that factors other than those related to the disease might have had an influence.

5. Conclusions

In conclusion, we clearly documented low SWL in the reasonable number of HS patients, which significantly correlated with numerous psychosocial parameters. Moreover, we found that different coping strategies were utilized by different HS subgroups. All measured modalities are patient-centered and assess both mental state, quality of life and coping with the disease. Taking into consideration the fact that the utilized tools are self-assessment scales, medicine is moving towards greater personalization and a holistic patient approach. Today patients' feelings and afflictions play a bigger role in care than raw test results. We think that further research in this area is required, particularly with a group of individuals who have more severe HS symptoms; it will provide a more accurate evaluation of how the condition affects both coping and overall SWL. Consequently, it is of great importance to establish interventions that can improve life with HS. Finding the psychological elements that affect coping appears to be essential. Reducing anxiety–depression comorbidities and encouraging optimum coping may be the main goals for these patients' improvements in the absence of a cure. However, long-term studies to assess coping efficacy and SWL in this patient population should be just as important.

Author Contributions: Conceptualization, J.E.R., J.M. and J.C.S.; methodology, J.E.R. and J.C.S.; software, P.K.K.; formal analysis, J.E.R.; investigation, J.E.R. and Ł.M.; data curation, J.E.R. and P.K.K. writing—original draft preparation, J.E.R.; writing—review and editing, J.M. and J.C.S.; visualization, J.E.R.; supervision, J.M. and J.C.S.; project administration, J.M. and J.C.S. All authors have read and agreed to the published version of the manuscript.

Funding: This research was funded by Wroclaw Medical University, grant number: SUBK.C260.23.042.

Institutional Review Board Statement: The project was approved by the Bioethical Committee of the Medical University of Wroclaw-KB number 910/2022. The study was conducted in accordance with the principles of Good Clinical Practice and the principles of the Helsinki Declaration of the World Medical Association.

Informed Consent Statement: Informed consent was obtained from all subjects that were involved in the study.

Data Availability Statement: Data supporting the reported results can be obtained on request, e-mail: julia.rymaszewska@umw.edu.pl.

Acknowledgments: The authors would like to express their gratitude to all participants of the study. Moreover, we thank Adam Reich, Department of Dermatology, Institute of Medical Sciences, Medical College of Rzeszow University for his valuable help in recruiting patients from his center.

Conflicts of Interest: The authors declare no conflict of interest.

References

1. Zouboulis, C.C.; Benhadou, F.; Byrd, A.S.; Chandran, N.S.; Giamarellos-Bourboulis, E.J.; Fabbrocini, G.; Frew, J.W.; Fujita, H.; González-López, M.A.; Guillem, P.; et al. What Causes Hidradenitis Suppurativa?—15 Years after. *Exp. Dermatol.* **2020**, *29*, 1154–1170. [CrossRef] [PubMed]
2. Sabat, R.; Jemec, G.B.E.; Matusiak, Ł.; Kimball, A.B.; Prens, E.; Wolk, K. Hidradenitis Suppurativa. *Nat. Rev. Dis. Prim.* **2020**, *6*, 18. [CrossRef] [PubMed]
3. Kaaz, K.; Szepietowski, J.C.; Matusiak, Ł. Influence of Itch and Pain on Sleep Quality in Patients with Hidradenitis Suppurativa. *Acta Derm.-Venereol.* **2018**, *98*, 757–761. [CrossRef] [PubMed]
4. Matusiak, Ł.; Szczęch, J.; Kaaz, K.; Lelonek, E.; Szepietowski, J.C. Clinical Characteristics of Pruritus and Pain in Patients with Hidradenitis Suppurativa. *Acta Derm.-Venereol.* **2018**, *98*, 191–194. [CrossRef]
5. Krajewski, P.K.; Matusiak, Ł.; Von Stebut, E.; Schultheis, M.; Kirschner, U.; Nikolakis, G.; Szepietowski, J.C. Pain in Hidradenitis Suppurativa: A Cross-Sectional Study of 1795 Patients. *Acta Derm.-Venereol.* **2021**, *101*, 1–4. [CrossRef]
6. Zouboulis, C.; Desai, N.; Emtestam, L.; Hunger, R.; Ioannides, D.; Juhász, I.; Lapins, J.; Matusiak, L.; Prens, E.; Revuz, J.; et al. European S1 Guideline for the Treatment of Hidradenitis Suppurativa/Acne Inversa. *J. Eur. Acad. Dermatol. Venereol.* **2015**, *29*, 619–644. [CrossRef]
7. Moltrasio, C.; Tricarico, P.M.; Romagnuolo, M.; Marzano, A.V.; Crovella, S. Hidradenitis Suppurativa: A Perspective on Genetic Factors Involved in the Disease. *Biomedicines* **2022**, *10*, 2039. [CrossRef]
8. Abu Rached, N.; Gambichler, T.; Dietrich, J.W.; Ocker, L.; Seifert, C.; Stockfleth, E.; Bechara, F.G. The Role of Hormones in Hidradenitis Suppurativa: A Systematic Review. *Int. J. Mol. Sci.* **2022**, *23*, 15250. [CrossRef]
9. Krajewski, P.K.; Matusiak, L.S.J. Adipokines as an Important Link between Hidradenitis Suppurativa and Obesity: A Narrative Review. *Br. J. Dermatol.* **2022**, *18*, 320–327. [CrossRef]
10. Ponikowska, M.; Matusiak, L.; Kasztura, M.; Jankowska, E.A.; Szepietowski, J.C. Deranged Iron Status Evidenced by Iron Deficiency Characterizes Patients with Hidradenitis Suppurativa. *Dermatology* **2020**, *236*, 52–58. [CrossRef]
11. Matusiak, Ł.; Bieniek, A.; Szepietowski, J.C. Hidradenitis Suppurativa Markedly Decreases Quality of Life and Professional Activity. *J. Am. Acad. Dermatol.* **2010**, *62*, 706–709. [CrossRef] [PubMed]
12. Głowaczewska, A.; Reszke, R.; Szepietowski, J.C.; Matusiak, Ł. Indirect Self-Destructiveness in Hidradenitis Suppurativa Patients. *J. Clin. Med.* **2021**, *10*, 4194. [CrossRef] [PubMed]
13. Głowaczewska, A.; Szepietowski, J.C.; Matusiak, Ł. Prevalence and Associated Factors of Alexithymia in Patients with Hidradenitis Suppurativa: A Cross-Sectional Study. *Acta Derm.-Venereol.* **2021**, *101*, 1–2. [CrossRef]
14. Cuenca-barrales, C.; Montero-vilchez, T.; Krajewski, P.K.; Szepietowski, J.C.; Matusiak, L.; Arias-santiago, S.; Molina-leyva, A. Sexual Dysfunction and Quality of Life in Patients with Hidradenitis Suppurativa and Their Partners. *Int. J. Environ. Res. Public Health* **2023**, *26*, 389. [CrossRef] [PubMed]
15. Matusiak, Ł.; Bieniek, A.; Szepietowski, J.C. Psychophysical Aspects of Hidradenitis Suppurativa. *Acta Derm.-Venereol.* **2010**, *90*, 264–268. [CrossRef]
16. Rymaszewska, J.; Krajewski, P.K.; Szczęch, J.; Szepietowski, J. Depression and Anxiety in Hidradenitis Suppurativa Patients: A Cross-Sectional Study among Polish Patients. *Adv. Dermatol. Allergol.* **2022**, *XL*, 35–39. [CrossRef]
17. Kirby, J.S.; Sisic, M.; Tan, J. Exploring Coping Strategies for Patients with Hidradenitis Suppurativa. *JAMA Dermatol.* **2016**, *152*, 1166–1167. [CrossRef]
18. Ovadja, Z.N.; Schuit, M.M.; van der Horst, C.M.A.M.; Lapid, O. Inter- and Intrarater Reliability of Hurley Staging for Hidradenitis Suppurativa. *Br. J. Dermatol.* **2019**, *181*, 344–349. [CrossRef]
19. Zouboulis, C.C.; Tzellos, T.; Kyrgidis, A.; Jemec, G.B.E.; Bechara, F.G.; Giamarellos-Bourboulis, E.J.; Ingram, J.R.; Kanni, T.; Karagiannidis, I.; Martorell, A.; et al. Development and Validation of IHS4, a Novel Dynamic Scoring System to Assess Hidradenitis Suppurativa/Acne Inversa Severity. *Br. J. Derm.* **2017**, *177*, 140. [CrossRef]
20. Juczyński, Z. *Polish Adaptation of the Satisfaction with Life Scale SWLS*; Diener, E., Emmons, R.A., Larson, R.J., Griffin, S., Eds.; Laboratory of Tests of the Polish Psychological Association: Warsaw, Poland, 2012; pp. 162–166.
21. Charles, S. Carver You Want to Measure Coping but Your Protocol's Too Long: Consider the Brief COPE. *Int. J. Behav. Med.* **1997**, *4*, 92–100.
22. Finzi, A.; Colombo, D.; Caputo, A.; Andreassi, L.; Chimenti, S.; Vena, G.; Simoni, L.; Sgarbi, S.; Giannetti, A. Psychological Distress and Coping Strategies in Patients with Psoriasis: The PSYCHAE Study. *J. Eur. Acad. Dermatol. Venereol. JEADV* **2007**, *21*, 1161–1169. [CrossRef] [PubMed]
23. Sterling, M. General Health Questionnaire-28 (GHQ-28). *J. Physiother.* **2011**, *57*, 259. [CrossRef] [PubMed]
24. Kroenke, K.; Spitzer, R.L.; Williams, J.B.W. The PHQ-9: Validity of a Brief Depression Severity Measure. *J. Gen. Intern. Med.* **2001**, *16*, 606–613. [CrossRef] [PubMed]
25. Spitzer, R.L.; Kroenke, K.; Williams, J.W.; Löwe, B. A Brief Measure for Assessing Generalized Anxiety Disorder: The GAD-7. *Arch. Intern. Med.* **2006**, *166*, 1092–1097. [CrossRef]
26. Thorlacius, L.; Esmann, S.; Miller, I.; Vinding, G.; Jemec, G.B.E. Development of HiSQOL: A Hidradenitis Suppurativa-Specific Quality of Life Instrument. *Ski. Appendage Disord.* **2019**, *5*, 221–229. [CrossRef] [PubMed]

27. Krajewski, P.K.; Matusiak, Ł.; Szepietowska, M.; Rymaszewska, J.E.; Jemec, G.B.E.; Kirby, J.S.; Szepietowski, J.C. Hidradenitis Suppurativa Quality of Life (HiSQOL): Creation and Validation of the Polish Language Version. *Postep. Dermatol. Alergol.* **2021**, *38*, 967–972. [CrossRef]
28. Díaz, D.; Rivera, A.; Otero, V.; Rueda, L. Epidemiology of Hidradenitis Suppurativa: Current Status. *Curr. Dermatol. Rep.* **2022**, *11*, 336–340. [CrossRef]
29. Bettoli, V.; Cazzaniga, S.; Scuderi, V.; Zedde, P.; Di Landro, A.; Naldi, L.; Cannavò, S.; Fabbrocini, G.; Marzano, A.V.; Mazzanti, C.; et al. Hidradenitis Suppurativa Epidemiology: From the First Italian Registry in 2009 to the Most Recent Epidemiology Updates—Italian Registry Hidradenitis Suppurativa Project 2. *J. Eur. Acad. Dermatol. Venereol.* **2019**, *33*, 4–6. [CrossRef]
30. Wierenga, K.L.; Lehto, R.H.; Given, B. Emotion Regulation in Chronic Disease Populations: An Integrative Review. *Res. Theory Nurs. Pract.* **2016**, *31*, 247–271. [CrossRef]
31. Machado, M.O.; Stergiopoulos, V.; Maes, M.; Kurdyak, P.A.; Lin, P.Y.; Wang, L.J.; Shyu, Y.C.; Firth, J.; Koyanagi, A.; Solmi, M.; et al. Depression and Anxiety in Adults with Hidradenitis Suppurativa: A Systematic Review and Meta-Analysis. *JAMA Dermatol.* **2019**, *155*, 939–945. [CrossRef]
32. Soliman, M.M. Feeling of Stigmatization and Satisfaction with Life among Arabic Psoriatic Patients. *Saudi Pharm. J.* **2020**, *28*, 1868–1873. [CrossRef] [PubMed]
33. Kowalewska, B.; Jankowiak, B.; Niedźwiecka, B.; Krajewska-Kułak, E.; Niczyporuk, W.; Khvorik, D.F. Relationships between the Acceptance of Illness, Quality of Life and Satisfaction with Life in Psoriasis. *Postep. Dermatol. Alergol.* **2021**, *37*, 948–955. [CrossRef] [PubMed]
34. Kulczycka, L.; Sysa-Jędrzejowska, A.; Robak, E. Quality of Life and Satisfaction with Life in SLE Patients-the Importance of Clinical Manifestations. *Clin. Rheumatol.* **2010**, *29*, 991–997. [CrossRef]
35. Nielsen, M.B.; Knardahl, S. Coping Strategies: A Prospective Study of Patterns, Stability, and Relationships with Psychological Distress. *Scand. J. Psychol.* **2014**, *55*, 142–150. [CrossRef]
36. Richards, H.L.; Ling, T.C.; Evangelou, G.; Brooke, R.C.C.; Fortune, D.G.; Rhodes, L.E. Evidence of High Levels of Anxiety and Depression in Polymorphic Light Eruption and Their Association with Clinical and Demographic Variables. *Br. J. Dermatol.* **2008**, *159*, 439–444. [CrossRef]
37. Iglesias-Rey, M.; Barreiro-de Acosta, M.; Caamaño-Isorna, F.; Rodríguez, I.V.; González, A.L.; Lindkvist, B.; Domínguez-Muñoz, E. How Do Psychological Variables Influence Coping Strategies in Inflammatory Bowel Disease? *J. Crohn's Colitis* **2013**, *7*, e219–e226. [CrossRef]
38. Schoenmakers, E.C.; van Tilburg, T.G.; Fokkema, T. Problem-Focused and Emotion-Focused Coping Options and Loneliness: How Are They Related? *Eur. J. Ageing* **2015**, *12*, 153–161. [CrossRef] [PubMed]
39. Ziarko, M.; Mojs, E.; Sikorska, D.; Samborski, W. Coping and Life Satisfaction: Mediating Role of Ego-Resiliency in Patients with Rheumatoid Arthritis. *Med. Princ. Pract.* **2020**, *29*, 160–165. [CrossRef]
40. Pokryszko-Dragan, A.; Chojdak-Łukasiewicz, J.; Gruszka, E.; Pawłowski, M.; Pawłowski, T.; Rudkowska-Mytych, A.; Rymaszewska, J.; Budrewicz, S. Burden of COVID-19 Pandemic Perceived by Polish Patients with Multiple Sclerosis. *J. Clin. Med.* **2021**, *10*, 4215. [CrossRef]
41. Blaževi, S.; Rubeša, G.; Brajac, I.; Vu, M.; Pavlovi, E. Satisfaction with Life and Coping Skills in the Acute and Chronic Urticaria. *Psychiatr. Danub.* **2016**, *28*, 34–38.
42. Lazarus, R.S. From Psychological Stress to the Emotions: A History of Changing Outlooks. *Annu. Rev. Psychol.* **1993**, *44*, 1–21. [CrossRef] [PubMed]

Disclaimer/Publisher's Note: The statements, opinions and data contained in all publications are solely those of the individual author(s) and contributor(s) and not of MDPI and/or the editor(s). MDPI and/or the editor(s) disclaim responsibility for any injury to people or property resulting from any ideas, methods, instructions or products referred to in the content.

MDPI
St. Alban-Anlage 66
4052 Basel
Switzerland
www.mdpi.com

Journal of Clinical Medicine Editorial Office
E-mail: jcm@mdpi.com
www.mdpi.com/journal/jcm

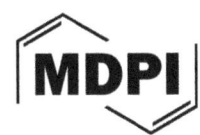

Disclaimer/Publisher's Note: The statements, opinions and data contained in all publications are solely those of the individual author(s) and contributor(s) and not of MDPI and/or the editor(s). MDPI and/or the editor(s) disclaim responsibility for any injury to people or property resulting from any ideas, methods, instructions or products referred to in the content.

www.ingramcontent.com/pod-product-compliance
Lightning Source LLC
LaVergne TN
LVHW070624100526
838202LV00012B/721

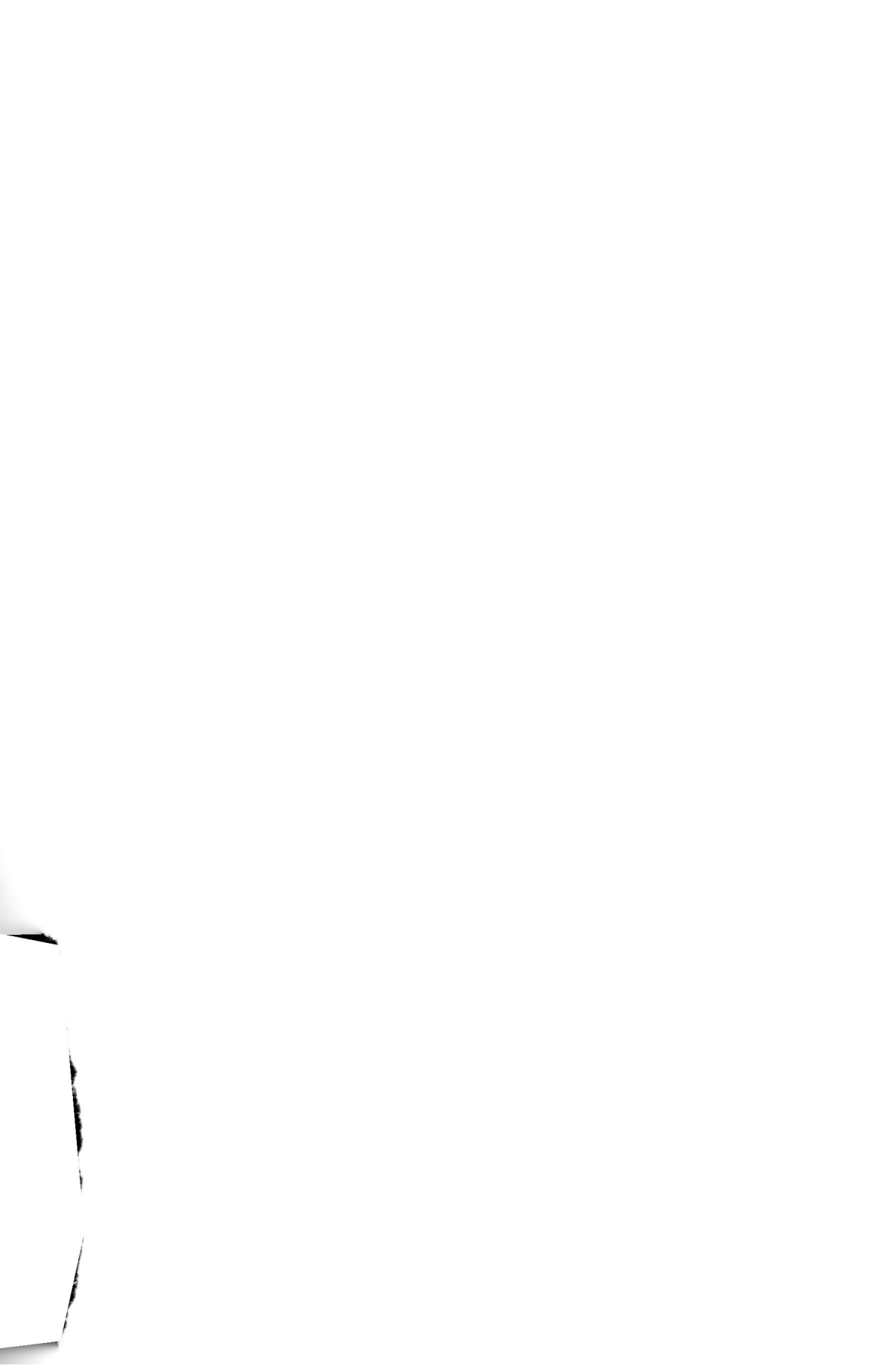

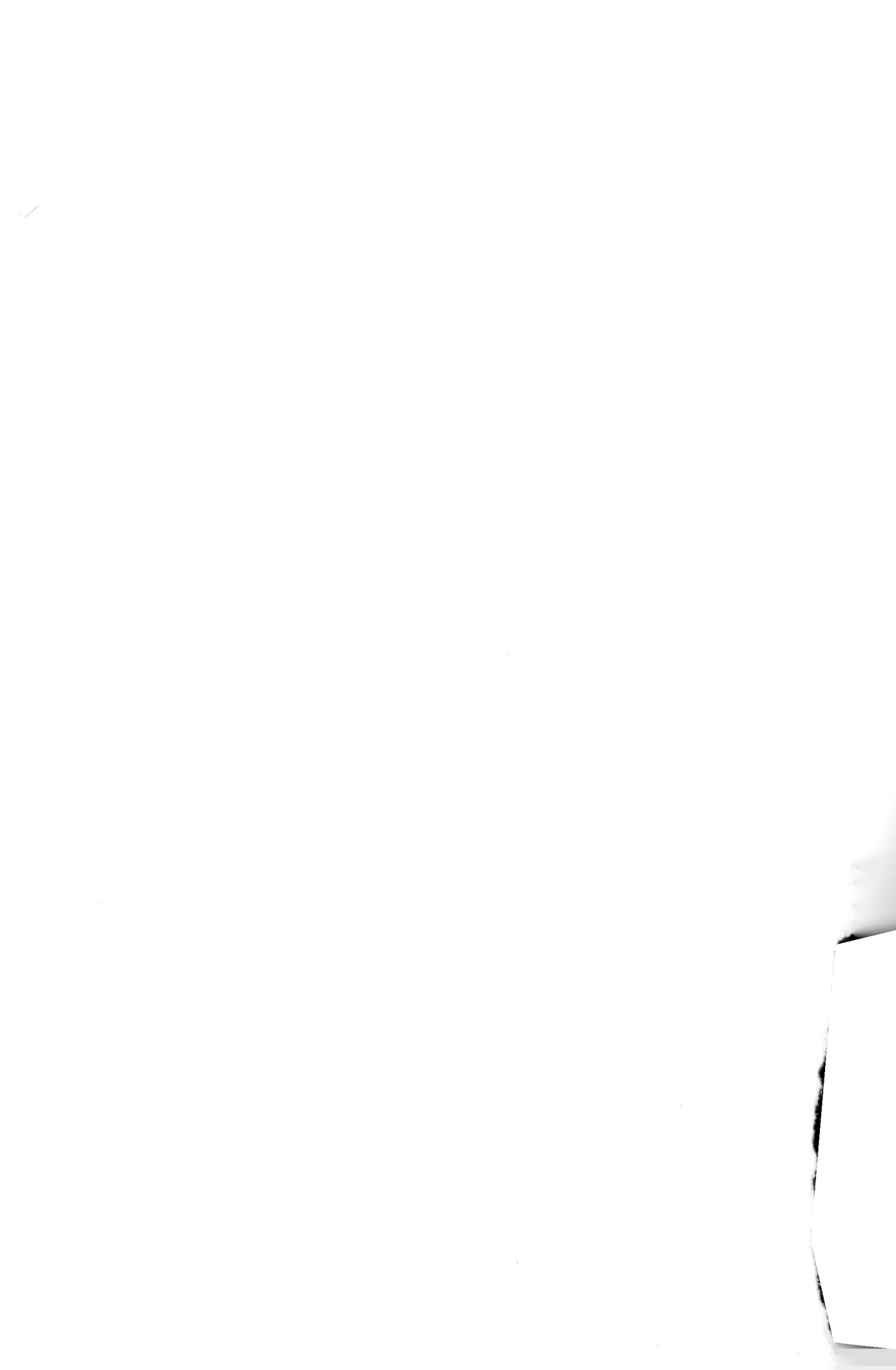